ESSENTIAL MEDICINE

For Churchill Livingstone:

Publisher: Laurence Hunter
Project Editor: Dilys Jones
Copy-Editor: Elif Fincanci-Smith
Production Controller: Lesley Small, Debra Barrie
Design: Design Resources Unit
Sales Promotion Executive: Marion Pollock

ESSENTIAL MEDICINE

Edited by

Alan E Read CBE MD FRCP
Emeritus Professor of Medicine, University of Bristol Medical School,
Bristol Royal Infirmary

John Vann Jones PhD FRCP
Professor, Department of Cardiology, Bristol Royal Infirmary

CHURCHILL LIVINGSTONE
EDINBURGH LONDON MADRID MELBOURNE NEW YORK AND TOKYO
1993

CHURCHILL LIVINGSTONE
Medical Division of Longman Group UK Limited

Distributed in the United States of America by
Churchill Livingstone Inc., 650 Avenue of the Americas,
New York, N.Y. 10011, and by associated companies,
branches and representatives throughout the world.

© Longman Group UK Limited 1993

First published 1993

ISBN 0 443 04595 X

British Library Cataloguing in Publication Data
A catalogue record for this book is available from the
British Library.

Library of Congress Cataloging in Publication Data
Essential medicine/edited by Alan E. Read, John Vann Jones.
    p.   cm.
  Includes index.
  ISBN 0-443-04595-X
  1. Internal medicine. I. Read, Alan Ernest Alfred.
II. Jones, John Vann.
  [DNLM: 1. Clinical Medicine. WB 100 E783 1993]
RC46.E875 1993
616–dc20
DNLM/DLC
for Library of Congress   93–2560
                      CIP

Printed in Singapore

CONTENTS

CONTRIBUTORS

Clive B Archer BSc MD PhD(Lond) FRCP
Consultant Dermatologist, Bristol Royal Infirmary

Montagu G Barker MB ChB FRCPEd FRCPsych DPM
Consultant Pyschiatrist and Clinical Director of Psychiatry,
United Bristol Healthcare Trust; Clinical Lecturer in
Mental Health, University of Bristol

Ralph E Barry BSc MD FRCP
Clinical Dean, Consultant Senior Lecturer in Medicine,
Bristol Royal Infirmary

James R Catterall BSc MRCP MD
Consultant Physician, Bristol Royal Infirmary

David P Coates LRCP MRCS MB BS FRCA
Consultant Anaesthetist, Bristol Royal Infirmary

Roger J M Corrall BSc MD FRCP FRCPE
Consultant Physician, Bristol Royal Infirmary

Iain T Ferguson MD FRCP
Consultant Neurologist, Southmead Hospital, Bristol

Stuart C Glover MB ChB (Hons) FRCP Ed FRCP
Consultant Physician and Specialist in Communicable and Tropical Diseases,
Southmead Hospital, Bristol; Honorary Lecturer in Medicine, University of Bristol

Martin Hartog DM FRCP
Reader in Medicine, University of Bristol; Honorary Consultant
Physician, Bristol and Weston, Southmead Health Districts

Richard F Harvey MD BS MRCS FRCP
Consultant Physician, Frenchay Hospital, Bristol

Kenneth W Heaton MA MD FRCP
Reader in Medicine, University of Bristol; Honorary Consultant
Physician, Bristol Royal Infirmary

Peter Hollingworth FRCP
Consultant Rheumatologist, Southmead Hospital, Bristol

John R Kirwan BSc MD FRCP
Consultant Senior Lecturer in Rheumatology, University Department
of Medicine, Bristol Royal Infirmary

Gabriel Laszlo MA MD FRCP
Consultant Physician, Bristol Royal Infirmary

Peter W Lunt MA MSc MB ChB MRCP
Consultant Clinical Geneticist, Bristol Royal Hospital for Sick
Children; Honorary Lecturer, University of Bristol

Howard G Morgan MD FRCP FRCPsych DPM
Norah Cooke Hurle Professor of Mental Health, University of Bristol

Anthony E G Raine BA BMedSc DPhil FRCP
Professor of Renal Medicine, St Bartholomew's Hospital; Honorary
Consultant Physician, St Bartholomew's Hospital, London

Alan E Read CBE MD FRCP
Emeritus Professor of Medicine, University of Bristol Medical School,
Bristol Royal Infirmary

Clive J C Roberts MD FRCP
Consultant Senior Lecturer in Clinical Pharmacology, Department
of Medicine, Bristol Royal Infirmary

Althea J Scott MB BS
Consultant in Genitourinary Medicine, Bristol Royal Infirmary

Geoffrey L Scott MA MD FRCP
Consultant Clinical Haematologist, United Bristol Healthcare
Trust, Weston Healthcare Trust, Bristol

David Stansbie BSc MB ChB PhD FRCPath
Consultant Chemical Pathologist, Bristol Royal Infirmary

Patrick K Taylor MRCS FRCOG
Consultant in Genitourinary Medicine, Bristol and Weston Health
Authority

John Vann Jones PhD FRCP
Professor, Department of Cardiology, Bristol Royal Infirmary

Gordon K Wilcock BSc DM(Oxon) FRCP
Professor of Care of the Elderly, University of Bristol;
Consultant Physician, Frenchay Healthcare Trust, Bristol

PREFACE

The purpose of this book is to provide a concise account of modern medicine in a format that is easy to read and to revise from. For younger medical students it provides the core, or essential, information about all the common medical conditions, while for more senior students it is designed to be compact but comprehensive. The layout is intended to be easy on the eye without long uninterrupted pages of text and using colour to highlight important points.

With one exception the chapters have all been written by consultants from the Bristol Hospitals. All contributors regularly teach medical students both at the bedside and in more formal surroundings. They have as a result an understanding of what the student needs to be competent in medicine and to be able to pass final examinations. Wherever possible, younger consultants were chosen for their enthusiasm and freshness of approach to teaching and writing.

The editors and publishers were very keen that the size and weight of this book should enable it to be taken in a pocket to the bedside or outpatient clinic and for it to be easy to refer to whenever appropriate.

Present-day medicine has to take into account demographic changes. Care of the elderly is an increasingly complex and respected specialty and we have included a brief separate chapter on this. Air travel has brought tropical and infectious diseases to our hospitals that we may not have seen a few years ago.

It is also commonplace for medical students to spend elective periods abroad, often in exotic places where the pattern of disease is different. We would hope that this book would travel conveniently with them and prove useful.

Genetics is a subject that is increasingly important and the treatment of many diseases in the future may depend on a good knowledge of this subject. Deliberate self-harm is increasing and it has been given extensive coverage in chapter 16, together with a comprehensive chapter on the psychiatric aspects of disease. All the conventional subjects such as neurology, cardiology, gastroenterology, respiratory medicine etc, have been covered in considerable detail but concentrating on the basic, or essential, facts.

In this day of increasing demands on student time – even to the extent of some subjects being dropped from the medical curriculum in some medical schools – we feel there is a place for a compact, comprehensive, readable account of general medicine as practised today. We hope we have achieved this with *Essential Medicine*.

AER
JVJ

Bristol
1993

ACKNOWLEDGEMENTS

Plate 1 is reproduced with the kind permission of Professor
Neil McIntosh. Plates 2 and 3 are reproduced from
Infectious Diseases by A. P. Ball and J. A. Gray,
Churchill Livingstone, 1992, by kind permission of the authors.

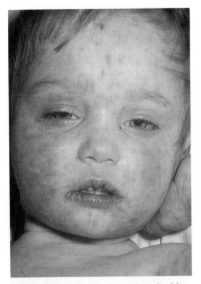

Plate 1 Measles rash. Reproduced with permission.

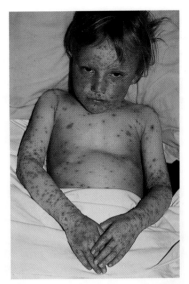

Plate 2 Varicella (chicken pox) rash. Reproduced with permission.

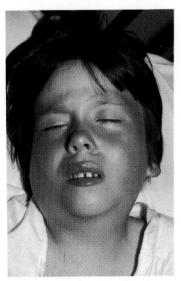

Plate 3 Mumps. Reproduced with permission.

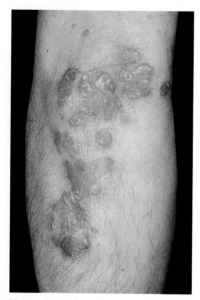

Plate 4 Psoriasis - red scaly plaques on the elbow.

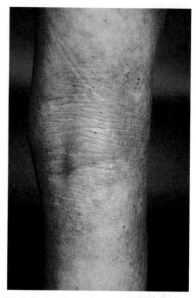

Plate 5 Atopic dermatitis - lichenified eczema affecting the popliteal fossa of a child.

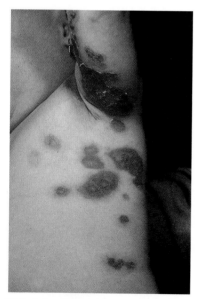

Plate 6 Impetigo - golden crusting and erosions in a baby.

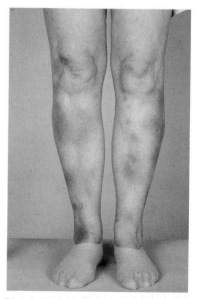

Plate 7 Erythema nodosum - painful red nodules on the shins, in this case associated with sacroidosis.

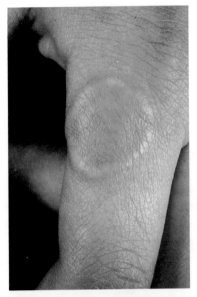

Plate 8 Granuloma annulare - a dermal circular lesion on the hand.

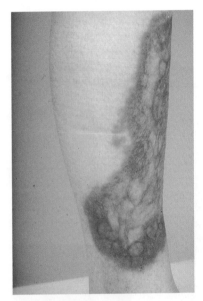

Plate 9 Necroblosis lipoidica - an extensive yellow- brown atrophic lesion on the shin of a patient with diabetes mellitus

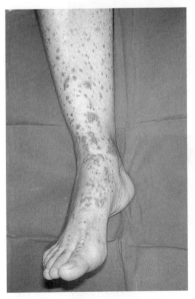

Plate 10 Vasculitis - palpable purpuric lesions on the lower legs.

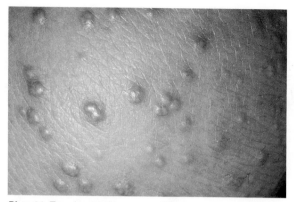

Plate 11 Eruptive xanthomata - reddish-
yellow lesions in a man with type
V hyperlipoproteinaemia.

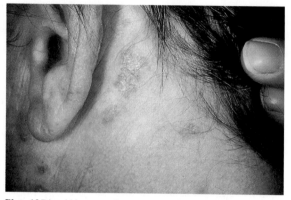

Plate 12 Discoid lupus erythematosus - red
hyperkeratotic and atrophic
plaques on a sun-exposed area.

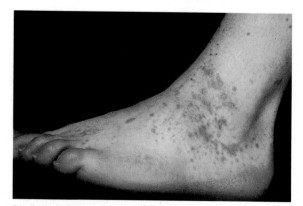

Plate 13 Lichen planus - reddish-brown
(violaceous) flat-topped papules
on the ankle.

1

DISEASES OF THE HEART AND CIRCULATION

John Vann Jones

Diseases of the heart are common the world over. In Western countries ischaemic heart disease predominates while in the Third World rheumatic heart disease remains a major problem. Heart disease often strikes in the prime of life; it is the commonest cause of death in males aged 34–65 in industrialised countries. Its treatment, and hopefully ultimately, its prevention remain a major health priority in all communities.

ISCHAEMIC HEART DISEASE

Ischaemic heart disease (IHD) is the commonest cause of death in the Western World. In males of working age it causes about 40% of all deaths. It remains relatively uncommon but is increasing in underdeveloped countries whereas it has started to decline in the industrialised nations. In the form of heart failure or angina, IHD also greatly contributes to morbidity.

Atheroma (fatty tissue) is deposited in the walls of blood vessels, and the coronary arteries seem particularly susceptible. A number of predisposing, or risk, factors have been identified for IHD. Some of these are potentially correctable, e.g. high blood pressure.

Risk Factors
Irreversible
Age. IHD increases with age. Not only is it more prevalent but it tends to be more devastating. Fewer elderly people survive their first heart attack when compared with younger patients.

Sex. Females have much lower rates of IHD before the menopause. Later the prevalence increases rapidly until females in their seventies have the same high risks for developing IHD as do males of equivalent age.

Family history. There are undoubtedly families with a strong history of IHD in whom none of the other risk factors can be identified. The offspring of such parents are at risk but it is common to find that the parents were heavy smokers or had hypertension and allowance must be made for this when ascribing a genetic influence to the likelihood of IHD.

The above are undoubtedly the major risk factors for the development of ischaemic heart disease. There are, however, many other factors that have been implicated.

Premature baldness, premature grey hair and the presence of an arcus senilis (thin line of fatty tissue at the outer edge of the cornea of the eye) before the age of 40 are said to carry some increased risk of IHD.

Reversible

High blood pressure. Hypertension seems to accelerate the atheromatous process and is the major potentially reversible risk factor for IHD. Sadly, anti-hypertensive therapy has had relatively little effect in preventing myocardial infarctions in the hypertensive population when compared with its effectiveness in preventing strokes.

Smoking. Inhaled tobacco smoke accelerates the atherosclerotic process. Heavy smokers are at roughly three times the risk of their non-smoking counterparts. All smokers are at substantially less risk if they do not inhale. Usually this means pipe or cigar smoking.

Hyperlipidaemia (elevated blood fat, or lipid, levels). An elevated blood cholesterol level seems to carry an increased risk of premature atherosclerosis which is linearly related over the range of cholesterols found in the population. Unless substantially elevated, triglycerides do not carry a risk of IHD but when both cholesterol and triglyceride levels are elevated together the triglycerides appear to contribute additionally to the risk. Increased high density lipoprotein (HDL) cholesterol levels may be protective.

Diet. Low-fat eaters do seem to live longer than those on more conventional diets. The relationship of this to IHD prevention in people with normal lipid levels has not been clearly established. Coffee excess and soft water drinking have also been linked with an increased risk of IHD.

Exercise. Regular exercise lowers both cholesterol levels and blood pressure and such people seem to live longer and have healthier lives.

Stress. The haemodynamic upset of stress can precipitate ischaemic chest pain in those with pre-existing atheroma, e.g. the racing heart and raised blood pressure following an argument. It is doubtful whether stress actually causes atheroma deposition although chronic stress can persistently raise the blood pressure in some people and may therefore have an indirect effect.

Obesity. Obese people have high blood pressure and often latent diabetes or glucose intolerance. When these are not present obesity does not carry a separate risk for IHD but if atheroma is already present these people will be more likely to get chest pain because of the physical exertion and therefore cardiac work involved in just getting themselves around.

Race. Racial influences are probably environmental, e.g. Japanese Americans have the same incidence of IHD as do white Americans whereas the Japanese

Table 1.1. Symptoms of heart disease

Dyspnoea (breathlessness)
>   Classified by the New York Heart Association as
>>   Grade 1 Uncompromised
>>   Grade 2 Slightly compromised
>>   Grade 3 Moderately compromised
>>   Grade 4 Severely compromised
>   Orthopnoea — dyspnoea occurring when the patient lies flat
>   Paroxysmal nocturnal dyspnoea (PND) — dyspnoea often acute and severe occurring during sleep. The patient awakens acutely breathless

Chest pain

Syncope

Palpitations

Fatigue and lethargy

---

in Japan have a low incidence of IHD. Similarly, as African people become urbanised there is evidence of increasing IHD which is virtually unknown in rural African communities.

Associated diseases

There are some specific medical conditions predisposing to IHD. The most noteworthy are hypothyroidism, diabetes and transplantation. These conditions will be considered in the relevant sections.

Symptoms and signs (Table 1.1)
Angina Pectoris

This is a descriptive term for a certain pattern and type of chest pain arising from the ischaemic heart. It is therefore a diagnosis that is heavily dependent on a well taken history. It describes the situation where retrosternal chest discomfort or pain comes on with exertion and settles within a few minutes with rest or easing back. It may also come on with emotion (which increases the work of the heart just like exercise) or excitement. Cold weather makes it worse and it may be more obvious shortly after meals. Often the patient is a little breathless (dyspnoeic) when he has his angina and at times the dyspnoeic aspect seems to be dominant.

The pain or discomfort of myocardial ischaemia may radiate to one or other or both arms but more usually to the left, to the jaw or teeth and more unusually through to the back. It is the relationship to exertion or exercise that largely makes the diagnosis but it is important not to confuse movement with exertion: a strained intercostal muscle can give a history that sounds like angina but it is movement rather than exercise that is causing the problem. Similarly, the site of pain or discomfort arising from the heart is never tender to the touch. It is evident that the history is of paramount importance in making the diagnosis of angina pectoris. Indigestion or gastro-oesophageal pain is the other type of

Table 1.2. Techniques used in the investigation of heart disease

Chest X-ray	
Postero-anterior (PA) to assess	Heart size
	Heart shape
	Specific chamber enlargement, e.g. left atrial size
	Lung fields
	Presence of calcification
Antero-posterior (AP) ⎤ Left lateral ⎬ Penetrated PA ⎦	Used in selected patients
Electrocardiogram (ECG)	Specific patterns, e.g. infarction
	Rhythm
	Cardiac axis
	Electrical conduction
Exercise Electrocardiography	Ischaemic heart disease
Echocardiography	Cardiac anatomy
	Left ventricular function
	Pericardial effusion
	Valve function

pain that is confused with angina and unsuspecting patients often initially think they have indigestion, especially as it may present following a meal. The patient with angina pectoris usually has no abnormal physical signs and therefore examination is unhelpful in confirming the diagnosis.

Investigations (Table 1.2)
Resting electrocardiogram (ECG) (Fig. 1.1). This is normal in up to 80% of people with quite classical angina. When it is abnormal, T wave changes predominate, e.g. inversion or flattening when they should be upright.
Exercise ECG (Fig. 1.2). As angina is an exercise-induced symptom it is rightly to be expected that an ECG recorded during exercise would be more helpful. Between 90 and 95% of people with angina will show changes on an exercise ECG, usually ST segment depression. Exercise tests are normally conducted in a standardised way using either a treadmill or a bicycle ergometer. It is possible to obtain false negative and, in females particularly, false positive results.

Not only is the ECG observed during an exercise stress test but so too are the patient and his symptoms. People with false negative exercise tests often give a good description of angina even when the ECG does not change.

Blood pressure should be measured at intervals during an exercise test. A drop in blood pressure usually reflects important myocardial ischaemia but people who are nervous or not used to exercise can develop near faints under

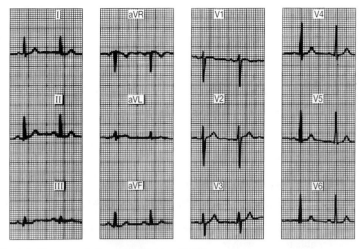

Fig. 1.1 The normal electrocardiogram (ECG)

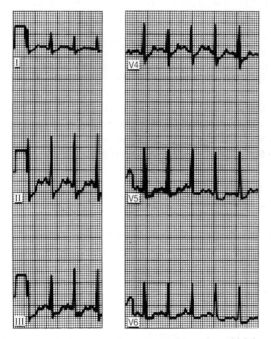

Fig. 1.2 Positive exercise test. There is ST segment depression which has developed with the increased cardiac work of exercise, seen here as a tachycardia

these circumstances and this, too, will drop the blood pressure without the sinister implications attributable to myocardial ischaemia itself. Exercise-induced arrhythmias or conduction abnormalities also generally reflect underlying ischaemia while those arrhythmias which disappear with exercise are usually benign.

Radioisotope studies. These can often be used to diagnose ischaemia when they are combined with an exercise test. They will further increase the diagnostic rate.

Coronary arteriography. X-ray studies of the coronary arteries are sometimes needed to finally establish a diagnosis. More usually, they are performed where the diagnosis has already been established by exercise ECG testing in order to obtain information prior to consideration for coronary artery surgery.

Treatment

Patients told they have angina naturally become anxious. Indeed they often start to notice chest pains which are clearly not coming from the heart and which they would have previously ignored. Correct management, therefore, includes:

A full explanation. Often when the patient understands his angina he is better able to cope with it.

Sensible limitation of activity. The patient should avoid strenuous exertion, e.g. rushing up stairs.

Addressing risk factors, e.g. smoking, high blood pressure, etc.

Reducing weight and getting fitter.

Prescribing glyceryl trinitrate (GTN). This drug is taken sublingually either in the form of a small tablet or of a spray with a metered dose. GTN dilates the coronary arteries and also reduces cardiac work by dilating the peripheral arteries and, especially, the veins. It is very potent in relieving angina and works extremely rapidly. The effect of each dose lasts 20–30 minutes.

Often, patients use GTN prior to situations which might precipitate their angina, e.g. before going out for a winter's walk, after Sunday lunch, etc. At this stage, many patients also start regular aspirin treatment for its anticoagulant effect. Narrowed coronary arteries are often finally blocked off by clotting and aspirin may help to prevent this.

Sustained anti-anginal therapy

If the above simple measures are inadequate in controlling the patient's symptoms then drugs are used to help reduce the frequency of anginal attacks. These include long-acting nitrate preparations, beta-adrenergic blocking drugs and the calcium channel blocking agents. They may be used singly or in combination. Patients with severe angina often take all three.

1. Long-acting nitrates. These are chemically related to GTN and are unpredictable in their response partly because tolerance develops and partly because they are extensively metabolised by the liver. The mononitrates are best. Like GTN they dilate coronary arteries and also, by dilating arteries and veins, they reduce cardiac work and lessen angina. Their principle side-effect is headache which often settles in a few days. GTN may itself be given percutaneously by means of patches applied to the skin. These preparations allow GTN to remain in the blood for many hours and patients find them highly acceptable.

2. Beta-adrenergic blocking agents (beta-blockers). These drugs modify the heart's response to exercise so that it works less hard for a given degree of exertion, i.e. the heart rate response to exercise is lessened as is the rise in blood pressure that also occurs.

In this way the patient's angina threshold is raised and activity is increased before discomfort begins. Beta-blockers can cause people to feel 'washed out' and lethargic because of a drop in cardiac output. They may also complain of cold limbs. These drugs are contraindicated in heart failure and asthma and relatively contraindicated in peripheral vascular disease, chronic obstructive airways disease and diabetes.

3. Calcium channel blockers. This is a heterogeneous group of drugs which prevent the normal movement of calcium in myocardial cells. They thus reduce energy requirements and oxygen utilisation and as such are effective in treating angina. Some of the drugs in this group are rather like beta-blockers in their actions on the heart, e.g. verapamil and diltiazem, whereas others appear to stimulate the heart, e.g. nifedipine. Flushing, headaches and fluid retention are the major side-effects.

Coronary angioplasty (percutaneous transluminal coronary angioplasty. PTCA)
Patients who fail to respond to medical therapy or who are unable to tolerate drugs may be considered for surgery but first a coronary arteriogram is needed. This sometimes shows relatively localised discrete lesions and in some cases these can be dilated at cardiac catheterisation using small inflatable balloons.

Coronary artery bypass grafting (CABG)
If the coronary arteriogram shows extensive disease, the patient is referred for surgery where grafts bypassing the coronary lesions will be constructed.

There are three factors which might potentially benefit from surgery.

1. Angina. The operation is very successful in relieving angina in patients where medicine has failed. Up to 95% of such patients will be substantially improved or free of angina.

2. Life expectancy. There is increasing evidence that surgery prolongs life. This is established where the proximal left coronary artery is diseased (left mainstem stenosis) and probably also when all three of the major branches are involved.

3. Cardiac function. The effects on cardiac function vary. Bypass grafting undoubtedly improves cardiac function in some patients but may reduce it in others. There is no consistent overall benefit.

Prognosis of angina pectoris
The mortality of these patients is 4% per year. The more extensive the disease, the worse the prognosis. It is also worse if the patient's blood pressure drops on exercise, the exercise test is strongly positive, the angina has developed following a myocardial infarct, or if there is heart failure. The prognosis is better if the

patient is a non-smoker, has not had heart failure, the resting cardiograph is normal and there is no history of previous heart damage.

Unstable angina

A few people will follow an accelerated course and may need urgent surgery despite full medical treatment. They are said to have unstable or pre-infarction angina.

Prinzmetal's angina (coronary artery spasm)

In some people the coronary arteries can go into spasm. It is very rare and the ECG usually shows gross ischaemic changes during an attack. Treatment is with nitrates and calcium channel blockers.

MYOCARDIAL INFARCTION

Most myocardial infarctions (MI) occur in relation to an occluded coronary artery. At post mortem 90% of patients will be found to have a clot blocking their artery where it is already narrowed by atheroma. In some, the vessel is still patent but the flow down it is so poor that the muscle downstream infarcts. In others haemorrhage into the atheromatous plaque is responsible for blocking the vessel.

Symptoms and signs

Chest pain situated behind the sternum is the most common presentation of myocardial infarction. It usually ranges from mild to agonising in its severity but some heart attacks are silent and not associated with significant pain (especially in the elderly and in those with diabetes).

The pain is usually crushing and may radiate to either arm but especially to the left and to the jaw and neck. The patient is often nauseated, may even vomit, is usually sweaty, and may be breathless particularly if the infarct has resulted in a degree of heart failure.

In an uncomplicated infarct, signs are remarkably few. The heart sounds may be soft and there may be an added third heart sound but often there is remarkably little to find unless a complication has set in. The complications giving rise to physical signs are:

Left ventricular failure. The patient is breathless, usually has a tachycardia and there are crepitations in the lung fields. Third or fourth heart sounds may be heard and give rise to a particular cadence when the heart is listened to which sounds like a horse galloping in the distance (gallop rhythm).

Cardiogenic shock. This occurs when the left ventricular damage is great. The patient is shocked with thready pulses, low blood pressure and tachycardia, and usually looks pale owing to constriction of the skin blood vessels (vasoconstriction), and is clammy and sweaty. Prognosis is poor.

Arrhythmias. A majority of patients in the minutes to hours after an MI have some form of heart rhythm disorder (arrhythmia). Treatment depends on the type of arrhythmia, its consequences, e.g. drop in blood pressure, and its duration.

Inflammation of the pericardium (pericarditis). Pericarditis is one of the causes of continuing pain after myocardial infarction and there is an associated pericardial rub. This is a superficial scratching sound caused by the surfaces of the inflamed pericardium rubbing together in time to the heartbeat. There is often a respiratory variation as well. It usually passes off within 1–2 days and the rub, in particular, can be very transient.

Mitral valve incompetence. Because the papillary muscles are often involved in the infarction, the mitral valve cusps then become out of alignment and allow degrees of mitral incompetence. In some cases the papillary muscles rupture and so allow free reflux through the damaged valve. A pansystolic murmur of varying intensity is heard over the mitral area. It is usually very loud and obvious if the papillary muscle has ruptured.

Ventricular septal defect (VSD). Occasionally the interventricular septum ruptures and allows a VSD to form. There is a pansystolic murmur at the left sternal edge. It can be quite difficult sometimes to differentiate between a VSD and mitral incompetence.

Emboli. These may occur either to the systemic side of the circulation and lead, for example, to strokes or to the pulmonary side giving rise to pulmonary emboli. They are especially common in relation to large infarcts on the anterior surface of the heart.

Investigations

ECG. This shows a characteristic pattern in MI. The dead muscle is no longer electrically active and so the recording leads 'look through' the infarcted area. This generally means that the electrical activity being recorded is moving away from the electrode and is therefore negative. This negative wave is called a Q wave. In the early stages there are usually ST segment changes (Fig. 1.3) as

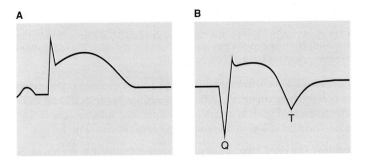

Fig. 1.3 The evolving ECG in myocardial infarction. (A) Acute stage shows ST segment elevation; (B) later stage shows less ST segment elevation together with appearance of Q waves. The T waves are also usually inverted.

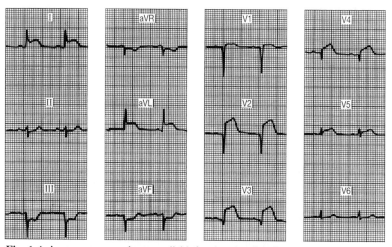

Fig. 1.4 Acute anteroseptal myocardial infarction showing Q waves and ST segment elevation in leads V_1–V_4. Reciprocal ST segment depression is seen in the inferior leads II, III and aVF

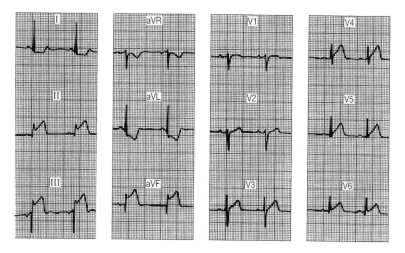

Fig. 1.5 Acute inferior myocardial infarction showing ST segment elevation in the inferior leads II, III and aVF. Q waves have not yet developed. There is reciprocal ST segment depression in I and aVL

well as various T wave abnormalities, e.g. T wave inversion. Different sites of infarction produce changes in different leads, i.e. leads II, III and aVF are for inferior infarcts (Fig. 1.4) and V_1–V_4 for anterior infarcts (Fig. 1.5). Partial thickness infarcts also give their own ECG appearances (Fig. 1.6).

Enzymes. The dead myocardial cells release enzymes into the blood. Some of those measured, lactate dehydrogenase (LDH) and alanine serum transaminase (AST), are not specific to the heart and may be released by other tissues, e.g. lung and liver. Creatinine phosphokinase (CPK) is released by damaged

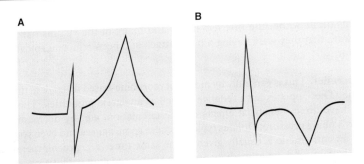

Fig. 1.6 The ECG in partial thickness (non Q-wave) myocardial infarction. (A) Tall peaked symmetrical T waves; and (B) sharp T wave inversion. This type of infarction is sometimes called subendocardial. Tall T waves may also be seen in ischaemia

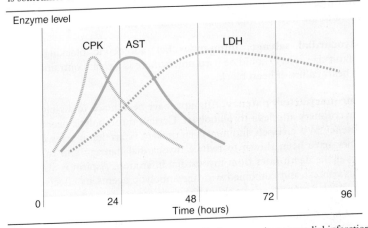

Fig. 1.7 Time course of the release of 'cardiac' enzymes in myocardial infarction. CPK = creatinine phosphokinase; AST = alanine serum transaminase; LDH = lactate dehydrogenase

muscle and is generally more useful in diagnosis but intramuscular injections, such as might be given for pain relief, can cause an elevation. Only the cardiac isoenzyme is specific for myocardial infarction but not many laboratories measure it routinely.

The time course of the release of the enzymes is variable and it can be useful to know this if the patient presents late (Fig. 1.7).

Temperature. This often rises for a few days.

Blood. The white cell count may be raised. The erythrocyte sedimentation rate (ESR) or viscosity may increase as in any major stressful illness. Similarly the blood glucose level may rise, often to quite high values.

Treatment

The four broad aims are pain relief, treatment of complications, salvage of the myocardium, and restoration of patency of the coronary arteries. The risk of dying from a heart attack is highest immediately following its onset. Most deaths occur within the first few hours and many of the victims have been unaware that they were having a heart attack and been reluctant to call their doctor.

Pain relief. This is generally by means of morphine-based drugs, e.g. diamorphine. These opiates have sedative as well as analgesic properties. They may also have direct beneficial effects on the circulation, e.g. by decreasing the heart's filling pressure. Opiates typically cause some nausea and even vomiting and an anti-emetic is usually given at the same time (e.g. prochlorperazine). Where pain is not an immediate problem simple sedation with diazepam may suffice to allay anxiety and should be given for 1–2 days even if the patient does not appear anxious.

Complications. These are treated as they arise, e.g. arrhythmia, heart failure, etc. and will be dealt with in other sections of this chapter.

Myocardial salvage. Intravenous beta-adrenergic blocking drugs limit infarct size. They should be used unless there is a clear contraindication such as heart failure or heart block.

Coronary artery patency. Attempts have been made to dissolve the clots in the coronary arteries—thrombolysis. Certain thrombolytic agents can restore patency to the vessels and may even prevent infarction if given early enough. They have been shown to reduce myocardial damage and to substantially lower the death rates from myocardial infarction. Aspirin is also effective in this context and combined with thrombolytic agents its effects are additive. Suspected infarct patients should be given aspirin as soon as possible.

Commonly used thrombolytic agents are streptokinase, anistreptase and tissue plasminogen activator (TPA). Streptokinase and anistreptase are much cheaper but because of antibody formation cannot be used again within 1 year. Under these circumstances TPA is then used.

Late care

Rehabilitation should include both physical training and psychological help. The evidence is that with this sort of support most MI patients achieve a better quality, and possibly quantity, of life.

The risk factors such as hypertension, smoking and hypercholesterolaemia should be tackled. The prognosis following an MI is worse if the patient continues to smoke.

Oral beta-blockers can also be used but it is the subject of debate as to how long this should continue post infarction. There is good evidence that it is still effective at 1 year and possibly at 3 years. All MI patients should be kept on lifelong aspirin treatment. Angiotensin converting enzyme (ACE) inhibitors are increasingly being used following anterior myocardial infarction.

ARRHYTHMIAS

Rhythm disorders of the heart (arrhythmias) are extremely common.

1. Most arrhythmias are benign. Their importance lies in the symptoms they cause, e.g. palpitations.
2. Some arrhythmias are more serious and can even be life threatening.
3. Arrhythmias are often intermittent and therefore identification can sometimes be very difficult.
4. Some arrhythmias represent underlying heart disease, e.g. atrial flutter, whilst some are commonly associated with otherwise normal hearts, e.g. ventricular ectopic beats.

Arrhythmias can be divided into those that are predominantly associated with rapid heart rates and those with slow heart rates. There is a third group where both fast and slow arrhythmias may occur in the same patient.

TACHYARRHYTHMIAS

With these arrhythmias the heart rate is fast. For convenience both ventricular and atrial ectopic beats are often included in this group. The patients are usually aware of palpitations and may notice the arrhythmia switching on and also switching off. They may notice sudden fatigue and dizziness and may sometimes become breathless. They seldom lose consciousness although this commonly occurs with ventricular tachycardia and inevitably with ventricular fibrillation but sometimes experience angina-like pain when the rate is very rapid and there is underlying IHD.

Often the cause of the arrhythmia is unknown but sometimes it can be brought on by excessive tea or coffee intake or by other cardiac stimulants such as cigarette smoking and alcohol.

Tachyarrhythmias are common with overactivity of the thyroid gland (thyrotoxicosis) or with valvular heart disease. They also occur with IHD and sometimes with high blood pressure. The tachyarrhythmias arising in the atria often occur for no known reason.

Sinus tachycardia

The rhythm is normal, the rate is in excess of 100 beats/min, and it is seen with exercise or excitement when it is physiological. Some patients are aware their hearts are beating under those circumstances and complain of palpitations.

In the history the palpitations are often noted to come on gradually and to increase in speed. With true arrhythmias the palpitations usually switch on extremely abruptly.

Sinus arrhythmia

This is a variant of normal sinus rhythm where the heart rate increases with inspiration and decreases with expiration. The change in rate can be particularly marked, especially in young people and is not to be confused with a true arrhythmia.

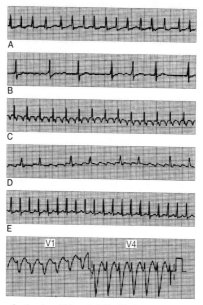

Fig. 1.8 Common arrhythmias: (A) atrial fibrillation with a rapid ventricular rate; (B) atrial fibrillation with a controlled ventricular response; (C) rapid atrial flutter with 2:1 ventricular response (block); (D) atrial flutter with variable block; (E) supraventricular tachycardia, (F) ventricular tachycardia

Supraventricular ectopic beats

Isolated beats arising from the atria are usually asymptomatic and generally benign. They need no treatment but can give rise to palpitations.

Paroxysmal supraventricular tachycardia (Fig. 1.8)

There are bursts of rapid regular atrial activity. The heart rate is up to 180 beats/min and it tends to occur in young people with basically healthy hearts.

Attacks may last from a few seconds to many days. When they occur frequently they can be a considerable nuisance and may require anti-arrhythmic treatment but more usually they are self limiting and certain manoeuvres which the patients can carry out themselves may terminate an attack. These include Valsalva manoeuvre (breath holding against a closed glottis), carotid sinus massage, rubbing an eyeball, taking a cold drink, and immersing the face in cold water. All of these cause activation of the vagus nerve but sometimes drug treatment and, very rarely, correction by means of an electric shock (cardioversion) are required. Few of these patients require long-term therapy.

Atrial fibrillation (AF) (Fig. 1.8)

AF is very common—one person in seven over the age of 70 is permanently in this rhythm—and it increases in frequency with age.

The atria do not contract properly (fibrillate) and transmit impulses down to the ventricle in a totally irregular manner. Clinically, the major problem is with the rapid rate and treatment is aimed either at correcting the arrhythmia or more frequently at controlling the heart rate. The latter is usually done by means of digoxin. When AF arises in an apparently normal heart it is worth while trying to convert it back to normal sinus rhythm either by drugs or electrically.

AF resistant to drug treatment is often associated with thyrotoxicosis.

Atrial flutter

This arrhythmia (Fig. 1.8) usually occurs in diseased hearts, e.g. in rheumatic heart disease. The atria are not contracting normally and again can transmit irregularly to the ventricles giving a clinical appearance similar to atrial fibrillation. However, the ECG shows much coarser waves in the atria called F waves.

Pre-excitation syndromes

Some people have abnormal tracts of tissue connecting the atria to the ventricles (bypass tracts). This allows the atrioventricular node and its heart rate modifying influence to be bypassed (pre-excitation). When these individuals develop atrial arrhythmias the resultant ventricular rate can be very fast, e.g. 220–250 beats/min. Such rates are potentially very dangerous. Bypass tracts occur in the Wolff-Parkinson-White (Fig. 1.9) and Lown-Ganong-Levine syndromes.

Ventricular ectopic beats

Here abnormal (ectopic) beats arise from the ventricles. The pulse feels as though beats are being missed. In fact, the beats are premature (Fig. 1.9) and do not allow the heart enough time to fill; hence no pulse is transmitted peripherally. The heart usually makes up the lost ground with the following beat so that the sensation to the patient can be one of pauses and thumps. In a small percentage these beats are caused by heart disease but generally they arise in an otherwise sound heart from one focus and, if of the benign variety, tend to go away with exercise. Those arising from diseased hearts tend to increase with the extra strain of exercise.

Benign ventricular ectopic beats seldom require treatment but they can occur up to 40 000 times per day in which case they can cause a lot of distress. The natural history is for them to come and go but over a matter of years they become more troublesome.

Ectopic beats arising near the T wave of the preceding QRS complex (R on T) or from several different foci can be associated with a risk of serious ventricular arrhythmias.

Ventricular tachycardia

Three or more ectopic beats occurring in rapid sequence is known as ventricular tachycardia (see Fig. 1.8). The rate is usually so rapid that cardiac output falls and ventricular tachycardia may go on and deteriorate to ventricular fibrillation. In an acute episode all patients must be restored to normal rhythm by

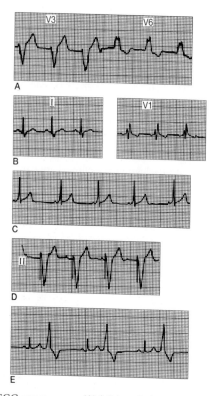

Fig. 1.9 Common ECG appearances: (A) left bundle branch block; (B) right bundle branch block; (C) Wolff-Parkinson-White syndrome, shows short PR interval and slurred upstroke to the QRS complex (delta wave); (D) pacing rhythm; (E) coupled ventricular ectopic beats

treatment if at all possible; if the episodes are short lived and self terminating, preventive drug therapy should be initiated. Ventricular tachycardia usually represents serious underlying heart disease and frequently follows an MI.

Ventricular fibrillation (VF)

This is one of the forms of cardiac arrest with the ventricles failing to contract. Cardiac output drops immediately. Within a few seconds the patient will be hypotensive and unconscious. Electrical cardioversion is required and preventive medical therapy (Table 1.3) instituted where the arrhythmia has been survived.

BRADYARRHYTHMIAS

These are rhythm disorders where the heart rate is excessively slow.

Sinus bradycardia

Usually defined as sinus rhythm slower than 50 beats/min, this can be quite normal in fit people, e.g. athletes. Drugs such as beta-blocking agents slow the

Table 1.3. Classification of anti-arrhythmic drugs

Class I	Membrane-stabilising agents, e.g. lignocaine, mexiletene, disopyramide, flecainide, propafenone
Class II	Beta-adrenergic blocking agents
Class III	Prolong action potential duration, e.g. amiodarone, sotalol (also class II agent), bretylium
Class IV	Calcium channel blocking agents, e.g. verapamil, diltiazem

Knowledge of this classification allows a rational approach to drug therapy of arrhythmias, e.g. two agents in the same class would not be used together.

Note digoxin is not classified as an anti-arrhythmic agent in this classification.

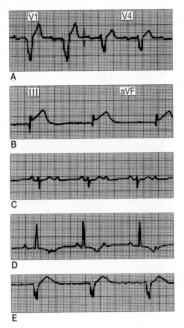

Fig. 1.10 Various types of conduction defect. (A) First degree heart block (long PR interval) with the QRS complexes showing left bundle branch block; (B) first degree heart block in acute inferior myocardial infarction; (C) second degree heart block (Mobitz type II; (D) third degree (complete) heart block; (E) complete heart block in atrial fibrillation. Note that here, despite the fibrillation, the QRS complexes occur at regular intervals

heart rate but, in the elderly, sinus bradycardia often reflects underlying problems with the conduction tissue.

Heart block (Fig. 1.10)

First degree heart block occurs when the PR interval on the ECG is prolonged.

Second degree heart block occurs when there is some dissociation between atrial and ventricular activity, e.g. two atrial contractions for every ventricular one (Mobitz type II). One particular form of second degree heart block occurs when the PR interval progressively lengthens until eventually one P wave is not followed by a QRS complex (Wenckebach phenomenon or Mobitz type I).

Third degree heart block occurs when there is no association between atrial and ventricular activity.

All three types are usually associated with abnormalities of the conduction tissue with the majority occurring as part of a degenerative process. IHD is another common cause. Generally, first degree heart block and the Wenckebach phenomenon do not need treatment but second degree heart block otherwise and third degree heart block may need treatment by means of pacemaker implantation. There is a rare form of congenital complete heart block where the overall heart rate is usually a little faster and pacing may not be required.

Sick sinus syndrome

This syndrome, which is being seen increasingly, is associated with periods of rapid heart rates and periods of slow heart rates. No intervention is required in asymptomatic patients but in some the rate is so slow that a pacemaker has to be inserted or so rapid that drug treatment is needed. It is not uncommon for both forms of treatment to be required. Generally the prognosis in sick sinus syndrome is good, and the patient is treated according to symptoms.

Cardiac pacemakers

These may be temporary, where the electrodes are inserted into the right ventricle, or permanent, where the electrodes are inserted into the right atrium, the right ventricle or both.

Temporary pacemakers are used while awaiting permanent pacing, e.g. in hospitals where only temporary pacing facilities are available, or where the conduction defects may reverse, e.g. heart block following an acute inferior MI.

Permanent pacemakers are used in the treatment of irreversible conduction defects. Anti-tachycardia pacemakers can be used to control or terminate rapid arrythmias.

VALVULAR HEART DISEASE

Valvular heart disease (Table 1.4) occurs when the valves become stenosed or incompetent or both. Valves may be affected primarily, as in mitral stenosis following rheumatic fever, or secondarily, as in papillary muscle damage with MI. Combinations of valve lesions can occur together but for learning purposes each lesion is best described separately.

MITRAL STENOSIS

Mitral stenosis usually develops many years after an attack of rheumatic fever (Table 1.5). It occurs more commonly in females but is now becoming rare as

Table 1.4. Aetiology of valvular heart disease

Mitral stenosis	Aortic incompetence
Rheumatic heart disease	Rheumatic heart disease
Congenital (very rare)	Congenital (often bicuspid valves)
Mitral incompetence	Hypertension
Rheumatic heart disease	Rheumatic diseases
Ischaemic heart disease	ankylosing spondylitis
papillary muscle dysfunction/infarction	rheumatoid arthritis
ruptured chordae tendinae	Infective endocarditis
Prolapsing valve	Marfan's syndrome
Myxomatous degeneration of the valve ring	Secondary to aortic dissection
Secondary to left ventricular failure/dilatation (functional mitral incompetence)	Syphilis and yaws
	Tricuspid stenosis
Rheumatic disease	Rheumatic heart disease
rheumatoid arthritis	Tricuspid incompetence
ankylosing spondylitis	Secondary to right heart failure (functional tricuspid incompetence)
Rupture of the chordae tendinae	Rheumatic heart disease
Infective endocarditis	Infective endocarditis (notably drug addicts)
Other rare causes	Pulmonary stenosis
ostium primum atrial septal defect	Congenital
hypertrophic cardiomyopathy	Pulmonary incompetence
Marfan's syndrome	Secondary to pulmonary hypertension
Aortic stenosis	Congenital
Rheumatic heart disease	
Congenital (often bicuspid valves)	
Degenerative (usually biscuspid valves)	

rheumatic fever dies out in developed countries. Rheumatic fever and subsequently rheumatic heart disease are still extremely common in underdeveloped countries. There is a rare form of congenital mitral stenosis presenting in very young children.

Symptoms

1. Dyspnoea.
2. Palpitations, from atrial fibrillation which may be intermittent at first but usually becomes permanent.
3. Frequent winter chest infections.
4. Haemoptysis.

Table 1.5. Diagnosis of rheumatic fever. This is made if two major, or one major and two minor, criteria are present

Major criteria	Minor criteria
Chorea (Sydenham's — called St Vitus' dance)	Raised ASO titre
	Other evidence of recent streptococcal infection
Carditis	Fever
Migrating polyarthritis	Raised white cell count (leukocytosis)
Subcutaneous nodules	Arthralgia
Erythema marginatum	Elevated ESR or viscosity
	Increased C-reactive protein
	Prolonged PR interval on the ECG

5. Effects of systemic emboli: clots form in the enlarged left atrium, especially if it is fibrillating, and may dislodge and result in strokes, ischaemic limbs, etc.

Signs

1. Malar flush (mitral facies), seen as a plethoric colour high on both cheeks.
2. The irregularly irregular pulse of atrial fibrillation.
3. Tapping apex beat. The stenosed mitral valve prevents blood from entering the left ventricle which is underfilled. As a result the apex beat feels like a tap on the chest wall.
4. A heave at the left sternal edge from right ventricular enlargement, found when pulmonary hypertension develops.
5. Loud first heart sound over the mitral area. It may even be palpable to the touch. There is also an opening snap audible in early diastole. Both are only heard if the valve is mobile and are lost when it becomes stiff and calcified.
6. Loud second heart sound in the pulmonary area when pulmonary hypertension develops.
7. Rumbling low pitched mid-diastolic murmur heard at the apex. It may be better heard after exercise or by turning the patient over to his left. It is caused by flow through the stenosed valve. Later in diastole if the patient remains in sinus rhythm the murmur may be accentuated due to atrial contraction—so called pre-systolic accentuation.

Investigations

ECG usually shows atrial fibrillation but there may be left atrial hypertrophy (P mitrale) if sinus rhythm persists. Sometimes right ventricular hypertrophy also occurs (R wave larger than S wave in V1 ± T wave inversion in leads V2 and V3).

Chest X-ray. There is usually cardiomegaly. The characteristic signs of left atrial enlargement are also evident, i.e. double shadow on the right heart border, enlargement of the left atrial appendage seen as a bulge below the left pulmonary artery (usually the border is concave here) and widening of the

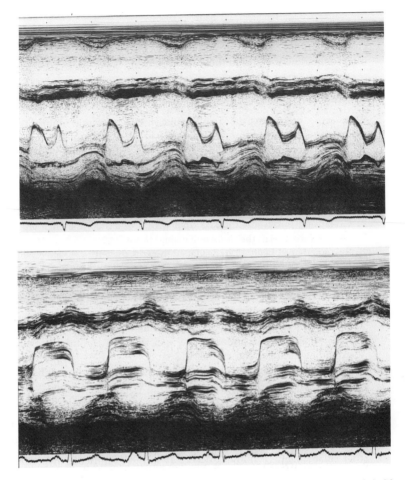

Fig. 1.11 Echocardiogram of normal mitral valve (top) showing the characteristic M shape. The lower trace is typical of mitral stenosis

bifurcation of the trachea. The upper lobe blood vessels may become more prominent as pulmonary congestion develops.

Echocardiography, now the most useful investigation for confirming the diagnosis and assessing its severity (Fig. 1.11)

Cardiac catheterisation, now largely restricted to preoperative assessment.

Treatment

Complications are treated medically. Digoxin for atrial fibrillation, diuretics for heart failure and anticoagulants to prevent clot formation and embolisation. The valve may be dilated (mitral valvotomy) or replaced surgically. There is also a new technique of stretching the stenosed valve with a balloon—mitral valvuloplasty. Its role has yet to be fully evaluated.

MITRAL INCOMPETENCE

Mitral incompetence has many causes (see Table 1.4) and is relatively common. It may develop rapidly, e.g. post MI when a papillary muscle ruptures, or gradually, e.g. after rheumatic fever.

Symptoms

With acute onset, dypsnoea and pulmonary congestion dominate. With chronic onset, the symptoms are very similar to those of mitral stenosis (see p. 18), palpitations are less common and emboli occur with a much lower frequency, especially if sinus rhythm is maintained.

Signs

1. Collapsing pulse, less marked than with aortic incompetence and sometimes referred to as the 'mini collapsing' pulse.
2. Sustained apex beat, often displaced towards the left.
3. Left parasternal heave of right ventricular hypertrophy develops with the onset of pulmonary hypertension.
4. Soft first heart sound at the apex as the cusps of the valve fail to come together properly.
5. Loud pulmonary second sound when pulmonary hypertension develops.
6. Pansystolic murmur heard at the apex and out towards the axilla and extending throughout the whole of systole.
7. As blood passes from the left atrium to the ventricle a further heart sound may be heard early in diastole over the apex (third heart sound).

Investigations

ECG usually shows sinus rhythm but can also show atrial fibrillation. Left atrial enlargement (P mitrale) occurs as will left ventricular hypertrophy in more severe cases (S wave in V_1 and R wave in V_5 or V_6, total > 35 mm).

Chest X-ray. Usually some degree of cardiomegaly is seen but signs of left atrial enlargement are less clearcut than they are with mitral stenosis. Upper lobe blood diversion may occur.

Echocardiography. Modern echocardiograms confirm the diagnosis and can give a good estimate of its severity.

Cardiac catheterisation. A left ventricular angiogram confirms the extent of the leak. It is largely restricted to preoperative assessment.

Treatment

Treatment may be medical, with digoxin for atrial fibrillation and diuretics for pulmonary congestion. There is debate as to whether these people should receive anticoagulants. Most cardiologists do this when there is evidence of left atrial enlargement and atrial fibrillation develops.

Surgery involves either replacing the valve (in most cases) or repairing it (in a few).

Functional mitral incompetence secondary to heart failure often improves as the heart failure is brought under control.

AORTIC STENOSIS

Aortic stenosis seems to be increasing as the population ages. The majority of stenoses are degenerative, occurring on previously bicuspid valves, and presentation is commonly in the later years of life. Some are congenital and may present at any age. Those secondary to rheumatic fever often also have mitral valve involvement and present in middle age.

Symptoms

1. Angina. The left ventricle hypertrophies and outgrows its blood supply while the aortic pressure, and hence coronary artery pressure, gradually falls as the valve stenosis develops.
2. Syncope due to heart block which develops as the valve and surrounding tissue calcify. Syncope on exertion (effort syncope) also occurs and is thought to arise from cardiac reflexes stimulated when the heart becomes overloaded.
3. Dyspnoea from pulmonary congestion.
4. Palpitations. Left atrial pressure may rise leading to atrial arrhythmias such as atrial fibrillation.
5. Occasionally sudden death occurs.

Patients with aortic stenosis are often asymptomatic because of the very considerable reserves of the left ventricle. The onset of symptoms is therefore very important and early investigation and treatment indicated.

Signs

A slow rising pulse is present. The blood pressure is low for the age together with a low pulse pressure. A sustained powerful apex beat is not generally displaced until heart failure develops. A thrill can sometimes be felt over the aortic area, in the carotid arteries or in the suprasternal notch.

The second heart sound is soft over the aortic area, especially when the valve becomes calcified and immobile. In younger people there may be an early systolic sound—the so-called ejection click. The murmur is quite characteristic. It is a harsh ejection systolic murmur which is crescendo–decrescendo in character. It is best heard over the aortic area and lower left sternal edge. It radiates well to the carotid arteries but poorly if at all to the axilla.

Investigations

ECG usually shows left ventricular hypertrophy and may also show ischaemia (so-called left ventricular strain pattern).

Chest X-ray shows a bulky but not grossly enlarged heart (Fig. 1.12). There is dilatation of the early part of the ascending aorta (post-stenotic dilatation).

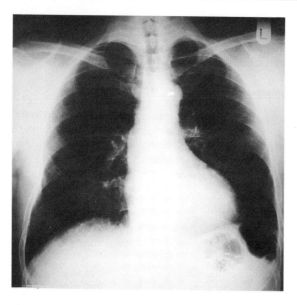

Fig. 1.12 Postero-anterior (PA) X-ray of the heart in aortic stenosis. The heart is not enlarged but looks bulky while the aorta is dilated just at its origin (post-stenotic dilatation)

In all patients the lateral chest X-ray almost invariably demonstrates heavy calcification in the valve. This is not seen in the postero-anterior (PA) film because of the overlying spine. When heart failure ensues the heart enlarges.

Echocardiography confirms the diagnosis and gives a reliable assessment of its severity.

Cardiac catheterisation is reserved for cases of doubt or for preoperative assessment.

Treatment

This is essentially surgical. When the patient becomes symptomatic an aortic valve replacement is needed. In some younger patients the valve may be split (aortic valvotomy). In a few elderly patients or in those too ill for surgery, balloon dilatation of the valve is occasionally performed (aortic valvuloplasty). Medical treatment is palliative until surgery can be performed.

AORTIC INCOMPETENCE

Symptoms

The symptoms of aortic incompetence are similar to those of aortic stenosis except that syncope occurs much less often. The heart seems to be able to cope with aortic incompetence well and judging the timing of valve replacement can be very difficult. Like mitral incompetence, aortic incompetence has many causes (see Table 1.4). Sometimes, there are also additional complicating features, such as aneurysms of the aorta in syphilis and Marfan's syndrome.

Signs

1. Collapsing or 'waterhammer' pulse.
2. Prominent arterial pulsations, e.g. the carotid arteries (Corrigan's sign).
3. High systolic and low diastolic blood pressure, i.e. wide pulse pressure.
4. Often, it is not possible to determine Korotkoff's fifth sound.
5. De Musset's sign (nodding of the head in time with the pulse) is seen in severe cases.
6. Quincke's sign (nailbed capillary pulsation).
7. Dancing retinal arteries (pulsating retinal vessels) may be observed on fundoscopy.
8. Pistol shot femorals. A crack is heard with light auscultation over the femoral arteries.
9. Durosiez's sign, a systolic bruit heard over the femoral arteries when the stethoscope is gently indented into the femoral artery.
10. Sustained apex beat which is displaced.
11. Soft aortic second sound.
12. High-pitched early diastolic murmur best heard at the lower left sternal edge and over the aortic area. It is classically described as blowing.
13. There may be an ejection systolic murmur over the same areas. This results from the large volume of blood having to be ejected at each systole and does not necessarily mean that the patient also has aortic stenosis.
14. Mid-diastolic murmur at the apex. The regurgitant jet of aortic blood may impinge upon the mitral valve resulting in a murmur there. This is the Austin-Flint murmur and, again, does not mean that the patient has mitral stenosis.

Investigations

ECG may show left ventricular hypertrophy and strain pattern if severe enough.

Chest X-ray shows cardiomegaly together with dilatation of the whole of the ascending aorta. It is more extensive and prominent that the post-stenotic dilatation of aortic stenosis.

Echocardiography confirms and can assess the severity of aortic incompetence.

Cardiac catheterisation. An injection of dye into the aorta (aortogram) at the time of cardiac catheterisation can also quantify the leak in the valve.

Aortic incompetence is well tolerated but if symptoms develop an aortic valve replacement is required.

TRICUSPID STENOSIS

Tricuspid stenosis is almost invariably secondary to rheumatic fever and as such occurs with rheumatic mitral or aortic valve disease which tend to dominate the clinical picture. There may be disproportionate venous and hepatic congestion and the liver may pulsate. It is often discovered coincidentally at echocardiography or cardiac catheterisation when the other valves are being investigated. Right atrial hypertrophy may be seen on the ECG and enlargement on the chest X-ray. Treatment is by tricuspid valvotomy and insertion of a supporting ring (annuloplasty). Valve replacement has not proved to be successful in tricuspid valve disease.

TRICUSPID INCOMPETENCE

Tricuspid incompetence is fairly common and usually secondary to right heart failure; it occurs when the right ventricle enlarges sufficiently to stretch the valve ring. The clinical picture is of dilated neck veins with prominent 'V' waves, a pulsatile enlarged liver and peripheral and sacral oedema and, if severe, ascites may also develop. It can disappear dramatically with resolution of the heart failure but annuloplasty may be required.

PULMONARY STENOSIS

Pulmonary stenosis is usually congenital. It is often asymptomatic, detected in the course of a medical examination. There may be a palpable thrill over the pulmonary area and a harsh ejection murmur radiating out into the lung fields. Even in mild cases the pulmonary arteries may be prominent on X-ray (from post stenotic dilatation). In severe cases the ECG shows right atrial and right ventricular hypertrophy. Echocardiography and, if needed, cardiac catheterisation confirm the diagnosis and give a reliable measure of its severity. Balloon dilatation is the treatment of choice although surgery may be needed in some cases.

PULMONARY INCOMPETENCE

Pulmonary incompetence is caused by pulmonary hypertension. The latter and its cause dominate the clinical picture and the pulmonary incompetence is largely a coincidental finding. Loud second heart sounds and an early diastolic murmur are heard in the pulmonary area and high left sternal edge.

INFECTIVE ENDOCARDITIS

This term now includes subacute bacterial endocarditis (SBE) and acute bacterial endocarditis (ABE).

SUBACUTE BACTERIAL ENDOCARDITIS (SBE)

Aetiology

Streptococcus viridans (the common dental organism). This now causes 30–50% of cases; in the past it was even more common. *Strep. epidermidis*, *Strep. faecalis*, *Staphylococcus aureus* and *Haemophilus influenzae* are other causative organisms.

In about 10% of cases the organism cannot be grown from the bloodstream and unusual infections, such as Q fever and those caused by chlamydia, anaerobes or fungi should be sought. The latter are particularly important where prosthetic valves have been inserted.

Symptoms and Signs

SBE usually presents very insidiously with weightloss, vague ill health and loss of appetite and energy. For these reasons diagnosis is difficult but eventually some helpful physical signs may appear, such as finger clubbing, small linear haemorrhages seen in the nailbeds of the hands and toes (splinter haemorrhages), painful nodules on the fingers (Osler's nodes), splenomegaly, small haemorrhagic spots seen in the optic fundi and probably resulting from arteritis (Roth's spots) and subconjunctival haemorrhages.

Haematuria is present in about 60% of patients; it is microscopic and only detected on testing of the urine.

On auscultation about 85% of the patients have a heart murmur and these are classically described as changing. Infective endocarditis typically develops on the valves of the heart but it may also occur on the heart wall, e.g. in the right ventricle opposite a ventricular septal defect.

If the valve is badly damaged heart failure may result. This can develop suddenly as valves perforate or are destroyed. SBE generally develops in relation to an underlying cardiac abnormality. It more usually occurs where there is high pressure turbulence, e.g. with a ventricular septal defect or in aortic stenosis. It is, therefore, relatively rare in mitral stenosis and atrial septal defects. Patients with a patent ductus arteriosus are particularly at risk. There must be bacteraemia for endocarditis to occur and this is particularly liable to happen with dental work or gastrointestinal surgery.

Investigations

Blood cultures must be taken before antibiotic treatment is started. Usually six blood cultures are sufficient (i.e. two batches of three).

A full blood count and ESR. These patients usually have a normocytic normochromic anaemia and a raised ESR. There is often a raised white cell count.

Circulating immune complex levels are high while complement levels are low. The haematuria is thought to be an immune response in the kidneys rather than to be caused by emboli.

Echocardiography detects vegetations on the valves. Absence of vegetations does not exclude infective endocarditis. Echocardiography can be extremely useful in monitoring progress of the condition and identifying the underlying cardiac abnormality.

Treatment

Antibiotics should be administered intravenously for up to 4 weeks. In some people a switch to oral antibiotics can be made before this time if the organism is very sensitive. Often, both penicillin and an aminoglycoside are used to potentiate each other. The blood levels of the antibiotics should be checked and titrated against their cidal (i.e. effective killing) levels of the organism isolated at blood culture. With prosthetic valves a slightly longer duration of treatment, perhaps up to 6 weeks, is advocated. During treatment it may become apparent that the infection is progressing remorselessly or that the valves, or, in some cases, renal function is deteriorating. All of these are indications for proceeding to surgery.

ACUTE BACTERIAL ENDOCARDITIS (ABE)

This is a much rarer condition and tends to be seen in people who are either immunosuppressed or subjected to overwhelming infection, e.g. drug addicts. Infection often develops on normal valves and the tricuspid valve can be affected here which is unusual with SBE. *Staph. aureus* is a common organism; it is highly destructive and associated with a high overall mortality.

CARDIOMYOPATHY

These are conditions that primarily affect cardiac muscle itself. Three types are described:
1. dilated or congestive cardiomyopathy
2. hypertrophic cardiomyopathy
3. restrictive cardiomyopathy.

DILATED CARDIOMYOPATHY

Some of these may represent a previous infection (myocarditis) of the heart muscle or may be due to end stage hypertension. In some cases they are alcohol induced and can occur with thyrotoxicosis. In the vast majority of people, congestive or dilated cardiomyopathy is of unknown aetiology. These people usually present with severely dilated hearts and heart failure.

Treatment is that of heart failure and removal of the cause, if possible. The majority deteriorate steadily and die within a few years of diagnosis.

HYPERTROPHIC CARDIOMYOPATHY

This used to be called hypertrophic obstructive cardiomyopathy (HOCM). The cardiac muscle hypertrophies in a disorganised way eventually obliterating the cardiac chamber. It is now known that this presents a major obstruction to filling of the heart whereas in the past the major problem was thought to be with cardiac emptying. It may be familial, with an autosomal dominant pattern, or be sporadic. The patients present with a full range of cardiac symptoms, namely rhythm disorders, breathlessness, heart failure, angina and syncope. The ECG is often grossly abnormal but the echocardiogram is characteristic showing asymmetrical hypertrophy, especially of the interventricular septum. This also results in a peculiar systolic anterior motion of the mitral valve (SAM). The aortic valve also closes early.

Treatment is with anti-arrhythmic agents, especially amiodarone. Beta-blockers and verapamil have also been used but when heart failure supervenes diuretics may be needed. In symptomatic patients, progress is often remorseless and life expectancy poor.

RESTRICTIVE CARDIOMYOPATHY

This is a rare form of cardiomyopathy and is usually caused by amyloid infiltration of the heart. It restricts movement of the left ventricle, hence the name. Clinically, the differentiation from constrictive pericarditis is important as this latter condition can be treated surgically whereas restrictive cardiomyopathy cannot.

DISSECTION OF THE AORTA

In patients with high blood pressure or atheromatous plaques of the aorta, blood can track into the aortic wall, travelling for a variable distance and then re-entering the aorta itself. A better term for this condition might be 'dissecting haematoma'. The outcome is decided by the distance, the re-entry point of the haematoma and the extent of the damage it causes en route. It may extend from just above the aortic valve all the way down beyond the renal arteries. Hypertension is the common predisposing factor but there are associations with Marfan's syndrome, coarctation of the aorta, bicuspid aortic valves and unfortunately with the third trimester of pregnancy. Three types have been described (Fig. 1.13):

1. Type 1 affects the ascending aorta and around the arch and is generally the most extensive.
2. Type 2 affects the ascending aorta.
3. Type 3 affects the descending aorta.

These are thoracic aneurysms but, of course, many aneurysms also occur in the abdomen. The treatment of choice for descending thoracic dissections is medical but surgical repair is required for types 1 and 2 and intra-abdominal aneurysms.

On examination all the arteries coming off the arch should be checked, i.e.

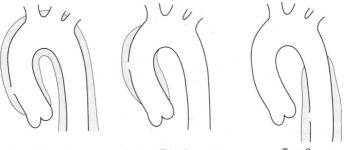

Type 1   Type 2   Type 3

Fig. 1.13 Types of aortic dissection

the radials and the carotids. Often the renal arteries are affected and the femoral arteries should also be checked. The dissection may cause the aortic valve to become incompetent and sometimes blood leaks into the pericardial sac or into the pleural space.

The chest X-ray shows a broad mediastinum and the various scanning techniques of the aorta such as ultrasound, CT or magnetic resonance imaging (MRI) may delineate the exact extent of the problem. Aortograms can be dangerous in this situation but are occasionally needed.

In all cases treatment is initially medical with bedrest, pain relief and lowering of the blood pressure but surgery may be required urgently for dissections involving other major arteries or the ascending aorta.

CARDIAC TUMOURS

Cardiac tumours are very rare. Any of the tissues in the heart may be involved in tumour formation. Myxomas are the most common, classically occurring in the left atrium and mimicking mitral stenosis. Occasionally they occur elsewhere in the heart and sometimes recur after surgical removal. They have a classical echocardiographic appearance. There is a high risk of embolisation of these tumours. They should be removed by surgery as soon as they are diagnosed.

MYOCARDITIS

Acute infection of the heart rarely leads to clinical problems. However, occasionally myocarditis mimics MI and it is thought that it can also progress to congestive or dilated cardiomyopathy in some patients.

In South America, Chagas' disease, caused by trypanosomiasis, is a common infection causing myocarditis and leading on to cardiomyopathy.

PERICARDITIS

Pericarditis may be acute or chronic. Acute pericarditis is usually the result of a viral infection and is self limiting. It can, however, be part of the clinical picture of MI and also occurs in uraemia.

Pericarditis classically causes a scratching sound over the heart. It is very superficial and occurs in time with the heartbeat. It may also be affected by the respiratory cycle.

In a classical case the ECG will show ST segment elevation which is concave upwards and present in most if not all of the leads.

In benign pericarditis the condition tends to be self limiting although anti-inflammatory drugs may occasionally be needed to ease the pain.

CONSTRICTIVE PERICARDITIS

In this condition the pericardium is thick and stiff and impairs cardiac filling. It may even be calcified and it used to be secondary to tuberculous infection.

Impaired filling of the heart may give rise to physical signs such as ascites and hepatomegaly. The venous pressure is usually raised and increases with

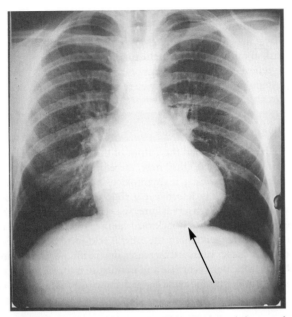

Fig. 1.14 Chest X-ray in constrictive pericarditis. The heart is large and very round in shape. Calcification (better seen on a lateral film) is noted on the diaphragmatic surface of the heart

inspiration (Kusmaul's sign). The heart itself may be largely impalpable which is out of keeping with the other physical signs, and a loud third heart sound may be audible (the pericardial knock).

The ECG is usually of low voltage and the chest X-ray shows a round heart (Fig. 1.14) often with calcium in the pericardium, more easily seen on a lateral film.

Likewise, the echocardiogram may show dense echoes around the heart. Tuberculosis is now rare and most cases are thought to be caused by trauma, rheumatoid arthritis, uraemia or to be secondary to neoplastic disease.

PERICARDIAL EFFUSION

Fluid may gather in the pericardial sac. This often follows pericarditis but is more commonly seen in heart failure or secondarily to neoplastic involvement. The pericardium is relatively inflexible and when fluid gathers the heart becomes compressed, resulting in pericardial tamponade. The physical signs represent those of impaired cardiac filling with a raised jugular venous pressure (JVP), a large liver, ascites and peripheral oedema, although all these findings are less common than with constrictive pericarditis.

Because of the impaired filling the normal inspiratory fall in blood pressure is more pronounced in the presence of a pericardial effusion. Although the fall in blood pressure occurs during inspiration it is called paradoxical. It is not really a paradox and usually exceeds 10 mmHg. Because of the fluid, the heart sounds are soft and distant.

The chest X-ray shows a round enlarged heart and there are low voltages on the ECG. Echocardiography is by far the best way of detecting and quantifying pericardial effusions. An echo-free space is seen behind the heart and also anteriorly if the effusion is large. Most effusions should not be drained because of the risk of infection but with the development of tamponade they may have to be to relieve the patient's symptoms. If the effusion is caused by neoplastic disease, tapping the effusion may be required to help with the diagnosis.

HEART FAILURE

Heart failure occurs when the output of the heart is incapable of meeting the demands of the tissues. There may, therefore, be high output failure when the demands are excessive, e.g. in thyrotoxicosis and anaemia, or low output failure where the heart itself is defective, e.g. following an MI. Many other terms have been used to describe heart failure, e.g. left heart failure, right heart failure, congestive cardiac failure, backward failure, forward failure, etc. In practice when either ventricle is failing, the other is seldom left unaffected. Failure of the left ventricle causes pressure increases upstream, i.e. in the lungs, which ultimately affect the right ventricle and may cause it to fail. When the heart fails, a number of endocrine and renal compensatory mechanisms are set in force.

Salt and water retention. Patients with heart failure retain fluid and it is this which gives rise to many of the physical signs, e.g. peripheral oedema or pulmonary crepitations and pulmonary oedema. The renin–angiotensin system is activated and aldosterone levels increase.

Vasoconstriction. In order to preserve the blood supply to the vital organs, the blood supply to the less important areas, i.e. the skin and muscles, tends to be reduced. Therefore the patient often looks very pale or even cyanosed. This is due to activation of the sympathetic nervous system. Knowledge of these various compensatory mechanisms, many of which in the long term can be disadvantageous, has allowed a rational approach to therapy.

Aetiology (Table 1.6)

Certain drugs depress myocardial contractility; for example beta-blockers can cause an impaired heart to fail. Others can cause fluid retention (e.g. steroids) or even damage the heart (e.g. some anti-cancer drugs).

Heart failure may also be secondary to other conditions such as hypothyroidism, hyperthyroidism, anaemia, diabetes, hypertension and obesity. However, ischaemic and valvular heart disease are by far the commonest causes.

Symptoms and signs

Assuming the patient does not have one of the rare forms of high output failure, both the symptoms and signs depend very much on whether failure predominantly affects the left side of the heart or the right.

Left-sided heart failure is associated with dyspnoea, tachycardia, and low blood pressure and thready low volume pulse. The patient is often pale, clammy and sweaty but in compensated heart failure most of these physical

Table 1.6. Aetiology of heart failure (low output)

Heart muscle disease	Arrhythmias*
Myocardial infarction/ischaemia	Atrial fibrillation
Cardiomyopathy	Atrial flutter
Myocarditis	Complete heart block
Pressure overload	Other causes
Hypertension	Constrictive pericarditis
Aortic stenosis	Pericardial tamponade
Volume overload	
Mitral incompetence	
Aortic incompetence	

* If they persist, even benign arrhythmias such as supraventricular tachycardia (SVT) can lead to heart failure.

signs are absent.

There may be crepitations in the lung fields and examination of the heart may reveal a cause for the failure, e.g. aortic stenosis. In other cases the heart may be enlarged, the quality of the heart sounds is generally poor, and there may be additional heart sounds, e.g. a third or fourth heart sound.

If failure is predominantly right sided, or if right-sided failure is present in addition to left-sided failure, venous pressure is usually elevated and can be seen as a raised JVP in the neck.

The liver may be enlarged and may be pulsatile. There is usually peripheral oedema in the lower limbs if the patient is upright and over the lower end of the back if the patient is confined to bed (sacral oedema).

Ultimately fluid may gather in the abdomen (ascites); this is a sign of very severe heart failure. Because the liver is enlarged and congested, these patients can often be jaundiced. The hepatic congestion may also make them feel nauseous, and the liver is often tender.

Investigations

These patients are often very unwell and investigation commonly follows treatment. The management of heart failure is fairly standard regardless of the cause but, of course, ultimately it may depend on the results of the investigations. In a patient with aortic stenosis, for example, who presents with heart failure, medical therapy will often resolve the heart failure but the long-term treatment depends on replacing the valve.

ECG. This is helpful in determining whether the patient may have had a myocardial infarct and also for showing any abnormal rhythm patterns. It may also demonstrate hypertrophy as occurs in hypertension or aortic stenosis.

Chest X-ray (Fig. 1.15) is occasionally helpful in determining the cause of heart failure but more usually simply confirms an enlarged heart with the

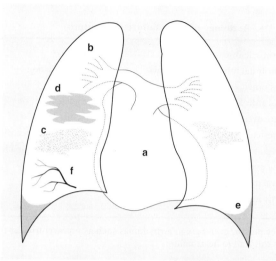

Fig. 1.15 The postero-anterior (PA) chest X-ray findings in heart failure. (**a**) An enlarged heart; (**b**) upper lobe blood diversion, i.e. prominent upper lobe pulmonary arteries; (**c**) fluid in the lung fields; (**d**) fluid in the lung fissures; (**e**) pleural effusions; (**f**) prominent lung lymphatics—Kerley B lines

appearance of fluid in the lung fields. Pleural effusions may be present.
Echocardiography is particularly useful in the assessment of left ventricular function and may also identify any valvular abnormality.

Cardiac catheterisation is needed in some cases, e.g. to exclude a left ventricular aneurysm.

Treatment

Treatment depends upon whether the onset of the heart failure is acute or chronic. In all forms of heart failure, symptomatic treatment is initiated to be followed by treatment of the underlying cause.

ACUTE LEFT VENTRICULAR FAILURE (LVF)

The onset of LVF is often extremely sudden. It may first occur in the middle of the night when redistribution of blood from the lower limbs to the chest is the final straw for the failing heart. Likewise, an acute onset of a rhythm disorder or undue physical exertion may be the precipitating factor. The patient is usually acutely breathless, very distressed and unable to communicate. Not surprisingly, most feel they are about to die.

Treatment

1. The patient should be sat upright and 100% oxygen administered. The upright position reduces venous return to the heart and also takes pressure off the diaphragm.

2. A loop diuretic, e.g. frusemide, is given intravenously.
3. Intravenous opiates, e.g. morphine; in addition to the psychological relief they bring, these drugs also benefit left ventricular function and have a mild diuretic effect.
4. Digoxin. Whether or not digoxin should be used in acute heart failure is arguable. It has a relatively slow onset of action and intravenously it can cause dangerous arrhythmias. It does, however, increase myocardial contractility without increasing oxygen demand.
5. Aminophylline has been used to dilate the airways. It also increases both heart rate and myocardial contractility but it may induce arrhythmias and has to be used carefully, if at all.
6. Some patients do not respond to the above measures and vasodilators can then be used. Glyceryl trinitrate (GTN) reduces both preload and afterload and can be used both sublingually or intravenously. Other drugs used occasionally in this context are sodium nitroprusside, hydralazine and prazosin.

CHRONIC LEFT VENTRICULAR FAILURE

Chronic LVF can range from mild to very severe. The former is often simply managed by diuretics. Sometimes digoxin is added and more recently the angiotensin converting enzyme (ACE) inhibitors have been used at this stage. Nitrates and the arterial vasodilators hydralazine and prazosin have also been used but tend to be reserved for more severe failure or for those in whom ACE inhibitors are contraindicated.

Bedrest is very important in heart failure. All patients with cardiac failure are well advised to have a siesta but in the more severe cases a few days in bed often reduces the work of the heart enough for it to at least partially recover. Additional extreme measures which may be used are to reduce sodium intake and restrict fluid intake. Certainly, all patients with heart failure should be encouraged not to add table salt to their food.

ACE inhibitors have been shown to improve both the quantity and the quality of life in people with chronic heart failure. The combination of a long-acting nitrate and hydralazine may do the same. Anyone with more than very mild heart failure ought to be given vasodilators if possible.

The treatment of the causes of LVF are described under the various headings, i.e. arrhythmia, MI, valvular heart disease, etc.

RIGHT VENTRICULAR FAILURE

Right ventricular failure (RVF) is almost always secondary to left ventricular failure although it can occur in its own right with pulmonary hypertension or pulmonary valve disease. Treatment is essentially similar to that of left ventricular failure.

HYPERTENSION

In Western societies blood pressure increases with age. In young women it is generally a little lower than in young men but crossover occurs in middle age so

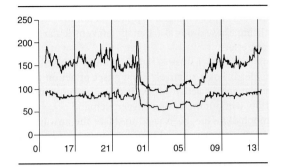

Fig. 1.16 Ambulatory intra-arterial blood pressure recording showing systolic and diastolic pressures over a 24-hour period. Note the wide variations in pressure that occur over this period with the characteristic fall during sleep

that elderly females have higher blood pressures than elderly men. Except for extremely low blood pressures, there is a linear relationship between the level of blood pressure and cardiovascular risk.

Blood pressure is very labile (Fig. 1.16) and it can fluctuate by 200–300% during the course of a day. For instance it is extremely high during sexual intercourse and may fall to one-third of those levels a few minutes later during sleep. Anxiety (the alerting response) can cause the blood pressure to be artificially elevated and it is well known that doctors can induce this response—white coat hypertension.

Many blood pressure measurements have to be taken before classifying a patient as hypertensive. As treatment for high blood pressure is generally lifelong, the diagnosis has to be secure before starting treatment. None the less, blood pressure is the most important determinant of life expectancy in Western societies and when high blood pressure is finally established this should be treated.

People who are diagnosed as having hypertension often develop symptoms which are attributed to it but, except for the malignant phase, hypertension is an asymptomatic disorder so when treatment is instituted it is important that it causes no symptoms. Lack of compliance is one of the great difficulties in managing hypertension. It is thought that about 10% of the population have significantly elevated blood pressures; very many of these are undetected and very many are detected but not managed properly. The quality of care in hypertension is all important to the outcome.

IDIOPATHIC HIGH BLOOD PRESSURE

In the majority of people, no cause can be found for the high blood pressure. This is called primary or essential hypertension and there is often a family history.

Obesity. Obese people have higher blood pressures in the main than slim people and substantial reductions in blood pressure can be obtained by weightloss.

Alcohol. There is a rough linear relationship between alcohol intake in units and blood pressure. Alcoholics have a higher incidence than normal of hypertension and the blood pressure drops when they abstain.

Salt intake. People with high blood pressure should be discouraged from adding salt to their food.

Exercise. Exercise is anti-hypertensive and a combination of increased exercise and weightloss can be very effective in reducing blood pressure.

A cause can be found for hypertension in 2–3% of middle-aged people. Even then, the treatment is very much as for essential hypertension with the result that extensive investigation of hypertension in middle and later life has largely been abandoned. In 20-year-olds, however, there is a 50% chance of detecting one of the causes of secondary hypertension and they should be investigated more exhaustively.

Symptoms and signs

History taking and physical examination are very important. Certain drugs can cause hypertension and enquiries should be made about them, e.g. the oral contraceptive pill which is often not regarded by the patient as a drug. Patients who have accelerated hypertension, i.e. those known to be normotensive a year or two ago and who are now significantly hypertensive, often have a renal cause for their high blood pressure.

The influence of high blood pressure on the target organs, e.g. the heart, the blood vessels, the kidneys and the brain, should be sought. The risk to the cardiovascular system of any given level of blood pressure is increased 4- or 5-fold in the presence of target organ damage.

Hypertension is usually asymptomatic. There may, however, be symptoms in malignant hypertension where fibrinoid necrosis of small blood vessels occurs. This gives rise to a systemic illness with weightloss, loss of appetite and general malaise. These patients have protein and blood in the urine with changes in the optic fundi and, untreated, their outlook is poor.

More usually the patient does not have malignant hypertension (occurs in only 1% of hypertensives) and the physical signs are more subtle.

1. The heart may be enlarged clinically but generally in pressure overload the heart hypertrophies concentrically inwards so that the apex is left ventricular in type but not displaced.
2. The optic fundi should always be examined as this is the only place in the body where arteries can be viewed directly. The classification of Keith and Wagener is used to describe them (Table 1.7).
3. The abdomen should be examined for masses (phaeochromocytoma) and the kidneys palpated.
4. Renal artery bruits may be heard on either side of the umbilicus or just below the ribs at the back in renal artery stenosis.
5. Femoral arteries should be palpated and in coarctation of the aorta the

Table 1.7. Retinal changes in hypertension (Keith–Wagener classification)

Grade 1	Arteries become straighter and reflect light due to thickening of their walls (silver wiring). They may also show some variation in calibre
Grade 2	In addition, the arteries (because they are thickened) compress the veins at points where they cross each other (arteriovenous (AV) nipping)
Grade 3	In addition, flame shaped haemorrhages are seen as are soft (cotton wool) white exudates
Grade 4	In addition, swelling (papilloedema) of the optic disc occurs

Points to note

Grades 1 and 2 may appear with advancing years. It is their premature appearance that is important

Grades 3 and 4 represent severe hypertensive change and often occur with malignant hypertension

Even in grade 4 hypertension there may be minimal or no upset in vision

Grades 3 and 4 changes usually resolve within a few weeks of successful anti-hypertensive treatment

femoral arteries are diminished and the pulse delayed. Abnormal blood vessels in coarctation may be detected over the back near the scapulae where they may be both felt and pulsations heard. In coarctation the blood pressure should be checked in both upper and lower limbs.

Investigations

Investigation of a middle-aged patient with hypertension is limited to chest X-ray, ECG, electrolytes, creatinine, mid-stream specimen of urine (MSU), full blood count and lipid profile.

Much of this will show any target organ damage, e.g. left ventricular hypertrophy on the ECG. Where a secondary cause for hypertension is suspected, there are specific tests as discussed below.

In a younger patient, routine investigation would also include assessment of urinary vanillylmandelic acid (VMA) and a hypertensive intravenous pyelogram (IVP). Some physicians may replace the IVP with a renal ultrasound examination.

SECONDARY CAUSES OF HYPERTENSION

Coarctation of aorta

In any young person presenting with high blood pressure, coarctation of the aorta should be suspected (see under Congenital heart disease, p. 44).

Endocrine causes

Cushing's syndrome

These patients usually present with the clinical picture of Cushing's syndrome and the hypertension is simply part of that picture (see p. 184).

Conn's syndrome

Resulting from an overproduction of aldosterone, some cases are due to adrenal tumours and others to hyperplasia of the adrenal gland. Despite the presence of a tumour, these people often respond well to an aldosterone antagonist (spironolactone) and surgery can be avoided. Conn's syndrome should always be suspected if an untreated patient with hypertension has a low potassium level. The diagnosis is confirmed by measuring the plasma aldosterone levels and by a CT scan of the abdomen. Clinically, there is weakness, headaches and thirst. It is important to remember that thiazide diuretics are the most important cause of hypokalaemia in the hypertensive population and if Conn's syndrome is suspected the patient should be off diuretics for at least 1 month prior to the electrolyte level being checked.

Phaeochromocytoma

This tumour arises in sympathetic nervous tissue, usually the adrenal gland, but in 10% it is found in sympathetic nervous tissue elsewhere. Approximately 10% of them are malignant. They should be suspected where the blood pressure is increasing rapidly or where there are associated symptoms such as flushing or attacks of pallor and sweatiness associated with hypertension. Although classically hypertension caused by phaeochromocytoma is described as intermittent, in fact it is more often sustained. All hypertensive patients under the age of 40 should be screened for this tumour.

Urinary VMA is checked in a 24-hour sample. If this is positive the urinary metanephrines and normetanephrines which are metabolites of adrenaline and noradrenaline respectively are checked. Some laboratories measure plasma catecholamines directly.

The tumour can sometimes be palpated in the abdomen although once detected it should not be repeatedly examined as catecholamines can be released into the circulation and cause major cardiovascular effects when handled. Sometimes the tumour shows up as calcification on a plain X-ray film of the abdomen. A CT scan is usually required to localise it. These tumours should be removed surgically.

Renal causes

Most renal diseases can cause high blood pressure. Chronic pyelonephritis or glomerulonephritis and polycystic kidney disease are common causes. Formerly, it was thought that pyelonephritis could be unilateral; however, the second kidney seldom escapes the infection and therefore unilateral nephrectomy has largely been abandoned.

Renal artery stenosis

Renal artery stenosis should be suspected with relatively recent onset of hypertension. A bruit may be heard in the abdomen but often there are no physical signs. In the younger patient fibromuscular dysplasia is the cause while in the older patient atheroma narrows the renal artery. In these older patients there may be evidence of atheroma elsewhere. Renal ultrasound will show a smaller kidney on the affected side. An IVP may show a delay in contrast medium appearance and clearance on the affected side. A renal arteriogram is performed to assess the anatomy, and renal vein renin levels may be elevated on the affected side.

In older patients the only reason for operating on renal artery stenosis is to preserve renal function but in younger patients either surgical correction of the stenosis is performed or dilatation by means of balloon angioplasty may be attempted. Very often the radiologist performing the renal arteriogram will go on to do the angioplasty at the same time if he detects a suitable lesion. About 50% of such people will have their hypertension cured by the procedure and another 35% will be easier to control medically.

Pregnancy

Eclampsia is a very serious condition with great risk to mother and child. Fortunately, it is rare, but much more common is pre-eclamptic toxaemia where the blood pressure is less severely elevated. There is usually ankle swelling and proteinuria and it is usual to treat the elevated blood pressure. Few drugs are recommended for use in pregnancy but propranolol, labetolol, hydralazine, methyl dopa and atenolol have all been shown to be relatively safe, as has nifedipine.

Pre-existing essential hypertension in pregnancy also presents an increased risk to mother and child and should be treated.

Drugs

The contraceptive pill

This is the commonest drug causing high blood pressure. Usually this is only a matter of a few mmHg but in some patients it can be greater. In females with pre-existing hypertension oral contraception is relatively contraindicated.

Corticosteroids

Usually steroids have to be given for important reasons, e.g. asthma, arthritis, etc., and cannot be stopped. The dose should certainly be titrated down to the lowest level possible and then the blood pressure treated if need be.

Liquorice derivatives

Carbenoxolone, which was used to treat peptic ulcers, can increase blood pressure.

Other drugs, e.g. the non-steroidal anti-inflammatory agents, can interfere with the action of some anti-hypertensive agents.

PATHOLOGICAL CONSEQUENCES OF HIGH BLOOD PRESSURE

High blood pressure itself is not a disease but predisposes to damage in the target organs. Before effective treatment, heart failure was the most common end point; now, it is MI and IHD. It is one of the enigmas of medicine that good blood pressure management has only little reduced the high incidence of IHD in hypertensive patients. The pathological sequelae of hypertension are myocardial ischaemia/infarction, cerebrovascular accident, renal failure, heart failure, and aneurysm formation with subsequent dissection or rupture.

Treatment

Treating people with severe hypertension is very effective in preventing subsequent morbid events. In the mild to moderate range of blood pressures, there is greater debate and the benefits are less clear cut. This is perhaps because of the difficulty in separating alerting responses from true hypertension but, of course, the risks for mild hypertension are lower than those for severe hypertension and many more people have to be treated before benefits emerge.

Irrespective of the cause of high blood pressure, all hypertensive patients (except for those with very severe or malignant hypertension) should be encouraged to take more exercise. They should also be encouraged to get down to their ideal bodyweight and to minimise their alcohol and salt consumption.

The philosophy behind treating hypertension has changed in recent years. It used to be advocated that if one drug did not work another should be added and so on. Now treatment is towards tailored care where if one drug does not work, another should be substituted rather than added. The commonly used first choice drugs are thiazide diuretics, beta-adrenergic blocking agents, calcium channel blocking agents and ACE inhibitors. To these may be added in due course the alpha-adrenergic blocking agents.

Thiazide diuretics (e.g. bendrofluazide, cyclopenthiazide, hydrochlorothiazide). These drugs are all effective anti-hypertensive agents. In the past they were used in high doses which increased the side-effects but not the anti-hypertensive effects. Hypokalaemia is the major side-effect but they also have adverse effects on blood lipids, blood glucose and uric acid levels. They may also cause excessive loss of sodium particularly in the elderly. Despite this they have been shown in general to be safe and effective in hypertension.

Beta-adrenergic blocking agents. A wide variety of beta-blockers are now available but cardioselective (i.e. largely working on the heart), agents should be used, e.g. atenolol, metoprolol. Beta-blocking agents can provoke bronchospasm and are contraindicated in asthma. They may also worsen heart failure and because of the drop in cardiac output the patients often feel disproportionately tired. Cold extremities have occasionally been severe enough to cause peripheral ischaemia and gangrene. Bad dreams are a strange but well recognised side-effect. Again, in the majority of patients they cause no problems and are good and effective anti-hypertensive agents.

Calcium channel blocking drugs. These constitute several different chemical types but basically all act as vasodilators. Some of them, e.g. verapamil, have a negative effect on cardiac contractility while nifedipine may even stimulate the heart. The side-effects include fluid retention and headaches. Many newer agents are being developed which have better side-effect profiles.

Angiotensin converting enzyme (ACE) inhibitors are well tolerated and, in the usual doses, seem to be safe. In people with high renin levels they can cause a precipitous fall in blood pressure. This is more likely to occur in people already on diuretics. ACE inhibitors should only be started under close supervision. Other than hypotension, an irritating dry cough is the principle side-effect.

Alpha-adrenergic blocking agents. These are now increasingly being used as first choice agents. The newer drugs do not cause the same postural hypotension as did the older alpha-blocking agents and they may have beneficial effects on blood lipids (e.g. terazosin).

Other anti-hypertensive agents. After these first choice drugs which can be used in practically any combination, additional drugs available include systemic arterial vasodilators, e.g. hydralazine, and centrally acting drugs such as methyldopa, clonidine and reserpine. All centrally acting drugs tend to have central side-effects such as sedation but clonidine can cause marked rebound hypertension after it is withdrawn while reserpine is said to cause depression. Impotence may also occur with these drugs.

Minoxidil is a potent vasodilator which is generally best reserved for hospital use. Its principal side-effect is hirsutism which makes it generally unsuitable for use in females.

Labetalol is a combined alpha- and beta-blocking drug which is predominantly alpha when used intravenously and beta when used orally. For some time it was widely used in pregnancy and in the management of malignant hypertension.

MALIGNANT HYPERTENSION

In about 1% of patients with hypertension the blood pressure follows an accelerated and worsening course. When necrosis of the small blood vessels (fibrinoid necrosis) occurs severe changes are found in the optic fundi and proteinuria and haematuria result. This is malignant hypertension and if untreated will lead to death, usually within 1 year.

Malignant hypertension may also present with hypertensive encephalopathy. In this condition there is raised intracranial pressure and the patient is confused and disorientated. Left ventricular failure can also result from malignant hypertension, as can dissection of the aorta.

In all forms of malignant hypertension the first essential is to reduce the blood pressure but not to normal levels. Any reduction in blood pressure represents a move in the right direction and certainly initially a systolic pressure of around 200 mmHg and a diastolic pressure of around 110 mmHg is an acceptable target. After that, in the ensuing days and weeks the blood pressure can be titrated further downwards. With dissection of the aorta more vigorous treatment is required, possible using intravenous drugs and monitoring in an intensive care unit. All patients with malignant hypertension should be admitted to hospital for treatment.

PERIPHERAL VASCULAR DISEASE

Aetiology

Smoking, hyperlipidaemia, hypertension and diabetes are the major causes.

Symptoms and signs

Cramp-like discomfort, usually in the calves or buttocks, on exertion. If disease is severe, the pain can occur at rest. If ulcers are present they can be very painful. There is coldness in the legs distally. The major signs are cold limbs (often difference between the two sides), hair loss, shiny pale skin, absent or poor pulses and possible ulcers or gangrene.

Management

The risk factors must be reduced, and the patient started on regular aspirin. Good skin and foot care, e.g. by a chiropodist, are essential. Regular exercise to encourage development of collateral (new) vessels should be encouraged. Treatment may be by balloon dilatation or surgical.

RAYNAUD'S DISEASE AND RAYNAUD'S PHENOMENON

Spasm occurs in the digital arteries, and the fingers become white and bloodless. It is much worse in colder weather and occurs in up to 5% of the population. It is more common in females and occasionally secondary to other diseases (Raynaud's phenomenon) but is usually of unknown aetiology (Raynaud's disease).

TEMPORAL ARTERITIS

Inflammation of the temporal arteries presents as headache with tenderness over the vessels. It may lead to sudden blindness and needs immediate treatment with large doses of corticosteroids, e.g. 60–80 mg prednisolone daily.

The blood viscosity and ESR are raised when the disease process is active.

Other types of arteritis:

TAKAYASU'S ARTERITIS

Arteritis of the vessels arising from and including the aortic arch eventually leads to loss of pulses (pulseless disease) and hypertension.

SYPHILIS

Syphilis causes aortitis which, in turn, may lead to aortic aneurysms, aortic valve incompetence and narrowing of the ostia of the coronary arteries.

VARICOSE VEINS

Seen in the lower limbs, varicose veins are usually of cosmetic importance only. Occasionally they cause pain and discomfort and may lead to ulcer formation. Treatment is by sclerosing injection or surgical removal.

SUPERFICIAL THROMBOPHLEBITIS

This usually occurs in the legs but may also involve the veins of the arms. The vein is inflamed and thrombosed and can be very painful and tender. It feels like a hard cord and is frequently seen at sites of intravenous infusions. Thrombophlebitis responds to simple symptomatic therapy, e.g. pain relief or anti-inflammatory drugs.

DEEP VENOUS THROMBOSIS (DVT)

There are a number of predisposing factors to DVT, including immobility (especially in hospital), increasing age, obesity, surgery, varicose veins, pregnancy, family history, contraceptive pill use and congenital defects. Malignancy also predisposes to deep venous thrombosis and should be suspected if the DVT is recurrent.

The patient may be asymptomatic but will often have calf pain, swelling of the leg with prominence of superficial veins and discoloration (cyanosis). The affected limb is usually warm and there is a risk of pulmonary embolism. DVT can be detected by ultrasound but more usually a venogram is performed. Anticoagulation is required for 3 months although if recurrent it may be for life. Support stockings and occasionally, if the thrombosis is massive, thrombolysis may be used (streptokinase).

It should be noted that venograms can be falsely negative and should not override the diagnosis in a clinically apparent case.

CONGENITAL HEART DISEASE

Congenital heart disease is found in 8 out of every 1000 children born. Many aborted fetuses are also found to have malformed hearts. If a couple already

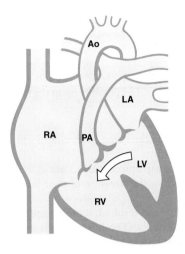

Fig. 1.17 Ventricular septal defect

has one child with congenital heart disease then the chances of the next or subsequent children being affected is increased to 25 per 1000 live births.

The aetiology of congenital heart disease is largely unknown but there are some associations:

1. chromosome abnormalities such as occur with Turner's or Down's syndromes
2. exposure to rubella virus in early pregnancy
3. drug exposure in the first trimester of pregnancy
4. ionising radiation.

NEONATAL CONGENITAL HEART DISEASE

The incidence and type of congenital heart disorders are quite different in this age group from those in the older child. These young patients present either with signs of heart failure or with cyanosis. They should all be referred for specialist investigation and treatment as soon as anything is suspected.

CONGENITAL HEART DISEASE IN OLDER CHILDREN

This is usually classified as cyanotic or acyanotic. The acyanotic forms greatly exceed cyanotic forms.

ACYANOTIC CONGENITAL HEART DISEASE

Ventricular septal defect (VSD) (Fig. 1.17)

There is a defect (sometimes multiple defects) in the interventricular septum.

Overall, VSDs constitute 25% of all cases of congenital heart disease and are the commonest malformation. Because the left side of the heart has higher pressures than the right, the flow-through the defect is in a left-to-right direction. The high pressure left ventricle can pump large quantities of blood through a ventricular septal defect and it is the quantity of such flow (or shunt) that determines the outcome; 30–40% of VSDs will close spontaneously, usually in the first year of life, but possibly up to the fourth decade.

Symptoms and signs

At any age, large VSDs can cause heart failure with dyspnoea, fatigue, failure to gain weight or to thrive.

Most children are asymptomatic but are closely followed up in case they develop heart failure or the pressure in their lungs starts to rise (pulmonary hypertension).

Unless heart failure has resulted, these patients appear normal but the heart may be enlarged clinically. The heart sounds are usually normal but if pulmonary hypertension is developing the pulmonary second sound (P2) is loud. There is a pansystolic murmur, best heard at the left sternal edge in the third and fourth intercostal spaces. A systolic thrill can often be felt in the same area.

Investigations

Chest X-ray shows an enlarged heart with increased lung markings due to the increased pulmonary blood flow, i.e. plethoric lung fields.

ECG is usually normal but T wave changes in lead V_1 in particular may indicate the onset of pulmonary hypertension in young children, i.e. the T waves

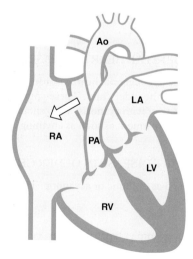

Fig. 1.18 Atrial septal defect

become flat or upright being normally inverted.

Echocardiography often demonstrates the defect in the interventricular septum and quantifies the size of the shunt.

Cardiac catheterisation can quantify the shunt and injection of contrast medium can identify its site.

Treatment
This should be medical if at all possible because of the possibility that the VSD may close spontaneously but some do need to be closed surgically.

Atrial septal defect (ASD) (Fig. 1.18)

There are two major types: ostium secundum defect, which is usually an isolated defect, and ostium primum defect, which forms part of the spectrum of abnormalities occurring when there is defective development of the endocardial cushions in the heart. As well as the atrial septum, the ventricular septum and both mitral and tricuspid valves may be defective. In the absence of the associated defects it can be impossible clinically to differentiate between the two types of ASD. However, they give quite different ECG and echocardiographic appearances.

Symptoms and signs
These patients are usually asymptomatic and the ASD is found coincidentally when a murmur is noticed. The second heart sound remains split either widely

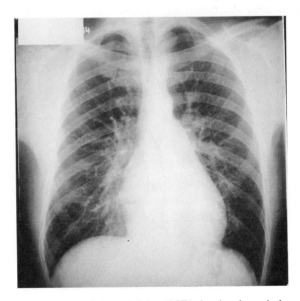

Fig. 1.19 Chest X-ray in atrial septal defect (ASD) showing the typical appearance of small aorta, enlarged pulmonary artery, increased heart size and lung vascularity (plethoric lung fields)

with some respiratory variation or more classically fixed splitting occurs.

Increased blood flow over the normal pulmonary valve results in an ejection systolic murmur. With ostium primum defects, there may be pansystolic murmurs of mitral reflux or of a ventricular septal defect (VSD) or both. If pulmonary hypertension develops the P2 may be loud.

Investigations

Chest X-ray shows a characteristic peardrop appearance. This arises because the aorta is small and the pulmonary artery is large. The lung fields look plethoric and the heart is slightly enlarged (Fig. 1.19).

ECG usually shows partial right bundle branch block (RBBB) pattern. There is shift of the heart's electrical access to the left in ostium primum defects (left axis deviation) and to the right in ostium secundum defects (right axis deviation). The PR interval may be prolonged in primum but not secundum defects.

Echocardiography identifies and quantifies the defect and is able to differentiate the two types.

Cardiac catheterisation can confirm the defect and quantify the degree of shunting.

Treatment

Large ASDs need to be closed if the pulmonary to systemic blood flow ratio is 2:1 or greater. Spontaneous closure does not occur. Small ASDs are best left alone. All patients with ASDs, whether open or operated upon, are liable to develop atrial arrhythmias, e.g. atrial fibrillation, in later life.

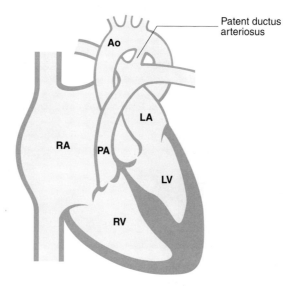

Fig. 1.20 Patent ductus arteriosus

Patent ductus arteriosus (PDA) (Fig. 1.20)

In utero the ductus arteriosus carries oxygenated blood from the placenta through into the aorta, bypassing the lungs. It normally closes at birth. When it remains open, it allows blood from the high pressure aorta to flow through into the pulmonary artery. The duct can vary in size from trivial to very large in which case it can cause heart failure early in life. It sometimes closes in response to indomethacin but surgical closure is simple and safe and this is often needed. In very young children the physical signs are limited to an ejection systolic murmur over the upper left sternal edge and there are usually prominent bounding pulses.

Older children are usually symptom-free and the ductus is found on routine examination. Physical findings include large volume pulses and the characteristic 'machinery' murmur which has systolic and diastolic components because of the continuous pressure gradient between the aorta and pulmonary artery. It sounds like the engine room of an old-fashioned steamer—hence the name.

The ECG and chest X-ray are often normal although the lung fields may be plethoric and the heart enlarged when the patent ductus is itself large. In this latter case the ECG may show right ventricular hypertrophy. Echocardiography can demonstrate the ductus and quantify the shunt. Cardiac catheterisation is seldom necessary. This lesion carries a high risk of infection (infective endocarditis) and is usually closed unless very small.

Aortic stenosis*

These patients may present with heart failure and a malformed valve in the neonatal period but aortic stenosis is detected much more commonly later in life when a murmur is heard. These abnormal valves often have only two cusps, i.e. are bicuspid, instead of the usual three, i.e. tricuspid.

Symptoms and signs
1. Usually asymptomatic and normal.
2. Unlike adult cases, angina and heart failure are uncommon.
3. Occasionally effort syncope occurs.
4. Low volume pulse.
5. Coarse ejection systolic murmur over the aortic area radiating to the neck. There may be a systolic thrill.
6. The chest X-ray is often normal, as is the ECG.
7. The diagnosis is confirmed at echocardiography.

Treatment is surgical in severe cases, by either splitting the valve (valvotomy) or replacing it.

Rare forms of aortic stenosis occur where the narrowing is either above the valve (supravalvular) or below it (subvalvular).

Coarctation of the aorta

This may present early in life with heart failure or be picked up later in well children. The aorta is narrowed just below the left subclavian artery. The pulses in the arms and legs are of different quality and the femoral pulses may be delayed and weak when compared with the radial pulses. Blood pressure in the upper limbs is elevated. An ejection systolic murmur is heard over the upper left sternal edge.

Collateral blood vessels may be both felt and heard over the scapula. These are blood vessels which have enlarged to carry blood by an alternative route to the lower limbs, bypassing the constricted aorta.

Sometimes, associated bicuspid aortic valves, aortic stenosis or aneurysms of the circle of Willis in the brain are present.

Investigations and treatment

The chest X-ray may show notching on the underside of the ribs from erosion by intercostal collateral vessels. The aorta is abnormal in shape, showing two bulges—the '3' sign. The opposite, the reverse 3 or 'E' sign, is seen in the oesophagus using a barium swallow X-ray.

Echocardiography may show the site of the coarctation. Cardiac catheterisation is often still needed to identify the site of the collateral vessels and establish whether or not significant aortic stenosis is present as well as demonstrating the site of the coarctation itself. Treatment is surgical but up to 50% of patients will still need anti-hypertensive therapy. If significant hypertension does not develop in the upper limbs then the coarctation is best left alone.

Pulmonary stenosis

This lesion is relatively common and may affect the pulmonary valve, or the stenosis may be just below the valve in the right ventricle itself. There is an ejection systolic murmur over the pulmonary area that radiates out clearly to the lung fields over the back. There is often a thrill at the second left intercostal space and with valvular stenosis a systolic sound—the ejection click—may be heard. The pulmonary second sound is widely split. If severe enough, balloon dilatation is the treatment of choice although surgery may sometimes be necessary.

Ebstein's anomaly

The tricuspid valve is seated low in the right ventricle so that part of the ventricle is atrialised (i.e. incorporated into the right atrium). The degree of this determines the functional end result, i.e. mild with no disability to severe with intractable heart failure from the inadequate right-sided structures.

CYANOTIC CONGENITAL HEART DISEASE

Tetralogy of Fallot

The tetralogy comprises pulmonary stenosis, VSD, right ventricular hypertrophy and over-riding of the aorta. It is the commonest form of cyanotic congenital heart disease after the first year of life. Much more rarely, there is an

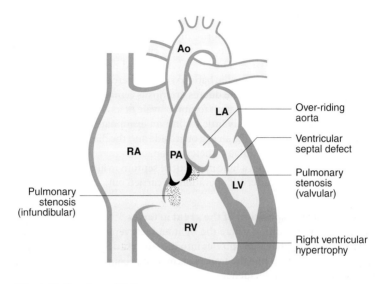

Fig. 1.21 Tetralogy of Fallot

associated ASD—Fallot's pentalogy. As with pure pulmonary stenosis, the pulmonary narrowing may either affect the valve, be just below the valve in the right ventricle or both (Fig. 1.21).

Symptoms and signs

Cyanosis, the degree of which may come and go, is present. Severe cyanotic episodes are known as 'spells' and are probably caused by spasm occurring in the narrow part of the right ventricle. Cyanotic spells may be precipitated by exertion or crying.

These children may frequently squat, especially after exercise. Cerebral thrombosis or abscesses may occur. The heart is not usually greatly enlarged and a pulmonary stenotic murmur is heard. A systolic thrill may be present in the pulmonary area.

Investigations

The chest X-ray shows a boot-shaped heart. There is a relative absence of the pulmonary arteries, and the lungs show diminished vascular markings (i.e. oligaemic lung fields). The ECG shows right ventricular hypertrophy. Echocardiography is diagnostic, showing the features of the tetralogy and especially the overriding by the aorta of the interventricular septum. Cardiac catheterisation may be needed to confirm the anatomy.

Treatment

Cyanotic spells are a medical emergency. These respond to morphine and also to beta-adrenergic blocking drugs. Digoxin should be avoided as it increases myocardial contractility and excitability. Surgery is eventually indicated in most patients.

Transposition of the great arteries

This is the most common form of cyanotic congenital heart disease in neonates. The aorta is connected to the right ventricle and the pulmonary artery to the left ventricle. Thus the systemic and pulmonary circulations are completely separate and for the baby to survive there must be some connection between the two. Usually the ductus arteriosus remains patent although these children also often have a patent foramen ovale or associated VSD.

There is usually relatively little to find on examination but the chest X-ray shows a heart that looks like an egg on its side and the diagnosis is confirmed by echocardiography or cardiac catheterisation.

The cardiologist tears a hole in the atrial septum to allow the child to survive and, later, one of a variety of operations is carried out.

Corrected transposition of the great arteries

This is a rare condition where the right and left ventricles have switched over such that the right atrium empties into the left ventricle which empties into the pulmonary artery. Thus the transposition has become corrected. Not surprisingly, there is a high incidence of associated defects, e.g. VSD.

PULMONARY HYPERTENSION

Elevation of the pulmonary artery pressure (pulmonary hypertension) occurs where there is increased pulmonary blood flow, caused by an ASD, a VSD or by PDA (i.e. left-to-right intracardiac shunting of blood), increased pulmonary capillary pressure resulting from increased back pressure from left heart disease, e.g. LVF, mitral valve disease, or increased pulmonary vascular resistance from chronic lung disease (e.g. chronic bronchitis, emphysema), recurrent pulmonary thrombo-embolism or primary pulmonary hypertension (see below).

The physical signs reflect the increased pulmonary and right heart pressures: loud pulmonary second sound, right ventricular enlargement, right heart failure, and a pulmonary valve incompetence (early diastolic) murmur may be audible.

The chest X-ray may reveal the cause, e.g. mitral stenosis, emphysema. In addition, the proximal pulmonary arteries are enlarged and the peripheral pulmonary arteries small and depleted in number. The ECG may show right atrial and right ventricular hypertrophy. Treatment is that of the underlying cause.

PRIMARY PULMONARY HYPERTENSION

This is a rare condition of unknown aetiology but it may lead to recurrent thrombosis of the pulmonary arteries. It predominantly affects young adult females and is remorselessly progressive with death within a few years. There is no effective treatment but anticoagulants are usually started and vasodilators have had limited success.

PULMONARY EMBOLISM

Pulmonary embolism ranges from small, with no clinical effect, to massive with sudden death (10%). The emboli usually arise from the leg or pelvic veins in people who have been immobile or had recent surgery/childbirth.

Symptoms and signs

Clinical features include chest pain or choking sensation, dyspnoea, syncope or collapse, haemoptysis and tachycardia and other signs of circulatory compromise, e.g. low blood pressure.

Investigations

The chest X-ray and ECG are often normal initially. Ventilation/perfusion (V/Q) scans are helpful (the lung is ventilated but not perfused). Venograms are sometimes performed to establish the source of the emboli; rarely, pulmonary angiography is required but this itself can be dangerous.

Treatment

1. Anticoagulation for 6 months in mild to moderate cases.
2. Clot lysis (thrombolysis) with streptokinase in moderate lesions causing some circulatory deficit.
3. Surgical removal of the embolus in severe cases with circulatory compromise or collapse.

If pulmonary emboli are recurrent then lifelong anticoagulation is required with or without surgical plication of the inferior vena cava or the insertion of a filter.

COR PULMONALE

Cor pulmonale is defined as right heart failure resulting from chronic lung disease or chest deformity, e.g. chronic bronchitis and emphysema, pulmonary fibrosis (fibrosing alveolitis), recurrent pulmonary thrombo-embolism, severe kyphoscoliosis, and rarely neuromuscular disease such as myasthenia gravis.

Treatment is that of the cause and of heart failure.

2

RESPIRATORY MEDICINE

Gabriel Laszlo, James R. Catterall

Lung disease is secondary only to heart disease as a cause of death in industrialised countries but is a greater cause of morbidity and loss of earnings. Cigarette smoking continues to cause carcinoma of the bronchus and to contribute significantly to chronic obstructive airways disease. Both tuberculosis and asthma are increasing in prevalence. Thus lung disease affects all age groups and all socioeconomic groups.

TESTS OF RESPIRATORY FUNCTION USED IN CLINICAL PRACTICE

1. Measurement of peak expiratory flow, vital capacity (VC) and the forced expired volume–time curve (Fig. 2.1 below).
2. Subdivisions of the total lung capacity.

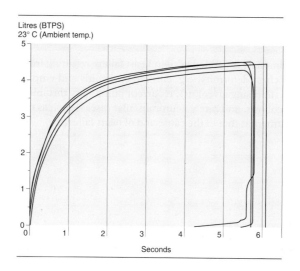

A

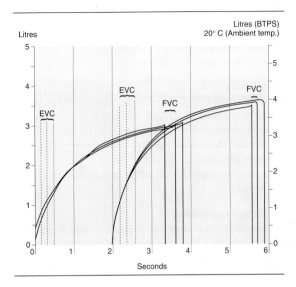

B

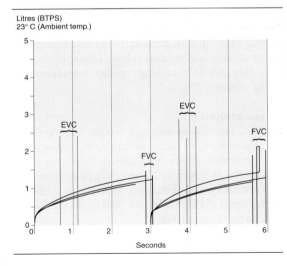

C

Fig. 2.1 Timed forced expiratory traces (curves) and expired vital capacities (vertical lines) in **(A)** a normal subject; **(B)** an asthmatic subject before and after administration of a bronchodilator; **(C)** a bronchitic subject before and after administration of a bronchodilator. The forced vital capacity (FVC) is the vital capacity during **rapid** forced expiration from full inspiration. The expired vital capacity (EVC; also known as the relaxed vital capacity) is the vital capacity during **slow** expiration from full inspiration. The vital capacity is usually taken as the higher of these values.

3. Partial pressure (or tension) of oxygen and carbon dioxide (PO_2 and PCO_2) in arterial blood.
4. Carbon monoxide (CO) transfer.
5. Tests of respiratory muscle power.

Vital capacity

This is the maximum volume of air that can be expired after full inspiration and may be reduced by:

1. Loss of inspiratory reserve (restrictive ventilatory defect: lung fibrosis, loss of alveoli, chest wall rigidity, respiratory muscle weakness). Total lung capacity is reduced.
2. Increased volume of residual air (airways obstruction). Total lung capacity is normal.

Time forced expiration

A full breath is exhaled as fast as possible into a spirometer. The most useful derived variable is FEV1, the volume of air expired in the first second of forced expiration. A value which is less than 75% of vital capacity indicates obstruction to airflow.

Peak (maximal) expiratory flow rate (PEF)

This is the flow rate at the beginning of a maximal forced respiration and is useful in detecting severe airflow obstruction and monitoring change in bronchial asthma.

Measurement of lung volumes

When vital capacity is reduced and the cause not obvious, measurements of total lung capacity and residual volume help to distinguish obstructive defects (reduced flow, normal total lung capacity) from restrictive disorders (reduced total lung capacity) (Fig. 2.2).

Blood gas analysis

High PCO_2 (ventilatory failure, 'alveolar hypoventilation') is seen in very severe lung disease, weakness or fatigue of respiratory muscles, and loss of intrinsic respiratory drive or CO_2 chemoreceptor sensitivity.

Low arterial PO_2 may be caused by hypoventilation, mismatching of pulmonary ventilation and perfusion or right-to-left cardiac shunt.

Normal limits of PO_2 may be predicted from the alveolar air equation which allows for alveolar ventilation

$$\text{Alveolar } PO_2 = \text{inspired } PO_2 - \text{Alveolar } \frac{PCO_2}{R}$$
$$\text{Where } R = CO_2 \text{ output/oxygen consumption}$$

The alveolar–arterial PO_2 difference should not exceed 20 mmHg or 3 kPa breathing air. A useful approximation is:

Arterial PO_2 should be more than $16 - $ arterial PCO_2 (kPa)
or Arterial PO_2 should be more than $120 - $ arterial PCO_2 (mmHg)

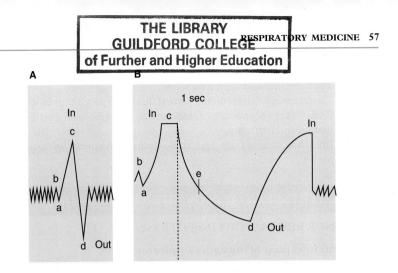

Fig. 2.2 (A) Spirometric trace (diagrammatic) to show subdivisions of the static lung volumes; ordinate = volume; abscissa = time. **(B)** Fast spirometric trace (diagrammatic) to illustrate timed ventilatory tests in a patient with airways obstruction. a = functional residual capacity (FRC); ab = tidal volume; ac = inspiratory capacity; c = total lung capacity; cd = vital capacity; d = residual volume; ce = forced expired volume in 1 sec (FEV_1).

Carbon monoxide (CO) transfer

Carbon monoxide binds rapidly to haemoglobin. The ability of the lungs to extract a trace of CO from inspired air can be used to test the distribution of inspired gas to the alveoli and the integrity of the alveolar capillary system. Clinically the test is most useful when vital capacity, FEV1/VC and haemoglobin are normal: then reduction of CO transfer to 80% of predicted normal or less indicates disease at the alveolar level.

Tests of respiratory muscle power

When the respiratory muscles are intrinsically weak or when some groups are paralysed, they are at risk of developing fatigue during exercise or acute respiratory infections.

The maximum pressure that can be generated from the mouth during inspiration or expiration through an obstructed tube is normally > 70 cmH_2O.

Bilateral diaphragmatic paralysis may be identified by a fall in VC > 25% on lying down. Diaphragmatic function is assessed by the measurement of pressures within the thorax and abdomen during inspiratory efforts (employing balloons swallowed into the oesophagus and stomach).

SPECIALISED INVESTIGATIONS

1. Examination of sputum

Microscopy of specimens stained for pyogenic organisms, acid-fast bacilli *(M. tuberculosis)* and malignant cells. New techniques include immunohistochemistry and DNA probes to identify micro-organisms. Culture of bacteria and fungi and sensitivity of organisms to antimicrobial agents.

2. Bronchoscopy

For visual examination of the bronchial tree, aspiration of bronchial and alveolar liquid by lavage and by bronchial or transbronchial biopsy.

3. Percutaneous needle biopsy for the diagnosis of solid tumours.
4. Thoracotomy and open lung biopsy.
5. Thoracentesis (aspiration of pleural fluid with or without biopsy).
6. Radioisotope scanning to determine the topographical distribution of ventilation and perfusion.
7. Bronchial arteriogram and embolisation (treatment of massive haemophysis).

ACUTE INFECTIONS OF THE AIR PASSAGES

MINOR RESPIRATORY INFECTIONS

Virus infections of the upper respiratory tract

Viruses cause a number of very common overlapping syndromes of upper respiratory infection: the common cold, pharyngitis and tonsillitis (sore throat, fever and neck stiffness from enlarged cervical glands), laryngo-tracheitis (hoarseness, painful cough, laryngeal obstruction in children ('croup'), and conjunctivitis (sore eyes).

Spread is by droplet infection, the incubation is short, infectivity high in the early stages and serious complications may occur in susceptible individuals. The virus may be isolated for up to 96 hours.

Complications include middle ear pain from eustachian tube obstruction with the retention of serious fluid while *Streptococcus pneumoniae, Haemophilus influenzae* and *Streptococcus pyogenes* may cause secondary bacterial otitis media. Osteomyelitis of the mastoid bones (mastoiditis), formerly a common complication, is now rare. Recurrent otitis media results in minor deafness, learning difficulties and under-achievement.

Tonsillitis

Streptococcal tonsillitis causes intense sore throat with pain, fever and malaise. It must be distinguished from infectious mononucleosis (p.402). Post streptococcal complications, including glomerulonephritis, rheumatic fever, chorea, scarlet fever and peritonsillar abscess, are now rare.

Oropharyngeal thrush

Candida albicans causes white plaques of fungus on the pharynx and palate which peel easily (thrush). Rare in healthy individuals, thrush complicates treatment with broad-spectrum antibiotics, oral and inhaled corticosteroid drugs and is also found when immunity is defective. The infection may spread to the oesophagus or the lungs. Eradication from the mouth and gastrointestinal (GI) tract is by oral non-absorbed antifungal antibiotics.

POTENTIALLY SERIOUS RESPIRATORY INFECTIONS

Diphtheria (See page 400)
Epiglottitis

Epiglottitis is a rare epidemic infection of children and adults with capsulated type B *H. influenzae* which invades and causes swelling of the epiglottis and epiglottic folds. There are microabscesses in the epiglottis. After minor respiratory symptoms, the patient rapidly develops sore throat, dribbling, dysphagia for saliva, muffling of the voice, restlessness and prostration. Depression of the tongue for examination is dangerous in children as it may cause complete airway obstruction. Parenteral antibiotics are needed with intravenous hydration in severe cases. The significant mortality rate is reduced by early treatment. Preventive vaccination is now available.

Bronchiolitis

This occurs mainly in children and is an acute infection of the respiratory tract with obstructive inflammation of the bronchioles. Most cases are caused by the respiratory syncitial virus. Presentation is with coughing, signs of airways obstruction, hyperinflation of the chest and limpness. Treatment consists of hydration and oxygenation with artificial ventilation if the PCO_2 rises.

Whooping cough (pertussis) (See page 401)

Influenza

An endemic, epidemic and occasionally pandemic illness causing fever, rigors and muscle pains with upper and lower respiratory symptoms of varying severity. The incubation period is 24–48 hours and the virus is excreted for up to 7 days. Complications include pneumonia, myocarditis, polyneuritis, myelopathy and encephalitis. There are three major strains (A, B, C) with epidemics of A and B occurring every 2–3 years. Crossimmunity between strains is light. Vaccination is only partially effective. The prophylactic administration of antiviral drugs is helpful in susceptible communities.

PNEUMONIA

Pneumonia is inflammation of the lung parenchyma resulting from infection. The term pneumonitis is reserved for lung inflammation caused by physical or chemical injury, e.g. irradiation.

Pneumonia remains an important cause of morbidity and mortality. In the UK, it causes ten times as many deaths as all other infectious diseases together, and in developing countries it is the most common cause of hospital admission in both adults and children.

The alveoli are normally kept sterile by local and humoral defences. Pneumonia occurs when these defences are overwhelmed by a sufficient number of virulent organisms or when the defences are impaired.

Community-acquired pneumonia usually occurs in previously healthy people or in patients with only slight impairment of lung defences. It is almost always caused by one of a small range of virulent organisms of which *Strep. pneumoniae* is the most common (Table 2.1). Pneumonias caused by *Mycoplasma pneumoniae, Legionella pneumophilia* and influenza virus often occur in epidemics.

Hospital-acquired pneumonia complicates many medical conditions and surgical operations and is usually from aspiration of gram-negative oropharyngeal organisms, especially in patients undergoing intensive care. Predisposing

Table 2.1. Community-acquired pneumonia. Clinical, radiological and haematological features associated with the most common causative organisms

Streptococcus pneumoniae	By far the commonest cause at any age
	Rigors, herpes labialis; lobar consolidation
Staphylococcus aureus	Influenza epidemics, drug addicts
	Bilateral cavitating pneumonia
Klebsiella pneumoniae	Alcoholics, elderly
	May have more gradual onset than pneumococcal pneumonia in some patients
	Upper lobes, 'bulging' out
Mycoplasma pneumoniae	Closed communities, e.g. army barracks
	Also larger epidemics
	Cold agglutinins positive in 50%
Chlamydia spp	Contact with sick birds not always elicited
Legionella spp	Outbreaks in hotels and hospitals (water-cooled air conditioning)
Influenza virus	In epidemics
	Diffuse bilateral shadowing on chest X-ray
	May be complicated by superinfection with *Staph. aureus*

factors are intubation, the use of H_2-receptor antagonists and the loss of fibronectin from upper respiratory tract epithelial cells.

Aspiration pneumonia occurs when large numbers of oropharyngeal flora reach the lower respiratory tract in patients with impaired upper airway defences. It is usually polymicrobial with gram-negative bacteria, gram-positive cocci and anaerobes all contributing.

Pneumonia in the immunocompromised patient. Patients with AIDS or haematological malignancies and patients receiving cytotoxic/immunosuppressive therapy are at greatly increased risk. Different forms of immunodeficiency predispose to different organisms. The range of pathogens is wide and includes fungi (Table 2.2).

Pathology

The organisms are usually inhaled. They excite an inflammatory response in the bronchioles and alveoli, which become filled with organisms, fluid and inflammatory cells, the bronchi remaining patent (consolidation). A whole lobe or segment may be densely consolidated (lobar/segmental pneumonia) or the inflammation may be patchy, affecting mainly the lower lobes (bronchopneumonia).

Table 2.2. Pneumonia in the immunocompromised host. Common causative organisms associated with different defects in host defences

Neutropenia (e.g. Cytotoxic chemotherapy, aplastic anaemia)	Bacteria Fungi
Defect in antibody production (e.g. splenectomy, myeloma, chronic lymphatic leukaemia)	Encapsulated bacteria, especially *Streptococcus pneumoniae*
Defect in cell-mediated immunity (e.g. Hodgkin's disease, AIDS, immunosuppressive therapy)	Viruses (CMV, HS, VZ) *Pneumocystis carinii* Fungi *Mycobacterium tuberculosis* and atypical mycobacteria

CMV = cytomegalovirus; HS = herpes simplex; VZ = varicella zoster

Symptoms

Systemic symptoms include fever, rigors, sweating, malaise, myalgia and headaches. Respiratory symptoms are cough, sputum (purulent when a pyogenic organism is present; absent, mucoid or watery in other patients), haemoptysis (often absent, and rarely marked; classically rusty in pyogenic infections), dyspnoea at rest, confusion (most common in the elderly, usually associated with hypoxaemia), and pleuritic pain (common in bacterial cases). Diaphragmatic pleurisy may mimic acute surgical conditions of the abdomen and also be referred to the shoulder (C4 dermatome).

Signs

The patient is usually ill, pyrexial and tachypnoeic, and sometimes cyanosed. There may be pleuritic pain. Blisters of labial herpes simplex may be present (reactivation of latent infection by fever).

Localising chest signs are not always present, especially in non-bacterial pneumonia and in early bacterial pneumonia, but in established pneumonia they result from bronchiolo-alveolar inflammation (fine/medium inspiratory crackles), consolidation (diminished chest movement on affected side, dullness to percussion, bronchial breathing, increased vocal resonance, whispering pectoriloquy), and pleural inflammation (pleural rub or effusion).

Investigations

Chest X-ray

The chest X-ray shows opacification without loss of volume. Any loss of volume of a lobe or lung affected by pneumonia should arouse suspicion of proximal bronchial obstruction (Fig. 2.3).

The pattern of opacification on chest X-ray indicates the extent of lung involvement and may give clues to the likely causal organism.

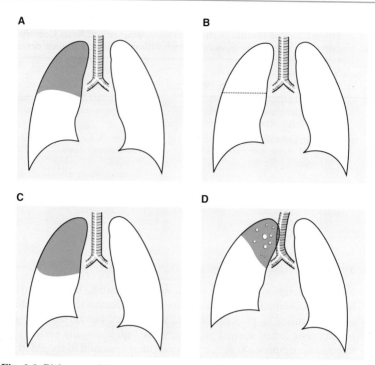

Fig. 2.3 Right upper lobe pneumonia. **(A)** and **(B)** Pneumococcal: resolution with pleural thickening, restoration of lung architecture. **(C)** and **(D)** Suppurative (e.g. *Klebsiella*): **(C)** bulging shadow; **(D)** resolution with fibrosis and cavitation.

Lobar or segmental pneumonia. Dense opacification of a whole lobe or segment, sometimes more than one, may indicate *Strep. pneumoniae* or *Klebsiella pneumoniae*.

Bronchopneumonia. Bilateral patchy opacification, mainly in the lower zones often indicates a mixed infection with *Strep. pneumoniae* and *H. influenzae* although bronchopneumonia can also occur with other organisms.

Diffuse bilateral shadowing is typical of viral and other non-pyogenic pneumonias, e.g. *M. pneumoniae*, *Pneumocystis carinii*.

Cavities are typically seen in pneumonia due to *Staph. aureus* or *Klebsiella pneumoniae* and also in tuberculosis.

Other investigations

Arterial blood gas tensions. To determine the severity of hypoxaemia; $PaCO_2$ is usually low.

Differential blood count. Neutrophil leukocytosis often occurs in bacterial infections but the white cell count may be normal or low in the severely ill. A low white cell count is typical of non-bacterial infections and in immunocompromised patients.

Blood cultures. Positive in 50% of fulminating bacterial pneumonias.

Culture and microscopy of sputum. More sensitive, less specific than blood cultures.

Acute and convalescent serum. For antibodies to viruses, *Legionella*, *Mycoplasma* and *Chlamydia*. Useful in epidemics and for retrospective diagnosis.

Broncho–alveolar lavage fluid. Infective agents may be identified; used in seriously ill patients.

Differential diagnosis

Other causes of consolidation are pulmonary infarct, pulmonary eosinophilia, pulmonary tuberculosis and malignancy. Non-infective causes of pneumonia are listed in Table 2.3. Bronchopneumonia can sometimes be confused with acute pulmonary oedema due to heart failure or adult respiratory distress syndrome.

In immunocompromised patients, the usual clues to infection (e.g. pyrexia, leukocytosis) are often absent. Non-infectious causes of pulmonary infiltrates in these patients include extension of the primary disease (e.g. in haematological malignancies), intrapulmonary bleeding in thrombocytopenia, lung damage caused by cytotoxic drugs/irradiation, and malignant disorders in AIDS.

Table 2.3. Non-infective causes of pneumonia

	Cause	Course
Exogenous lipid pneumonia	Inhalation of oily droplets	Chronic
Radiation	Radiotherapy	Subacute 1–20 weeks after treatment Lasts several weeks Good resolution, functional impairment
Acute chemical burns	Inhalation injury by toxic chemical fumes	Bronchial hyperreactivity May heal with bronchiolar fibrosis, chronic airflow obstruction
Eosinophilic pneumonia	Aspergillosis, hypersensitivity to drugs or cryptogenic	Recurrent, responds to oral corticosteroids
Cryptogenic organising pneumonia	Variant of cryptogenic fibrosing alveolitis	Recurrent, responds to oral corticosteroids

Complications

Pleurisy and serous pleural effusion are much more common after bacterial than viral pneumonia. Empyema (pus in the pleural cavity) should be evacuated. Resolution of pneumonia may be poor, leading to abscess formation or fibrosis.

Treatment

Antibiotics

Treatment should be started without delay, i.e. before the results of cultures are known. The choice of antibiotic will depend on the likely organism, taking into account the clinical, radiological and haematological findings.

Community-acquired pneumonia. In mild pneumonia, amoxycillin or erythromycin or another macrolide. In severe pneumonia, cefuroxime and erythromycin should be given, both parenterally, at least until the causative organism has been identified. Flucloxacillin should be added if staphylococcal pneumonia is suspected or if the pneumonia occurs during an influenza epidemic. If these antibiotics have failed, a third generation cephalosporin or aminoglycoside should be included. When a specific pathogen is identified, the antibiotic therapy may need to be modified.

Aspiration pneumonia. Cefuroxime and metronidazole.

Hospital–acquired pneumonia. Broad-spectrum agents to cover gram-negative organisms are included. Empirical treatment is with cefuroxime or ceftazidime.

Pneumonia in the immunocompromised patient. The choice of antibiotic depends on the clinical situation, e.g. gentamicin plus azlocillin i.v. in neutropenia, high-dose cotrimoxazole i.v. for suspected *P. carinii* pneumonia in AIDS.

Supportive treatment

Supportive treatment consists of administering oxygen (aiming to keep the $PaO_2 > 60$ mmHg; 8kPa), fluids (parenteral if necessary, to maintain adequate hydration) and analgesia for pleuritic pain.

Prognosis

Prognosis depends on the underlying health and age of the patient, the causative organism and whether bacteraemia or complications like hypotension, leukopenia and renal failure occur. The overall mortality for pneumococcal pneumonia is 5–13%. In most patients who survive, resolution is remarkably complete.

LUNG ABSCESS

A necrotic area of lung, secondary to aspiration of anaerobic and aerobic bacteria often from the mouth. Differential diagnosis: tuberculosis, carcinoma.

TUBERCULOSIS

An infection by the tubercle bacillus (*Mycobacterium tuberculosis*) in the lungs and elsewhere. Tuberculosis is characterised by granulomatous lesions which tend to become necrotic and heal by fibrosis.

New cases are now notified in England and Wales at a rate of 10–20/100 000 per year with a low mortality, deaths occurring mainly in the elderly and in occasional undiagnosed cases.

Patients with HIV infection (p. 403) are particularly susceptible to a wide variety of mycobacterial strains. Where overcrowding and poor nutrition and alcoholism persist, the incidence and mortality remain high and tuberculosis is a significant cause of mortality in the young worldwide (India, South East Asia, Africa, the Pacific Islands). Resistance to infection is lowered by malnutrition, alcoholism, diabetes mellitus, smoking, corticosteroids given in high doses long term, immunosuppression, silicosis, pregnancy, old age and diseases associated with reduced immunity.

Microbiology

The acid–alcohol-fast bacillus may be stained in smears of sputum or bronchial lavage fluid, concentrated urine and cerebrospinal fluid and may be cultured on special media in 6 weeks. Rapid identification by DNA amplification is possible.

PRIMARY TUBERCULOUS INFECTION

This usually occurs in childhood in places where the disease is common. There is a minor inflammatory reaction at the site of entry (lungs, tonsils, small intestine) with rapid spread to regional lymph nodes. Most commonly there is a small area of consolidation (Ghon focus) in the periphery of the middle and lower lobes of the lungs with hilar adenopathy. Cervical and mesenteric node tuberculosis are less common than formerly. Clinical manifestations may be absent or include mild malaise, weightloss or failure to grow, a brief febrile illness, cough, erythema nodosum or phlyctenular conjunctivitis. In the great majority of cases uncomplicated healing and calcification occur.

Complications of primary tuberculous infection (Fig. 2.4)
Complications include: obstruction of lobar bronchi by enlarged nodes, bronchial seeding with confluent pneumonia, pleural effusion (a common cause of unexplained pleural effusion in patients under 30 years old), pericardial effusion, blood-borne spread to the kidneys, bone, meninges, adrenals. Widespread macroscopic lesions throughout the body are called **miliary tuberculosis.** These phenomena occur within 12 weeks to 1 year of primary infection (or when immunity is impaired).

Post-primary tuberculosis

Post-primary tuberculosis arises by direct progression of a primary lesion (rarely before puberty in Europeans), reactivation of a dormant lesion,

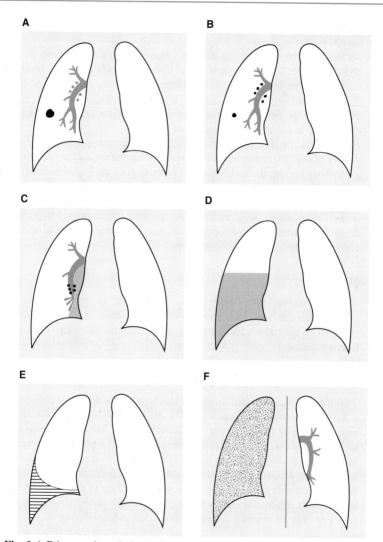

Fig. 2.4 Primary tuberculosis and its consequences. **(A)** Primary complex; **(B)** calcified (healed primary) complex; **(C)** bronchiectasis; **(D)** pneumonia; **(E)** pleural effusion; **(F)** miliary TB (2-mm nodules obscure the pulmonary blood vessels).

haematogenous spread to the lungs or re-infection. The illness has a slowly progressive course.

Pathology

Usually the upper lobes are affected. The organisms are contained within caseating granulomata surrounded by areas of inflammation. Healing is by fibrosis. Disease may spread to the pleura, the larynx, the tongue and the intestines, or cause miliary tuberculosis.

Symptoms and signs

These may be inconspicuous initially. There is lassitude, loss of weight, pyrexia 37–39°C, anorexia, cough (dry or with purulent sputum), haemoptysis and amenorrhoea.

The patient may look wasted but with high colour. In advanced cases there are signs of cavitation with amphoric breathing, consolidation, collapse and fibrosis with post tussive inspiratory crackles.

Investigations

1. Chest X-ray appearances depend on severity and include patchy irregular opacities centred on one or both upper lobes, cavities within such lesions, streaks of fibrosis radiating from the hilum, calcification and solitary round shadows (Fig. 2.5).
2. Advanced cases show anaemia, raised plasma viscosity, raised erythrocyte sedimentation rate (ESR) and acute phase proteins. Leukocytosis is unusual.
3. Search for *M. tuberculosis* in sputum or in bronchoscopic aspirate if sputum is not available.
4. *Tuberculin* or *Mantoux* or *Heaf test* detects previous BCG (Bacille Calmette–Guerin) vaccination or previous or present tuberculosis infection. Tests are very occasionally negative with active disease.

Complications

Hyponatraemia, tuberculous empyema or pericarditis, tuberculous pneumonia, miliary tuberculosis, massive haemoptysis, amyloidosis.

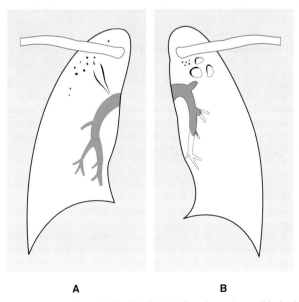

A   **B**

Fig. 2.5 Pulmonary tuberculosis. **(A)** Early infiltration = 'consolidation'; **(B)** extensive consolidation, lobar contraction, cavity formation. There is peribronchial thickening and fibrosis extending to the hilum.

Differential diagnosis

Bronchial asthma, pyogenic lung abscess, pneumonia, drug-induced lung infiltrates, Wegener's granuloma, resolving pulmonary oedema.

Treatment of infection with M. tuberculosis

Combinations of antimycobacterial chemotherapeutic agents are given to prevent the emergence of resistant strains. A regimen consisting of rifampicin, isoniazid and pyrazinamide for 2 months, followed by rifampicin and isoniazid for 4 months has been shown to sterilise most infections. Other drugs are available. The best regimens result in a relapse rate of less than 1%; results are worse if compliance is poor.

Miliary tuberculosis

This usually present with pyrexia and weightloss. Miliary shadowing on the chest X-ray and tubercles on the choroid, visible on ophthalmoscopy, are classic hallmarks. Usually there are no localising features so diagnosis is difficult. Liver biopsy may show granulomata, and mycobacteria may be isolated from bronchial secretions, urine or bone marrow culture. A therapeutic trial of antituberculous therapy may be necessary.

Prevention of tuberculosis

1. Screening. Infective cases should be identified by screening individuals from high risk areas and contacts of cases using chest X-rays and tuberculin tests.

2. BCG vaccination. An attenuated tubercle bacillus is used as a vaccine to produce a positive tuberculin test. It was highly effective in England and Wales from 1965–1970 in reducing the incidence from 5% to 0.5% in those before the age of 20 with the virtual abolition of life-threatening miliary or meningeal tuberculosis. High-risk individuals, including healthcare workers and travellers, are vaccinated. BCG vaccination is ineffective in many parts of the world, including India and the USA; the reasons are unknown but probably relate to genetic and nutritional differences.

A strongly positive tuberculin test in an unvaccinated subject indicates current or recent infection. Chemotherapy may be advisable.

SOME PULMONARY MYCOSES

Actinomycosis

Actinomyces species may cause chronic segmental pneumonias, occasionally distal to carcinomas, sometimes discharging through the chest wall. They are often diagnosed at thoracotomy. Prolonged treatment of at least 6 months is necessary. *Actinomyces* respond to penicillin, *Nocardia* to sulphonamides.

Histoplasmosis

Endemic in central and northern USA, *Histoplasma capsulatum* is a dimorphic fungus causing acute and chronic granulomatous disease, similar to primary tuberculosis and chronic sarcoidosis. The condition responds to intravenous amphotericin B given for 14 days. Adrenal failure is common in the disseminated form of the disease. Serological tests are available.

Cryptococcosis

Cryptococcus neoformans, a ubiquitous yeast, causes chronic pulmonary disease and infects skin and bones. Acute or subacute meningitis is the commonest syndrome, often presenting as obscure pyrexia. Amphotericin B is given for several weeks.

Aspergillosis (Table 2.4)

The fungus *Aspergillus fumigatus* occurs as hyphae. It spores throughout the year but mainly around October. In most patients, disease is due to an immune hypersensitivity to the spores. In some situations the inflammatory reaction creates a favourable environment for growth of the organism in its filamentous

Table 2.4. Clinical syndromes caused by *Aspergillus fumigatus*

Syndrome	Skin prick test Specific IgE	Precipitins	Complications	Treatment
Asthma	+	+ or −		As for asthma Maintenance
steroids				often needed
Fleeting lung shadows with blood eosinophilia	+	++		Corticosteroids by mouth
Bronchiectasis of proximal airways	+	++	Secondary infection	
Bilateral upper lobe fibrosis	+	++	Chronic airflow obstruction	Corticosteroids, postural drainage
Recurrent lobar collapse with aspergillus growing in bronchi and mucus plugs	+	+		
Mycetoma: ball of fungal hyphae in lung cavity	+	++	Haemorrhage	Excision sometimes practicable Corticosteroids to reduce systemic symptoms
Invasive pneumonia, sinusitis, endocarditis, septicaemia, pulmonary	+	+	Fatal unless treated	Intravenous amphotericin

form. It causes hypersensitivity syndromes and may cause pneumonia and septicaemia, complicating diabetic ketoacidosis, intensive care and immunosuppression.

CHRONIC AIRFLOW OBSTRUCTION

Chronic diffuse airflow obstruction occurs in chronic bronchitis and emphysema, chronic bronchial asthma, obliterative bronchiolitis and bronchiectasis (including cystic fibrosis).

These conditions are characterised by chronic inflammation and damage to the bronchi and lungs, with reduction of expiratory flow rate and breathlessness. In some, usually older, patients, these conditions coexist or become indistinguishable from each other, and the general terms chronic obstructive lung disease (COLD), chronic obstructive pulmonary disease (COPD) and chronic obstructive airways disease (COAD) are used.

CHRONIC BRONCHITIS AND EMPHYSEMA

Chronic bronchitis consists of chronic mucus hypersecretion, causing regular expectoration of sputum, especially in the winter months, and narrowing and obliteration of small airways. Emphysema is a pathological term meaning dilatation of the air spaces distal to the terminal bronchioles with destruction of their walls.

These conditions usually coexist and are almost always caused by smoking. Chronic bronchitis alone is occasionally caused by occupational dusts and by the use of irritant fuels indoors. Emphysema with or without chronic bronchitis is occasionally caused by alpha-1-antitrypsin deficiency.

Pathology

Bronchial mucous glands are hypertrophied and goblet cell numbers increased. There is no excessive secretion of mucus. Squamous metaplasia, with desquamation and loss of the ciliated columnar epithelium, results in pooling of sputum and retention of inhaled organisms. Damage to the intact airways results in first colonisation and then invasion of the lower respiratory tract by upper respiratory organisms, notably *H. influenzae* and *Strep. pneumoniae*. Inflammatory cells accumulate within respiratory bronchioles and cause breakdown of adjacent alveolar walls by the liberation of proteases.

Physiopathology

Physiological consequences of bronchiolar and alveolar damage consist of reduction in airflow during forced expiration, gas trapping and hyperinflation. This causes:
1. increased work of breathing,
2. impaired gas exchange with alveolar hypoxia,
3. secondary changes in pulmonary arteries leading to pulmonary hypertension,

4. right ventricular hypertrophy—'cor pulmonale'—in which fluid retention further damages the lungs with worsening of pulmonary gas exchange,
5. secondary polycythaemia, with predisposition to pulmonary artery and vascular thrombosis.

Epidemiology

Epidemiological studies have shown:
1. a major effect of cigarette smoking, related to dose,
2. a marked interaction between smoking and living in towns,
3. a rise in mortality associated with severe air pollution,
4. decreased mortality in privileged sections of the community,
5. predisposition caused by childhood respiratory infection, prematurity, asthma and certain occupations.

50% of smokers admit to morning cough and sputum; 25% of these develop progressive dyspnoea caused by chronic airflow obstruction. For a lifelong smoker, symptoms become important at the age of 50, and mortality is advanced to a median of 65 years.

Symptoms and signs

In patients with predominantly chronic bronchitis the main symptoms are cough and sputum which precede dyspnoea. When emphysema is dominant, patients present with dyspnoea on effort, inexorably progressive over several years. Very breathless patients often lose weight.

The main signs are a large chest with horizontal ribs, low diaphragm, reduced cricosternal distance and symmetrical reduction of chest expansion, absent cardiac and hepatic dullness, increased use of accessory muscles of respiration, expiration through pursed lips, quiet breath sounds and rhonchi.

'Pink puffers' and 'blue bloaters'. Some patients with severe chronic airflow limitation are able to maintain relatively normal oxygenation by hyperventilating. These patients (pink puffers) are constantly very breathless and tend to lose weight but they are not cyanosed and do not develop cor pulmonale or secondary polycythaemia. In contrast, other patients (blue bloaters) develop central cyanosis, hypoxaemia, CO_2 retention, secondary polycythaemia and cor pulmonale with elevation of the jugular venous pressure and peripheral oedema. The reasons for these different clinical patterns are poorly understood and most patients lie within these two extremes.

Investigations

1. Respiratory function tests. PEF, FEV1 and FEV1/VC are low. Total lung capacity is normal or high. In emphysema, CO transfer is reduced. FEV1 response after bronchodilator therapy is < 20%. VC, blood gases and exercise tolerance vary with the clinical state.
2. Chest X-ray to exclude other diseases.
3. CT scan demonstrates distribution of macroscopic lesions of emphysema.

4. Alpha-1-antitrypsin estimation to detect hereditary deficiency.

CHRONIC BRONCHIAL ASTHMA (See p.74)

Patients with asthma, especially those who smoke, are prone to develop irreversible progressive bronchiolar obliteration. The prognosis is said to be better in these patients if they take prophylactic medication and do not smoke. They may be identified by a diagnosis of asthma prior to the development of chronic changes, by a history of variability of symptoms unrelated to infective episodes, the presence of other atopic disorders, by physiological tests and by the lack of characteristic emphysematous changes on CT scan.

The degree of shortness of breath is related to airflow obstruction. Hypoxaemia and secondary pulmonary hypertension occur late in the disease. Wheezing is common, especially after exertion, and partially relieved by the inhalation of bronchodilator drugs.

OBLITERATIVE BRONCHIOLITIS

This is a rare cause of irreversible airflow obstruction characterised by fibrosis and obliteration of bronchioles without asthma or emphysema. It sometimes complicates rheumatoid arthritis, severe viral bronchiolitis or inhalation of chemicals and is a manifestation of rejection after lung transplantation.

A proportion of patients with fibrosing lung diseases, notably sarcoidosis and extrinsic allergic alveolitis, develop bronchial inflammation and narrowing. The course and progress is similar to that of chronic bronchitis, except that associated lung fibrosis results in reduced lung volumes for the same degree of airflow limitation. Characteristic radiographic changes are generally present, and thick walled, distorted bronchi are particularly well seen on CT scans.

TREATMENT OF CHRONIC AIRFLOW OBSTRUCTION

1. *Assessment of reversibility.* Irreversible chronic bronchitis is difficult to distinguish from untreated or partially treated asthma. A 3-week trial of oral prednisolone, with serial tests of ventilatory function and subjective symptom scoring, identifies these patients.
2. Symptomatic improvement in respiratory discomfort and walking distance may follow the use of bronchodilators, even when simple ventilatory tests are not improved.
3. Peripheral oedema indicates generalised fluid retention, and diuretics may relieve dyspnoea as well as oedema.
4. In patients with chronic airflow obstruction, with FEV1 < 1.0 litre and PO_2 < 55 mmHg (7.5 kPa), long-term oxygen therapy at home (2.0 l/min via a nasal cannula for at least 15 hours daily) may improve quality of life and reduce hospital admissions.
5. Marginal benefits may be obtained from supervised exercise re-training and endurance may be increased by availability of portable oxygen therapy.
6. In cases of severe dyspnoea at rest, the use of respiratory depressants may provide relief in the terminal phase of the illness.

7. Some but not all patients benefit symptomatically from regular antimicrobial treatment of lower respiratory infection identified by culture of purulent sputum.

EXACERBATIONS OF CHRONIC AIRFLOW OBSTRUCTION

Minor respiratory infections may result in worsening of lung function, respiratory distress, increased wheezing and shortness of breath, worsening pulmonary gas exchange and the development of respiratory muscle fatigue (see p. 98). In patients with fluid retention, exacerbations may be precipitated by an increase in lung water. In either case, proliferation of lower respiratory organisms follows with the development of purulent sputum.

Treatment is with antibiotics active against *H. influenzae* and *Strep. pneumoniae*, the usual respiratory pathogens. Regular bronchodilators relieve dyspnoea. Systemic corticosteroids may have an anti-inflammatory effect during acute exacerbations but must be withdrawn if not shown to have long-term benefit. Oxygen therapy and the treatment of respiratory failure are discussed on page 103.

BRONCHIECTASIS

This is a localised or generalised dilatation of the bronchi with susceptibility to increased sputum production and recurrent bronchopulmonary infection.

Most cases result from chest infections in childhood (notably measles, whooping cough or adenovirus infections), allergic asthma, allergic bronchopulmonary aspergillosis, cystic fibrosis, defective cilia (rare), obstruction to a bronchus, extrinsically (e.g. tuberculous lymphadenopathy) or intrinsically (e.g. inhaled foreign body), or as a complication of congenital or acquired IgG_2 deficiency.

Pathology

Lung fibrosis causes traction on adjacent bronchial walls. The dilated bronchi lack cilia, leading to pooling of secretions and chronic bronchial infection. *H. influenzae*, *Staphylococcus aureus* and *Pseudomonas aeuruginosa* are common pathogens. Bronchopulmonary vascular anastomoses may rupture causing haemorrhage.

Symptoms and signs

Severe. Sputum greater than 30 ml per 24 hours, purulent and offensive; cough on lying down or exercise; haemoptysis of fresh blood; dyspnoea with restrictive or obstructive ventilatory disturbance; episodes of pneumonia with fever, pleuritic pain and sometimes vomiting during expectoration; clubbing of fingers and toes; coarse expiratory crackles over the affected lobes heard throughout inspiration; cyanosis and respiratory failure when ventilatory function is reduced.

Mild. The patient may have no signs between chest colds or have a tendency to expectorate sputum in small volumes daily. There may be a few persistent crackles but no clubbing or gross pulmonary dysfunction.

Investigations

1. Sputum culture for antimicrobial sensitivity.
2. In severe cases, bronchiectasis can be seen on the plain chest X-ray as cystic changes and/or 'tramline shadows' of thickened bronchial walls. In most patients however, CT scanning is required. Bronchography is justified only in localised disease or if complications are suspected.
3. Vital capacity and FEV1 with PO_2 and PCO_2 in severe exacerbations, are a guide to the effectiveness of treatment.
4. Immunoglobulin levels.

Complications

Cerebral abscess, amyloidosis and life-threatening haemoptysis are the main complications.

Differential diagnosis

Congenital abnormalities of the respiratory tract.

Treatment

Exercise and postural drainage help to reduce the volume of retained sputum and resident organisms. Antibiotics, if necessary in high doses, are given until lung function is optimised. Relapsing infections sometimes respond to regular maintenance chemotherapy if they relapse immediately. Localised disease may be resectable surgically.

Prognosis

Severe cases progress to respiratory failure and chronic obstruction in the fifth or sixth decade regardless of any remission as a result of surgical treatment. Mild or moderate cases have a normal lifespan.

ASTHMA

Bronchial asthma is defined as widespread narrowing of the airways which changes its severity over short periods of time either spontaneously or with treatment. It is common and increasingly reported, affecting 5–10% of children and 2–5% of adults.

The essential feature of asthma is bronchial hyperreactivity, i.e. airway narrowing in response to a variety of stimuli (trigger factors) which cause little or no narrowing in normal subjects.

It is possible to measure bronchial hyperreactivity by measuring FEV1 after inhaling concentrations of histamine or methacholine, but this is rarely helpful in clinical practice. Bronchial hyperreactivity to pharmacological agents is not synonymous with asthma, as it can occur in chronic bronchitis, emphysema and cystic fibrosis, and sometimes transiently following respiratory tract infections.

The pathological basis of bronchial hyperreactivity is airway inflammation. The airways of all asthmatics are infiltrated with inflammatory cells, mainly neutrophils and eosinophils, and these appearances improve in parallel with symptoms when asthmatics are treated with inhaled corticosteroids.

Although many trigger factors can be shown to provoke asthma (Table 2.5), most patients are affected by only a few, and usually no definite trigger can be identified. The trigger factors affecting an individual may also change over time. Brief exposures to allergens, infection and occupational chemicals worsen asthma.

In two-thirds of patients, asthma worsens in the early hours of the morning. The reasons are not fully understood but include overnight falls in circulating adrenaline and cortisol levels, and increases in airway vagal tone.

Bronchoconstriction occurs after short periods of intensive exercise and during longer periods of sustained exercise. It is caused by airway cooling and drying (Fig. 2.6).

Table 2.5. Factors precipitating bronchoconstriction

Factors causing bronchoconstriction in all subjects, to which asthmatics are highly susceptible	Trigger factors causing asthma in susceptible subjects
Acetylcholine*	Diurnal variations of bronchial calibre
Histamine*	Episodes of respiratory infection
Burning plastics	Inhaled or ingested allergens
Cigarette smoke	Proteins, e.g. house dust mite, pollen, animal fur, moulds, egg, shell fish, horse serum
Formaldehyde	
Sulphur dioxide	Sensitisers, e.g. aspirin, isocyanates
Foggy atmospheres	Exercise (worse in cold air)
Inert dusts	Cold air (worse with exercise)
	Change of humidity
	Hyperventilation, repeated forced expirations
	Psychological stress

*Methacholine and histamine are used in laboratory tests of bronchial reactivity

Note: All above factors interact. Thus, exercise-induced bronchoconstriction or marked diurnal variation may occur only when the airways are sensitised, e.g. during the pollen season.

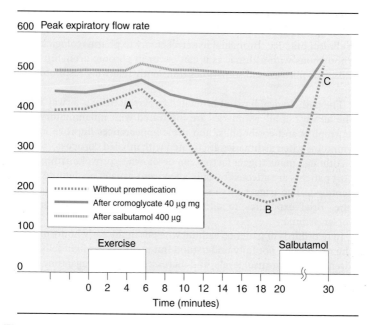

Fig. 2.6 Measurements of PEFR before, during and after exercise-induced asthma. **(A)** Transient rise of PEFR at start of exercise; **(B)** fall after exercise. This fall takes place more rapidly in children than in adults and is shown here beginning to resolve spontaneously after 20 minutes. **(C)** The attack is terminated rapidly by the administration of a bronchodilator aerosol.

Airborne allergens, which may be seasonal (e.g. grass pollen), non-seasonal (e.g. house dust mite) or occupational (e.g. urinary proteins from laboratory animals) cause immediate (10–120 min) and late (8–48 h) reactions.

Respiratory infection, usually with viruses or *H. influenzae*, may lead to exacerbations which last several days.

Classification and aetiology

Three main clinical subgroups of asthma are recognised: atopic, non-atopic and occupational. This classification is largely based on aetiology but it is imperfect and highlights our limited understanding of the underlying causes of asthma.

Atopic asthma (also called juvenile-onset asthma, extrinsic asthma). There is a strong association between atopy and asthma, but the relationship between them is incompletely understood. In susceptible individuals, inhaled allergens cause IgE-mediated antigen–antibody reactions which in turn lead to bronchial hyperreactivity and the clinical features of asthma. However, other factors must be involved because only a proportion of atopic individuals have asthma.

Most young asthmatics are atopic. There is often a family history of asthma, hay fever or infantile eczema, and the presence of specific IgE antibody can be detected by radioimmunoabsorbent tests on blood or by skin prick tests. In most asthmatics, a number of different allergens give positive results, the most important ones in the UK being the house dust mite, pollens, animal danders and moulds, especially *Aspergillus fumigatus*.

Non-atopic asthma (also called late-onset asthma, intrinsic asthma). This presents in adult life. Skin prick tests to allergens are negative and IgE levels usually within the normal range. The underlying causes of bronchial hyperreactivity in this group are not known.

Occupational asthma. Exposure to allergens or chemicals at work can cause asthma. It can occur in atopic or non-atopic individuals, and it is not clear why some individuals develop asthma while others involved in the same work do not. The term occupational asthma is used when the allergen or chemical at work is believed to be the underlying cause of the bronchial hyperreactivity. It does not apply to patients with pre-existing asthma who have exacerbations at work due to non-specific irritants. The number of recognised causes of occupational asthma is increasing (Table 2.6).

Rarely asthma is a manifestation of polyarteritis nodosa and the Churg Strauss syndrome (p. 97).

Pathology

Airway narrowing is caused by constriction of airway smooth muscle, oedema of the bronchial wall, and tenacious sputum (mucus plugs) in the airway lumen. Inflammatory cells are present, especially eosinophils and T lymphocytes, and the ciliated airway epithelium is disrupted.

Symptoms

Symptoms consist of episodic wheeze and/or dyspnoea and/or cough. In many patients symptoms resolve between asthma attacks but in chronic asthma it is common for symptoms to persist in a less severe form between exacerbations. Points to note in the history include the following:

Table 2.6. Some causes of occupational asthma

Sensitizing agent: Isocyanates	Found in: Spray paints, varnishes, plastics, packing, printing
Epoxy resins	Hardeners in plastic adhesives
Colophony fumes (pine resin)	Soldering
Animal urine and insect droppings	Research laboratories
Flour and grain	Milling, baking

1. Symptoms are usually worse at night or in the early morning. This is often the first evidence of an impending severe attack.
2. Cough is common and may be the only symptom.
3. Trigger factors cannot always be identified.
4. Intolerance of cigarette smoke is common. However, some asthmatics smoke.
5. Sputum is typically thick and jelly-like, sometimes with thick plugs or small spirals.
6. A family history of atopy (i.e. asthma, hay fever and/or eczema) is common.
7. Occupational asthma should be suspected when symptoms improve at weekends and/or on holiday.

Signs

Between attacks there may be no abnormal findings, although some patients may have coexistent nasal obstruction or eczema.

During periods of bronchoconstriction, wheeze (usually multiple, sometimes audible without a stethoscope, sometimes only heard on forced expiration,) prolongation of expiration, hyperinflation of the lungs and tachycardia may be present.

In severe attacks, increasing tachycardia, often > 120/min, pulsus paradoxus from large swings of intrathoracic pressure, increasing distress, often with marked agitation, use of accessory muscles, and eventually exhaustion are seen. The latter is an ominous sign, leading to diminished breath sounds (as less air is moved with each breath), confusion and coma caused by hypoxaemia and CO_2 retention.

Investigations

Demonstration of reversible airflow obstruction is crucial to the diagnosis of asthma. Airflow obstructions show spontaneous variability and reversibility to bronchodilators. The former is best demonstrated by peak flow measurements at home 2–3 times daily, including a measurement on waking. Most patients with asthma show a 'morning dip' in peak flow (Fig. 2.7). In suspected occupational asthma, measurements should be made 2-hourly while awake.

Reversibility to bronchodilators will show a >15% rise in peak flow, FEV1 or VC 10–20 min after inhaling a beta-adrenergic agent.

Skin prick tests to common allergens help to identify atopic individuals and occasionally point to specific allergens. Nasal, bronchial and food challenge may help the expert in difficult cases.

Chest X-ray, performed mainly to exclude other disease, is often normal, although it may show hyperinflation. A chest X-ray is crucial in severe asthma to exclude pneumothorax.

Arterial blood gas tensions are usually normal and measured only in severe asthma. $PaCO_2$ should be low during acute attacks. A 'high normal' $PaCO_2$ is a very serious sign, suggesting the onset of ventilatory failure.

A blood count may show eosinophilia which is suppressed by systemic steroids.

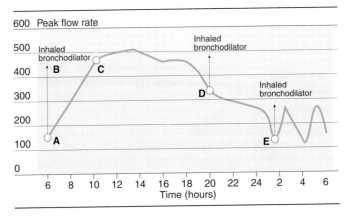

Fig. 2.7 Diurnal variation of PEFR in an asthmatic. Exercise-induced asthma may be superimposed upon this variability which occurs spontaneously. **(A)** Morning dip; **(B)** relief by bronchodilator; **(C)** near normality during the day; **(D)** fall during the evening; **(E)** nocturnal awakening.

Differential diagnosis

Chronic bronchitis and emphysema. Most patients with chronic bronchitis and emphysema have irreversible airflow obstruction. Those who do show reversibility should be treated in the same way as asthmatics.

Infection. Wheeze may occur in chest infections, and purulent sputum in asthma attacks. The main difficulty arises in children in whom 'recurrent bronchitis' usually turns out to be asthma.

Central airway obstruction. Occasionally laryngeal or tracheal tumours, or aspiration of a foreign body, can simulate asthma. However, the main sign is stridor, a mainly inspiratory sound, and not wheeze which is mainly expiratory. The spirometric trace is characteristic. Acute laryngeal oedema occurs as part of generalised anaphylactic reactions.

Psychogenic 'laryngospasm' (adduction of true or false cords) may cause difficulty. Blood gases are usually, but not invariably, normal. Diagnosis is by direct laryngoscopy.

Acute left ventricular failure. This can mimic (or exacerbate) asthma by causing nocturnal dyspnoea. Other features of cardiac disease usually make the distinction simple.

Complications

These include ventilatory failure, pneumothorax and allergic bronchopulmonary aspergillosis—a form of pulmonary eosinophilia, often with mucus plugging of bronchi and lobar collapse which can lead to bronchiectasis. Treatment with oral steroids is recommended, and may prevent the bronchiectasis.

Treatment

Routine treatment

Avoidance. Beta-blockers should be avoided by all patients, as should occupational chemicals known to cause asthma. Allergens, food stuffs and drugs to which there is an idiosyncratic reaction (e.g. aspirin) need be avoided only if they cause symptoms. Patients with occupational asthma may be entitled to compensation.

Drugs. Most asthmatics require medication. Short-acting inhaled beta-agonists are available for symptomatic relief, and in very mild asthma may be the only treatment needed. However most asthmatics (including all with nocturnal wheeze) should also be treated with a regular inhaled anti-inflammatory agent—usually inhaled corticosteroids, although sodium cromoglycate may suffice in children. Long-acting inhaled beta-agonists, inhaled anticholinergic agents and oral theophyllines are second line agents. Oral corticosteroids are vital during acute exacerbations, but they should be used as a last resort for maintenance treatment because of their many adverse long-term effects. Nebulised high-dose bronchodilators may be self-administered by selected patients with severe airflow obstruction.

Inhaled therapy is generally preferable to oral therapy, being more effective at lower dosage. A variety of inhaler devices are available (Fig. 2.8) and almost all patients should be able to use at least one, with tuition. Inhaler technique must be checked regularly, poor technique or the use of an inappropriate device being a common reason for inadequate control of asthma.

Peak flow monitoring. Response to treatment, and the need for changes in treatment, can be assessed by peak flow readings made at home. This is especially important in unstable asthma and in patients who have difficulty perceiving bronchoconstriction.

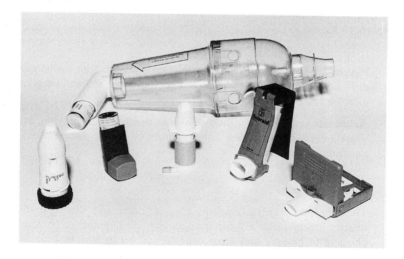

Fig. 2.8 A selection of devices for the administration of inhaled bronchodilators.

Education

This takes time and should include simple explanation of asthma, correct use of inhaler device and peak flow meter, principles of drug therapy, especially prophylactic versus symptomatic treatment, and recognition of worsening asthma and specific instructions on appropriate action.

Recognition and management of worsening asthma

Recognition. Patients should be aware that the following are warning signs of an impending attack:

1. increase in nocturnal waking due to asthma,
2. failure of symptoms to resolve by midmorning,
3. progressive deterioration day by day,
4. a cold which 'goes down to the chest'.

Treatment. Prompt action can often abort an asthma attack. Mild exacerbations (morning PEF > 70% predicted) can usually be managed by doubling the dose of inhaled steroid, but more severe attacks (morning PEF 50–70% predicted) should be treated with oral prednisolone. Patients should contact their general practitioner, but ideally they should be able to start treatment on their own immediately. A morning peak flow remaining above 50% predicted, usually avoids hospital admission.

Recognition and management of acute severe asthma

Recognition. In a distressed or exhausted asthmatic patient, indications for emergency hospital treatment are inability to speak in full sentences, pulse rate > 120/min (140/min in a child), pulsus paradoxus > 20 mmHg (absence of pulsus paradoxus does not exclude acute severe asthma), central cyanosis, PEF well below the patient's usual value, and no relief from the patient's usual or beta-agonist therapy. Exhaustion, diminished breath sounds, mental confusion and a high or high–normal $PaCO_2$ are signs of life-threatening asthma.

Treatment. As soon as possible (in the house or ambulance) the patient should receive a beta-agonist, ideally via a nebuliser or large-volume spacer device, oxygen and hydrocortisone 200 mg i.v.

Nebulised beta-agonist treatment should be repeated on hospital admission if necessary and then continued 3–4 hourly, with the addition of nebulised ipratropium if bronchoconstriction is severe. In addition, oxygen (to maintain PaO_2 > 60 mmHg 8 kPa) and hydrocortisone, 100 mg i.v. 6-hourly, should be given.

Arterial blood gas tensions, chest X-ray, to exclude pneumothorax, and serum electrolytes, to exclude hypokalaemia, will be required.

If severe bronchoconstriction continues despite 5–10 mg (two doses) of nebulised salbutamol and 0.5 mg (one dose) of nebulised ipratropium, an intravenous infusion of aminophylline (0.5 mg/kg/h) should be started provided that oxygenation is adequate. If the patient might have taken slow-release theophylline before admission, the serum level should be checked before starting.

IPPV is only rarely necessary. Exhaustion and inability to maintain adequate oxygenation are the main indications.

Prognosis

Most patients have a normal lifespan, with exacerbations of asthma occurring at unpredictable intervals. Between exacerbations most patients are relatively free of symptoms provided that they are treated appropriately. However, some adults with chronic asthma develop irreversible or partially irreversible airflow obstruction, with symptoms even between exacerbations. Decline of lung function over time is greater in adult-onset asthma. A few patients need maintenance oral prednisolone with consequent side-effects.

Children with asthma often become symptom-free at puberty but at least 50% have asthma in adult life. Children at greatest risk of having adult asthma are those with severe disease, those whose asthma started at an early age and those with severe infantile eczema.

Death from asthma is uncommon considering the prevalence of the disease. However, some 2000 deaths from asthma occur in the UK each year. Retrospective studies have shown that most deaths occur outside hospital, half resulting from under-estimation of the severity of attacks by patients and doctors.

CYSTIC FIBROSIS

Cystic fibrosis (CF) is an autosomal recessive condition caused by one of a number of mutations on chromosome 7. One individual in 25 is a carrier. A defective membrane transfer protein affects chloride ion transport in mucosa. Many of the symptoms are explicable by obstruction of tubules by mucus. Pancreas, lung, sinuses, bile ducts and seminiferous tubules are affected. Severe cases present in infancy with intestinal obstruction, failure to thrive, steatorrhoea and associated vitamin deficiency, or with recurrent respiratory infection leading to bronchiectasis and progressive respiratory impairment. Hepatic cirrhosis, sinusitis and pneumothorax are frequent problems. Diabetes mellitus occurs. Most males have azoospermia but girls are fertile.

Symptoms and signs

Failure to thrive, steatorrhoea, recurrent or chronic bronchial infection with purulent sputum, progressive shortness of breath, and haemoptysis, often severe.

Clubbing of fingers and toes is nearly always present. Chest deformity, usually hyperinflation, sometimes restrictive, respiratory crackles over the upper lobes, and respiratory failure are seen.

Investigations

Sweat [Na^+]. In children, > 59 mmol/l is diagnostic. In adults, 70–90 mmol/l is borderline, > 90 mmol diagnostic.

Chest X-ray. Bronchiectasis, cysts and nodular changes in upper and middle zones, fibrosis and recurrent consolidation, and abscess formation are present.

Sputum. *H. influenzae, Staph. aureus* and *Ps. aeruginosa* are the common pathogens occurring in that order during the lifetime of the patient, unless eradicated by antibiotic treatment.

Pancreatic function is impaired (p. 276). Adequacy of pancreatic replacement is monitored in children by stool fats and by height and weight, and in adults by serum levels of fat-soluble vitamins (A, E and D) and calcium.

Lung function. Airflow obstruction is progressive, with falling FEV1 and usually hyperinflation. PO_2 is reduced during exacerbations. Elevation of PCO_2 occurs late. Infective pulmonary exacerbations cause transient falls of VC.

Complications

These include heat exhaustion (loss of sodium in sweat), pneumothorax, haemoptysis, abdominal pain, constipation and intestinal obstruction (meconium ileus equivalent, distal intestinal syndrome).

Treatment

Adequate calorie intake must be ensured. Oral pancreatic supplements are given before meals and snacks in doses sufficient to control steatorrhoea. H_2 antagonists reduce gastric breakdown of pancreatic enzymes. Vitamins A, D and E supplements are needed.

Exercise is beneficial, postural drainage and forced expiratory physiotherapy aid expectoration. Long-term flucloxacillin, up to 4 g per 24 hours prevents staphylococcal lung infection.

Acute exacerbations are treated for as long as necessary with appropriate antibiotics. Frequent recurrences are treated with nebulised antibiotics. Indwelling intravenous lines may be needed. Antibiotics are given for fever, acute pneumonic illness, increasing sputum or progressively falling VC. Consistent carefully explained management by a skilful team and easy access to expert care are essential. Bilateral lung or heart/lung transplantation is increasingly available.

Prognosis

Life expectancy is improving and is currently around 30 years in all but the most severely affected cases. It is dependent on the severity of respiratory disease.

SARCOIDOSIS

Sarcoidosis is a systemic disease of unknown cause with non-caseating granulomata in lymph nodes and other sites, usually having a benign course. Its prevalence varies according to population, ranging from 27 to 200/100 000. Clinically indistinguishable disorders may be caused by chronic exposure to industrial beryllium (berylliosis) and by tattooing. The characteristic pathological lesion is the granuloma, a reaction to an insoluble antigen, which may heal with no residue or with fibrosis. CD4 (helper) T lymphocytes are concentrated in active sites such as the lung, which results in reduced immunoreactivity elsewhere (delayed hypersensitivity tests may become negative). T cell function is normal, as is resistance to infection.

Symptoms and signs

Acute sarcoidosis presents with a febrile illness, erythema nodosum and bilateral enlargement of the hilar lymph nodes in the chest. Prognosis is good with more than 80% recovering spontaneously. A few patients develop pulmonary infiltrations and may become breathless. The lung changes may progress to a chronic destructive fibrotic disease which may occasionally be fatal. Afro-Caribbeans are more commonly prone to severe forms.

Chronic sarcoidosis may present in a variety of ways. Pulmonary sarcoidosis presents with rapid or slow progression of cough, dyspnoea or chest pain and may be detected at a routine chest X-ray. Cardiac sarcoidosis (rare) causes arrhythmias, sudden death and congestive cardiomyopathy.

Examination reveals some of the manifestations listed (Table 2.7). Inspiratory crackles are usually scanty or absent. Cor pulmonale may result from progression to severe fibrosis.

Investigations

1. Characteristic histology of affected node or site—liver, bronchus, lung, labial gland—is diagnostic.
2. Kveim test. Installation of 0.1 ml of antigen from sarcoid spleen intra dermally will result in a granuloma in 6 weeks (confirmed by biopsy).
3. Chest X-ray may show hilar adenopathy and diffuse lung shadows, especially in upper and middle zones. Later, upper zone or generalised pulmonary fibrosis will be seen with generalised cyst formation (honeycomb lung) and 'eggshell' calcification of hilar nodes. CT and magnetic resonance scans will show the extent of adenopathy and pulmonary involvement.
4. Blood. Raised ESR and plasma viscosity occur in most patients with erythema nodosum. Serum calcium levels are elevated in 10%. Abnormal liver function and elevated angiotensin converting enzyme level (acute phase protein) may be detected. Most patients with lone pulmonary sarcoid have no blood abnormality.
5. Lung function tests do not mirror exactly the severity of radiological granulomatosis but show good correlation with the degree of dyspnoea. Reductions of VC and CO transfer occur with alveolar wall fibrosis. Fibrotic disease or bronchial stenosis causes chronic airways obstruction. Hypoxaemia and respiratory failure occur late.
6. Bronchoscopy may show granulomata, bronchial stenosis and characteristic histology.

Table 2.7. Systemic manifestations of chronic sarcoidosis

Eye	Anterior uveitis: glaucoma Posterior uveitis Kerato-conjunctivitis (occasionally dryness) Lachrymal gland enlargement
Salivary exocrine glands	Parotid and other salivary glandular enlargement, dry mouth
Skin	Recurrent erythema nodosum (rare) Papules and nodules: 'lupus pernio' Hypertrophic scars are common
Joints	Polyarthralgia: polyarthritis Bone cysts (accompanied by skin changes)
Central nervous system	Neuropathy, especially cranial Meningomyelitis Posterior pituitary lesions, diabetes insipidus
Gastrointestinal tract	Hepatomegaly, splenomegaly with portal hypertension
Ear, nose and throat	Nasal laryhgeal granuloma
Lung	Bronchial inflammation, stenosis Lung granuloma and fibrosis, rarely pleural Hilar adenopathy
Heart	Cardiomyopathy Heart block Sudden death
General	Hypercalcaemia and renal complications Enlarged lymph nodes Fever (rare)

7. Gallium radioisotope scan shows positive images at active sites in the lungs and salivary glands.
8. Hand X-rays show cysts in bone.

Differential diagnosis

Hilar adenopathy and erythema nodosum: usually sarcoid, very rarely tuberculosis. All organs may be involved in sarcoidosis.

Prognosis

Prognosis is variable; 50% become chronic with a marginally reduced life expectancy and a few progress rapidly. The disease is more aggressive in patients of African descent.

Treatment

Active sarcoidosis responds to corticosteroids which, given early, suppress granuloma formation and prevent progression to fibrosis but do not alter the prognosis for eventual remission or relapse. Powerful immune suppressants have little advantage over moderate doses of prednisolone (5–17.5 mg per 24 hours for 4 weeks). There is no known radical cure.

Absolute indications for corticosteroid therapy include anterior uveitis (drops are effective), posterior uveitis, hypercalcaemia, dyspnoea, and cardiac and CNS involvement (efficacy variable).

Corticosteroids should be considered where skin lesions are disfiguring, for nasal disease and symptomatic lymphatic or glandular swellings or for drying of salivary secretions.

TUMOURS OF THE LUNG

Almost all tumours of the lung are malignant or potentially malignant. By far the most common is bronchial carcinoma.

BRONCHIAL CARCINOMA

Bronchial carcinoma is responsible for more male deaths in the developed world than any other cancer, with more than 30 000 deaths/year in the UK. The principal cause is cigarette smoking. The death rate in the UK seems to have reached a plateau in men. It is less common but rising in women and now rivals breast carcinoma as the most common malignant disease, reflecting a 4-fold rise in cigarette consumption by women between 1940 and 1975. The excess risk approximately halves every 5 years after smoking is stopped. Pipe and cigar smokers have a smaller increased risk. Passive smoking may carry a significant risk. Patients with asbestosis also have an increased risk of bronchial carcinoma.

Pathology

Most tumours originate in the larger bronchi where they may cause partial or total obstruction. They spread to the mediastinum, pleura and chest wall by direct invasion, and to the hilar, mediastinal and supraclavicular lymph nodes via the lymphatics. The most common sites for blood-borne metastases are the brain, liver and bones. The histological subtypes (Table 2.8) vary in prognosis.

Table 2.8. Characteristics of different cell types in bronchial carcinoma

Cell type	Frequency	Growth	Metastases
Squamous	40%	Slow	Early
Small cell	25%	Rapid	Early
Large cell undifferentiated	20%	Intermediate	Intermediate
Adenocarcinoma	15%	Intermediate	Intermediate
Alveolar cell carcinoma	<1%	Rapid	Late

Symptoms and signs

Local effects of tumour in a bronchus
1. Cough (frequently ignored because most smokers regard a morning cough as normal), sometimes changing in character.
2. Haemoptysis, which should always be investigated.
3. Bronchial narrowing—dyspnoea, stridor (if the narrowing affects the trachea or main bronchi), fixed rhonchus, distal infection with peripheral obstruction.
4. Distal collapse—dyspnoea, mediastinal shift to the affected side, diminished expansion, dullness to percussion, diminished breath sounds and diminished vocal resonance all on the affected side.
5. Weightloss, usually with anorexia.
6. Finger clubbing is seen in 30% of patients. Note that chronic bronchitis and emphysema do not cause clubbing.

Spread to mediastinum
1. Left recurrent laryngeal nerve paralysis leads to hoarse voice, bovine cough.
2. Superior vena caval obstruction causes headache, sometimes aggravated by bending forward, plethora and peripheral cyanosis of the face and conjunctivae, engorged non-pulsatile neck veins, and distended collateral veins on the chest wall.
3. Dysphagia from compression of the oesophagus by either the tumour or lymph nodes.
4. Phrenic nerve paralysis results in elevation and paradoxical movement of the diaphragm; this causes dullness and diminished breath sounds but is usually easier to detect radiologically than clinically.
5. Pericardial invasion causes a blood-stained pericardial effusion and arrhythmias.

Spread to pleura and chest wall
1. Malignant pleural effusions are usually blood stained. Pleural effusion in bronchogenic carcinoma is not always the result of local invasion but may be secondary to infection.
2. Chest wall pain—constant and often severe.
3. Apical (superior sulcus, Pancoast) tumours often erode the first rib and involve the brachial plexus and cervical sympathetic nerves. They may cause pain in the inner aspect of the arm (T1 dermatome), wasting of the small muscles of the hand and Horner's syndrome.

Spread to lymph nodes
1. Hilar lymphadenopathy can cause bronchial narrowing by extrinsic compression. Enlarged hilar lymph nodes can also cause retrograde obstruction of pulmonary lymphatics—lymphangitis carcinomatosa—which presents with cough and dyspnoea.
2. Mediastinal lymphadenopathy can compress and invade other mediastinal structures.
3. Supraclavicular lymphadenopathy is detectable clinically and should always be sought on examination.

Distant blood-borne metastases

1. Bone—pain, pathological fractures, including vertebral collapse, and hypercalcaemia. Hypercalcaemia can also result from squamous growths. Symptoms include malaise, nausea, confusion, thirst, polyuria and constipation.
2. Liver—hard, irregular hepatomegaly, sometimes tender.
3. Brain—epilepsy, localising neurological defects, headache, papilloedema.
4. Adrenal glands—usually asymptomatic but can rarely cause Addison's disease.
5. Skin—painless nodules.

Non-metastatic (paraneoplastic) complications

1. Pulmonary hypertrophic osteoarthropathy—painful wrists or ankles.
2. Endocrine syndromes caused by products of tumour cells which mimic hormones—Cushing's syndrome (ACTH), dilutional hyponatraemia (ADH), hypercalcaemia (parathyroid hormone), gynaecomastia (oestrogens).
3. Neuromuscular syndromes—peripheral neuropathy, cerebellar dysfunction, dermatomyositis and a form of myasthenia (Eaton-Lambert syndrome).

Investigations

Chest X-ray is the commonest clue to diagnosis. Sometimes the tumour is detected on routine X-ray. Radiological appearances include slight enlargement or distortion of a hilar shadow or an obvious hilar mass, an area of pulmonary collapse with or without a hilar shadow, unresolved pneumonia, pleural effusion, lung abscess, a peripheral mass, and occasionally lymphangitis carcinomatosa.

The sputum can be examined cytologically but a negative result does not exclude the diagnosis.

Bronchoscopy with biopsy establishes the diagnosis and the position of the tumour in the bronchial tree in over 70%.

Screening for liver and bone metastases is by determining alkaline phosphatase, aspartate aminotransferase and serum calcium levels. Liver scan (ultrasound or CT) and radiological investigation for bone metastases (plain X-rays with or without isotope bone scan) or brain metastases (CT scan) are indicated only if there is a clinical or biochemical suspicion of metastases.

CT scan (or magnetic resonance images (MRI)) of the thorax determines the extent of a bronchial carcinoma, demonstrating invasion of the mediastinum and chest wall, enlargement of hilar and mediastinal lymph nodes, and other pulmonary lesions.

Mediastinoscopy is required to biopsy enlarged mediastinal lymph nodes, and pleural biopsy and cytology of the pleural fluid to diagnose most malignant effusions.

FEV1, VC, $PaCO_2$ and effort tolerance need to be determined. Respiratory failure will probably ensue if, after resection of the tumour, FEV1 is less than 1.0 litre.

Surgical excision may be necessary for diagnosis of resectable peripheral masses of uncertain cause.

Differential diagnosis

The differential diagnosis is wide and depends on the mode of presentation. The respiratory diseases which resemble bronchogenic carcinoma radiographically are pneumonia, lung abscess, tuberculosis, pulmonary infarction and pulmonary metastases. For lymphatic carcinomatosis and alveolar cell carcinoma, the differential diagnosis also includes cryptogenic fibrosing alveolitis and other causes of diffuse pulmonary fibrosis.

Treatment

Surgery. Removal of the affected lobe or lung is the treatment of choice, as it provides the best chance of cure. However, most patients are unsuitable for surgery at the time of presentation, either because the tumour has spread to the pleura, mediastinum or beyond, or because the patient is generally unfit for major thoracic surgery owing to cardiorespiratory disease or advanced age. Approximately 20% of patients are considered suitable for surgery, and of these 25–50% survive 5 years, the best results being obtained with squamous carcinoma. Resection of an apparently localised small cell tumour is usually followed by chemotherapy because of the likelihood of undetected metastases being present at diagnosis.

Radical radiotherapy. Occasionally localised lung cancer can be cured by radiotherapy. The results are not as good as with surgery, and the high doses of radiation necessary to achieve a cure damage surrounding lung tissue. The most radiosensitive tumours are small cell tumours but these are rarely, if ever, cured by radiotherapy because they have already spread at diagnosis. Squamous carcinoma is radiosensitive, adenocarcinoma is relatively insensitive, and the radiosensitivity of large cell undifferentiated carcinoma is very variable.

Palliative radiotherapy. Low-dose radiotherapy can greatly improve the quality of life, whatever the cell type. It is particularly useful for localised bone pain caused by either local spread or metastases, superior vena caval obstruction, stridor and impending bronchial obstruction, dysphagia from oesophageal compression, severe haemoptysis or cough and cerebral metastases.

Chemotherapy. Chemotherapy is not yet curative, but in small cell lung carcinoma, combination chemotherapy can prolong life (currently by 6–12 months in the 70% of patients who respond) and relieve symptoms. In other types of lung carcinoma chemotherapy is usually ineffective. Whenever appropriate, patients receiving chemotherapy should be asked to enter large clinical trials, which are essential to document the effectiveness of different regimens.

Palliation. Palliation is often achieved by radiotherapy (see above). For pain, regular analgesia is an alternative, with non-steroidal anti-inflammatory drugs and opiates. Occlusion of major airways by the tumour can be relieved by laser therapy and/or the insertion of a stent. Malignant pleural effusions causing breathlessness should be aspirated, followed by chemical pleurodesis. Hypercalcaemia is treated with fluids ± diphosphonates.

Counselling. Allocation of time for this by physicians, general practitioners and specialist nurses is of overriding importance.

OTHER PRIMARY LUNG TUMOURS

Bronchial adenomas

These uncommon tumours usually present with haemoptysis, recurrent infection or lobar/segmental collapse. The majority can be seen at bronchoscopy; 90% are **carcinoid tumours,** the remainder being **cylindromata.** Malignant change and local invasion are uncommon, metastases and the carcinoid syndrome rare. The treatment of choice is surgical excision unless there is evidence of metastasis. The outlook is excellent unless there is malignant change in the excised tumour.

Hamartomas

These rare benign tumours are fetal rests which grow in middle life. They may calcify. They resemble peripheral carcinomas and are usually removed by segmental resection.

Lymphomas

Occasionally, a lymphoma arises in the lung in the absence of disease elsewhere. More often, however, pulmonary involvement occurs when there is generalised disease with involvement of other organs.

SECONDARY TUMOURS OF THE LUNG

Blood-borne pulmonary metastases are common and can arise from malignant tumours anywhere in the body. The most common primary sites are breast, kidney, ovary, testes and gastrointestinal tract. They are usually multiple and sometimes appear as well defined round opacities, so called cannonball secondaries. They usually cause few respiratory symptoms unless lung tissue is extensively replaced by tumour or pleural effusion develops. Lymphatic carcinomatosis (see above) can also occur as a result of metastases, often from breast carcinoma.

DIFFUSE PULMONARY INFILTRATION AND FIBROSIS

A number of conditions cause diffuse infiltration of the alveolar walls with inflammatory cells, with or without alveolar exudate and fibrosis. The bronchioles may be involved. These present either as acute illnesses or insidiously, with breathlessness. Fine basal crackles are often present and some patients have finger clubbing. VC and lung volumes and/or gas transfer are reduced and there is variable hypoxaemia with hyperventilation. They progress to 'honeycomb lung' in which areas of the lung are replaced by cysts formed from dilated bronchioles surrounded by fibrosed and obliterated alveoli. Radiological change may be obvious but is not necessarily proportional to the functional abnormality.

Some characteristic causes are listed in Table 2.9. Most of these conditions are uncommon and only the important ones will be discussed.

CRYPTOGENIC FIBROSING ALVEOLITIS (SYNONYM:INTERSTITIAL PNEUMONIA)

This is a progressive condition of unknown cause characterised by acute or insidious inflammation of the alveolar wall leading to fibrosis.

Pathology

In acute cases, there is desquamation of type II alveolar cells with macrophages into the alveolar spaces and lymphocytic infiltration of alveolar walls. There may be obliteration of bronchioles and patchy consolidation. In chronic cases, fibrosis within alveolar walls may obliterate whole lobules.

There is overlap with the systemic autoimmune diseases and conditions resembling cryptogenic fibrosing alveolitis occur in rheumatoid arthritis, systemic sclerosis, chronic active hepatitis, Sjögren's syndrome and renal tubular acidosis.

Symptoms and signs

Most patients present between the ages of 40 and 70. The acute form presents with the rapid onset of dyspnoea at rest or on slight exertion with a non-productive cough. Fine inspiratory crackles are heard at the bases. Cyanosis or clubbing are present in the minority. Over half remit or respond to corticosteroids.

The more common chronic form presents with an insidious onset of exertional dyspnoea and variable, and usually, non-productive cough. Examination reveals fine inspiratory crackles, sometimes localised, heard at the end of inspiration. Clubbing occurs in over 50%. Only 10% respond to corticosteroids; more than half will die within 5 years of diagnosis.

Complications

These include bronchial infection, respiratory failure, pulmonary hypertension and pulmonary thrombo-embolic disease.

Investigations

A chest X-ray shows, progressively, fine nodulation, basal fibrosis and generalised 'honeycombing'.

Acute cases have elevated plasma viscosity, ESR and circulating immune complexes. Anti-DNA antibodies may be present.

VC and residual volume of lung volumes are low, expiratory flow rates normal, and CO transfer factor reduced (the earliest abnormality in insidious cases). PO_2 varies with clinical state but may be only slightly reduced in early cases. PCO_2 is low except terminally.

Bronchioalveolar lavage and transbronchial biopsy show all types of inflammatory cells including lymphocytes, neutrophils and eosinophils, to be present in excess. (Lymphocytosis is said to be associated with steroid responsiveness; neutrophilia and eosinophilia with a poor prognosis.) Histology of small samples is unreliable because of the patchy nature of the disease but characteristic changes may be detected.

Thoracotomy and lung biopsy yield histological diagnosis but are invasive. Pulmonary fibrosis and lung cysts are characteristic on CT scans.

Differential diagnosis (See Table 2.9)

Acute cryptogenic fibrosing alveolitis has to be distinguished from viral pneumonia.

Treatment

Treatment is currently unsatisfactory. Corticosteroids in high doses generally improve function in acute cases and are reduced to maintenance doses as clinical improvement occurs. Relapse is common. In a few cases, steroid doses may be reduced by the concomitant use of immunosuppressant agents such as cyclophosphamide. Most patients respond only transiently to anti-inflammatory medication.

EXTRINSIC ALLERGIC ALVEOLITIS

Numerous organic agents may cause acute or chronic bronchial and pulmonary lymphocytic infiltration, granulomas and fibrosis in susceptible subjects (Table 2.10).

Acute exposure leads to fever, malaise, cough and dyspnoea within 48 hours. The symptoms of chronic exposure are similar to those of chronic airflow obstruction. Lung function tests show a predominantly restrictive pattern with hypoxaemia. Stippling, diffuse lung fibrosis, often apical, will be seen on chest X-ray.

DISEASES CAUSED BY MINERAL DUSTS (PNEUMOCONIOSES)

Minerals inhaled at work or as a result of environmental pollution may cause clinical disease and/or radiographic change. Inhaled dust is transported out of the lungs by the mucociliary escalator and the alveolar macrophage system which transports the dust to the bronchi or to the lymph nodes. Toxic dusts damage macrophages with the liberation of cytokines resulting in an inflammatory response reflected in radiographic and functional changes. Molecular weight determines radiodensity (iron oxide, barium sulphate, tin oxide are opaque but inert). With heavy exposure, the lymphatics become blocked so

Table 2.9. Some of the disorders leading to diffuse pulmonary fibrosis

Disorder	X-ray lung fields	Inspiratory crackles	Clubbing	Histology
Cryptogenic fibrosing alveolitis				
Acute	Widespread nodular shadows	Present	Absent	Inflammation, desquamation of pneumocytes, fibrosis
Chronic	or basal fibrosis or none	Early sign	Often	Inflammation and fibrosis
Asbestosis	Basal fibrosis plus pleural disease	Early sign	Often	Inflammation and fibrosis
Silicosis	Nodular, confluent shadows	Late, rarely profuse	Late	Typical nodules near bronchioles, massive fibrosis
Coalworkers' pneumoconiosis	Nodular shadows	Absent	Absent	Carbon nodules
Sarcoidosis	Nodular shadows Hilar adenopathy	Few, late	Rare	Granuloma, fibrosis Lymphocyte infiltration
Eosinophilic granuloma	Nodular shadows	Absent	Sometimes	Eosinophilic granuloma, 'honeycomb lung'
Extrinsic alveolitis	Adenopathy sometimes A few progress to reticulation Variable nodulation: upper zone	Acute	Late	Inflammation Variable granuloma, bronchiectasis
Systemic sclerosis	Basal reticulation	Variable	Rare	Dense fibrosis
Radiation fibrosis	Variable	Variable	Rare	Vasculitis, fibrosis
Drugs (amiodarone, cytotoxic drugs, nitrofurantoin, sulphasalazine)	Variable	Present	Sometimes	Inflammation, eosinophilia, lymphocyte infiltration, fibrosis
Paraquat poisoning	Progressive basal reticulation	Usual	Absent	Fibroblast proliferation within alveoli
Recurrent pulmonary oedema	Sequence of films showing incomplete resolution	During acute attacks	Sometimes	Diffuse fibrosis
Disseminated secondary carcinoma, lymphoma leukaemia and bone marrow transplantation may also cause diffuse pulmonary infiltration				
Disseminated secondary carcinoma	Nodulation or lymphatic obstruction	Variable	Rare	Malignant cells
Lymphoma	Large or fine nodules	Late	Rare	Round cells (in alveolar walls)
Leukaemias	Nodular or linear infiltrates	Usual	Rare	Fibrosis after therapy

Table 2.10. Examples of extrinsic allergic alveolitis

Disease	Cause	Precipitin test
Farmer's lung Mushroom worker's lung	Spores of thermophilic actinomycetes	Usually positive but 10% false negative, 20% false positive among farmers
Pigeon fancier's lung	Pigeon serum in excreta	20% false positive among breeders
Budgerigar fancier's lung	Budgerigar droppings	Usually positive
Malt worker's lung	*Aspergillus clavatus* spores	Usually positive
Grain handler's lung	Grain weevil	Numerous antigens, no test available
Pituitary snuff taker's lung	Animal antigens	No test available
Humidifier fever	Thermophilic actinomycetes Saprophytic amoebae	Poor correlation between presence of antibodies and disease

that highly fibrogenic dusts are more toxic when they are mixed with inert particles.

Pneumoconioses result from a fibrous reaction to dusts retained in the lung, the severity of the condition depending on the inhaled dose, the size of the particles and their toxicity to macrophages.

Chronic bronchitis and emphysema are additional hazards, although their industrial incidence has been difficult to evaluate because of the small numbers of non-smoking men working in the industries concerned.

Coalworkers' pneumoconiosis

Simple pneumoconiosis refers to the nodular lesions affecting the lungs of coalminers caused by carbon deposition and associated with focal emphysema. The lesions are situated near the respiratory bronchioles and have a minor effect on lung function. In *complicated pneumoconiosis*, sheets of fibrotic tissue, yielding appearances resembling those of lung tumours on X-ray, are known as progressive fibrosis and are associated with dyspnoea. Miners with rheumatoid arthritis are especially prone to rheumatoid nodules within the lung (Caplan's syndrome).

The prevalence of the disease among coalminers led to an extensive system for identification and compensation of these cases. Improved mining methods have drastically reduced the incidence of this disorder.

Silicosis

This pneumoconiosis, caused by the inhalation of finely particulate silica, complicates mining of precious metals, tin, copper, graphite, mica and anthracite, quarrying and dressing of slate, granite and sandstone, road drilling and sandblasting, pottery and ceramics manufacture, boiler scraping, and grinding (new techniques avoid silica). Silica is more fibrogenic than coal. Progressive fibrosis may occur.

Silicosis causes dyspnoea with recurrent respiratory infections. Characteristic chest X-ray changes include multiple fine nodules in the upper and middle zones, with peripheral 'eggshell' calcification of mediastinal lymph nodes. Massive fibrosis within the lungs may cavitate and the right ventricle may enlarge.

Functional changes include reduction of VC and the preservation of the FEV1/VC ratio. The differential diagnosis includes sarcoidosis, miliary tuberculosis and other causes of diffuse pulmonary mottling.

Diseases related to asbestos exposure

Asbestos (*Gr.* 'indestructible') is a natural fibre consisting of aluminium, calcium, iron, nickel and magnesium silicates. It resists high temperatures. Several forms exist, mainly chrysotile (white asbestos) and the amphiboles particularly crocidolite and tremolite (blue asbestos).

Asbestos fibres measure 20×3 μm. They are distributed axially in the airstream to the lower lobes and deposited subpleurally, being transported through lymphatic channels to the parietal pleura,

Conditions caused by asbestos:

1. **Asbestosis** is a form of diffuse mainly basal pulmonary fibrosis clinically and radiologically similar to fibrosing alveolitis but with pleural involvement. It usually occurs 10–30 years or more after first exposure, the risk being related to the amount and duration of exposure.
2. **Pleural plaques,** which may calcify. Usually painless, they do not affect lung function.
3. **Non-malignant recurrent pleural effusion** with dense pleural thickening.
4. **Mesothelioma of pleura.** This is a malignant pleural tumour presenting with chest wall pain or pleural effusion. Local spread is more common than metastasis. It is usually fatal within 2 years; 90% of cases have been exposed to asbestos but in some cases the exposure has been low. Crocidolite is particularly implicated. The *peritoneum* may be involved.
5. **Carcinoma of the bronchus.** There is a marked interaction between cigarette smoking and asbestos in causing bronchial carcinoma.

Compensation

In many countries, compensation is available and litigation is commonplace. Until 1975 there was widespread ignorance among employers as to the necessary precautions; this is surprising because legal measures to control exposure were first introduced around 1930.

PULMONARY OEDEMA

The presence of oedema fluid in the pulmonary alveoli is caused by either transudation (cardiogenic, related to altered vascular pressure) or exudation (noncardiogenic, related to vascular permeability).

Pulmonary transudation is usually caused by left ventricular failure or mitral stenosis (see p. 18.) High altitude travel and raised intracranial pressure (ICP) which are rarer causes of pulmonary oedema operate by altering vascular pressures in the presence of normal cardiac function.

Acute non-cardiogenic pulmonary oedema occurs in intensive care units (adult respiratory distress syndrome ARDS). This complicates hypotension, oxygen toxicity, trauma and bloodloss, fat embolism, lung contusion and haemorrhage, viral pneumonias and inhalation or injection of certain toxic or therapeutic agents.

Management involves oxygenation and artificial ventilation as well as treatment of the underlying condition with circulatory support when necessary.

Chronic pulmonary oedema occurs in uraemia.

PULMONARY INVOLVEMENT IN SYSTEMIC DISEASES

Rheumatoid arthritis (see p. 368)

This is a multisystem disorder. Lung involvement includes fibrosing alveolitis (characterised by inspiratory crackles, gas transfer defect and respiratory symptoms in a proportion of such patients), 'necrobiotic' nodules which can cavitate and may be single or multiple, pleural effusion or painful pleural inflammation, recurrent bronchopulmonary infection, acute pleuropericarditis, pulmonary hypertension, and obliterative bronchiolitis.

Systemic lupus erythematosus (SLE) (see p. 383)

Acute manifestations which respond to steroids are recurrent pleural effusions, a syndrome like acute pulmonary oedema, small volume lungs, dyspnoea with reduced VC and CO transfer (possibly related to pulmonary vasculitis), diffuse pulmonary fibrosis (rarely typical fibrosing alveolitis), and respiratory muscle weakness, including impairment of diaphragm function in chronic SLE. Several of these conditions may coexist. There is generally a good symptomatic response to treatment with steroids and other agents, but some residual damage is usually detected by lung function tests.

Scleroderma (systemic sclerosis) (see p. 385)

Advanced cases show progressive basal alveolar and pulmonary vascular fibrosis, sometimes progressing to pulmonary hypertension. Dyspnoea and defects of pulmonary gas transfer precede X-ray changes. Respiratory muscles may be involved. Chest expansion may be affected by thickening of the skin.

Systemic vasculitis

Each specific variant of this group of disorders shows a number of pulmonary manifestations. Wegener's granuloma is an acute multisystem disease, classically causing malaise with a destructive vasculitis and granulomatosis of the nose, sinuses and lungs, associated with glomerulonephritis. Pulmonary changes may mimic pneumonia or pulmonary tuberculosis, or may consist of widespread infiltrates or solitary nodules resembling tumours. Secondary infection occurs with *Staph. aureus*. Diagnosis is by histology and the presence of anti-neutrophil cytoplasmic antibody in serum. Treatment is with corticosteroids and immunosuppressants and has reduced the mortality from 100% to a small fraction.

Churg Strauss syndrome consists of tumours within the lung and head and neck showing a characteristic granulomatous histology, associated with sinusitis, allergic rhinitis and bronchial asthma. The kidneys are not involved. The condition responds to corticosteroids. Asthma, eosinophilic pneumonia, pleurisy and pericarditis may form part of polyarteritis nodosa. Bronchial asthma and chronic airways obstruction occur in association with cranial arteritis.

All these disorders may affect blood vessels in skin, peripheral nerves, heart, skeletal muscle and elsewhere.

Thyroid disease

Breathlessness in thyrotoxicosis may be caused by severe respiratory muscle weakness or by impaired cardiac function. Pleural effusions occur in severe hypothyroidism.

DRUG-INDUCED LUNG DISEASE

Various syndromes are produced by drugs (Table 2.11).

Paraquat poisoning

Ingestion of paraquat leads to painful oropharyngeal and oesophageal ulceration, renal failure and progressive bronchopulmonary fibrosis.

THORACIC CAGE DISEASE

Kyphoscoliosis

Impaired expansion of the thoracic cage causes increased work of breathing and also maldistribution of pulmonary ventilation and perfusion. Scoliosis causes greater impairment than kyphosis. Ventilatory failure, with cor pulmonale and congestive heart failure, may occur between the ages of 30 and 50 but most patients survive into old age. The prognosis correlates with vital capacity and depends not only on the degree of kyphoscoliosis but also on the condition of the underlying lung and whether there is associated neurological disease.

Ankylosing spondylitis

Fusion of costovertebral joints yields a fixed chest with diaphragmatic ventilation. Inspiratory capacity is reduced by up to 30% but this does not cause

Table 2.11. Drug-induced lung disease. Various syndromes are produced by drugs. This list is incomplete. Some regimens are obsolete and are indicated with★

Drug-induced systemic lupus erythematosus (SLE)	Hydralazine in high doses★
	Phenytoin
	Procainamide
Pulmonary eosinophilia	Nitrofurantoin (with small pleural effusions)
	Sulphonamides (usually without pleural effusions)
Diffuse pulmonary fibrosis, acute and chronic	Amiodarone
	Nitrofurantoin
	Azopropazone, other non-steroidal anti-inflammatory drugs
	Gold
	Busulphan, bleomycin, other cytotoxic agents especially with radiotherapy
Pulmonary oedema	Amitriptyline overdose
Pleuro-pulmonary fibrosis	Long-term practolol★
	Methysergide
Asthma–Anaphylaxis	Aspirin and non-steroidal anti-inflammatory agents
	Penicillin
	Sera (e.g. antitetanus)★, desensitising courses of pollen and other extracts (rarely)

blood gas disturbance or dyspnoea. Bilateral upper zone fibrosis complicates this condition (cause unknown). Patients may develop respiratory failure when diaphragm function is impaired, e.g. after abdominal surgery or if they smoke or develop other lung diseases.

Paresis of respiratory muscles

Causes include acute polyneuritis, poliomyelitis, spinal cord injury and many chronic neuromuscular disorders.

Patients present with recurrent chest infections, orthopnoea and nocturnal dyspnoea. Paralysis of the diaphragm with intact intercostal muscles causes a 50% reduction of VC, worse on lying down. Loss of respiratory innervation below C2, with preservation of sternomastoids, yields a VC of under 1.0 litre with a loss of automatic breathing during sleep. In general, reduction of VC below 2.0 litres results in dyspnoea and below 1.0 litre is associated with a risk of ventilatory failure, especially if PO_2 is reduced by lung damage, e.g. repeated aspiration. Muscular weakness causes impairment of coughing.

The outlook has been improved by assisted nocturnal ventilation via a nasal mask.

PLEURAL DISEASE

Spontaneous pneumothorax

This is the entry of air into a pleural cavity through a spontaneous rupture of the pleural surface of a lung. Partial or complete retraction of the lung, hyperinflation of the hemithorax and movement of the mediastinum towards the normal side follows entry of air into the pleural cavity. If the defect on the surface of the lung is small, it seals with spontaneous resolution. If the tear acts as a check valve allowing more air to enter the pleural space during inspiration, positive pressure builds up thus causing 'tension pneumothorax'.

Most cases occur in healthy young men who are often tall and thin. Most older patients have emphysema or have previously had tuberculosis. Rare predisposing causes include Marfan's syndrome, cystic fibrosis, 'honeycomb lung', lung abscesses, infarcts and ectopic endometriosis.

Symptoms and signs

Sudden chest pain, usually on the side of the pneumothorax but occasionally central, with shortness of breath in some instances, is the main symptom.

Signs may include diminished breath sounds on the affected side, increased respiratory rate, diminished movement on the affected side which may be larger than the other, increased resonance to percussion on the affected side, and a precordial sound in time with the heart beat.

Tension pneumothorax causes very severe breathlessness, distended neck veins and hypotension, secondary to the obstruction to the venous circulation.

Investigations

Chest X-ray shows the pneumothorax. The pleural edge is separated from the rib cage and lung markings are absent peripherally.

Complications

These include tension pneumothorax, bilateral pneumothorax, haemothorax occasionally profuse, mediastinal air in pneumothorax (pneumomediastinum), persistent bronchopleural fistula, chronic pneumothorax.

Treatment

Shallow pneumothoraces may be left to resolve spontaneously; this process is speeded by breathing 28% oxygen for 2–3 days.

Large pneumothoraces or those causing dyspnoea are aspirated. One attempt may be made with an intravenous cannula and a 3-way tap. Otherwise an intercostal catheter (16 French gauge or larger), is connected to an underwater seal. Excessively rapid expansion causes transient pulmonary oedema. This procedure is carried out in the ward or in the accident department as an emergency, but premedication with atropine and an opiate is advisable and good pleural analgesia essential.

Intercostal catheters are usually inserted in the axilla, but the second anterior space may be convenient. Haemothoraces should be drained and antistaphylococcal chemotherapy given.

After resolution, the intercostal tube is clamped and removed if there is no recurrence. Large bronchopleural fistulae require suction with a pump that, for safety, cannot generate more than 30–40 cm of negative pressure above the water-seal and thus within the pleural cavity (not suction apparatus).

Occasionally, pleurodesis or pleurectomy is necessary for persistent or recurrent pneumothorax.

Tension pneumothorax is a medical emergency requiring the insertion of a wide-bore needle into the pleural space to relieve compression of the great veins, followed by intercostal drainage.

Traumatic pneumothorax follows penetrating stab wounds, fracture of the ribs with penetration of the lung, chest operations and artificial ventilation and high pressures. Haemothorax is common and may rarely implicate spontaneous pneumothorax. Up to 3 litres of blood may be lost into an haemothorax.

Pleural effusion and pleurisy

Pleural effusions complicate a number of conditions, of which they may be the principal manifestation. They usually consist of serum, but blood, pus and occasionally lymph may be found.

Serous effusions may be transudates caused by alterations in the balance of colloid osmotic pressure and lymphatic and vascular pressures. These pressures favour resorption under normal conditions. The protein content of these effusions is low (typically < 20 g/l). Transudates are caused by congestive cardiac failure or left ventricular failure of any cause and hypoproteinaemia, especially the nephrotic syndrome. Rare causes include myxoedema and ovarian fibroma (Meigs' syndrome).

Inflammation or neoplasia of the pleural lining may result in pleural exudates in which capillary permeability is high and protein content approaches that of serum (typically > 35 g/l). Inflamed pleural surfaces not separated by effusion result in the typical pain of pleurisy.

Exudates may be caused by acute infection, e.g. bacterial pneumonia which may be serous or purulent (empyema), chronic infection, (e.g. tuberculosis), toxoplasmosis, subphrenic infection, pulmonary infarction, malignant disease (bronchial carcinoma, metastatic pleural carcinoma or pleural mesothelioma) and autoimmune disease (rheumatoid arthritis, SLE, systemic vasculitis).

Chylous effusions contain fat and lymphocytes. They are rare and caused by lymphatic obstruction or trauma to the thoracic duct.

Most chronic pleural effusions occupying more than half the hemithorax are caused by malignancy or tuberculosis.

Symptoms and signs

Symptoms are pleural pain and dyspnoea, usually relieved by separation of the pleural surfaces when the effusion enlarges.

Signs are increased respiratory rate, shift of mediastinum towards the unaffected side, dullness on percussion, diminished breath sounds and signs of consolidation adjacent to the effusion.

Investigations

Chest X-ray will be required. Needle aspiration shows the presence and nature of fluid (Fig. 2.9). Blood-stained effusions are usually malignant or thromboembolic. Cytology and culture may reveal the cause. Malignant cells or pus

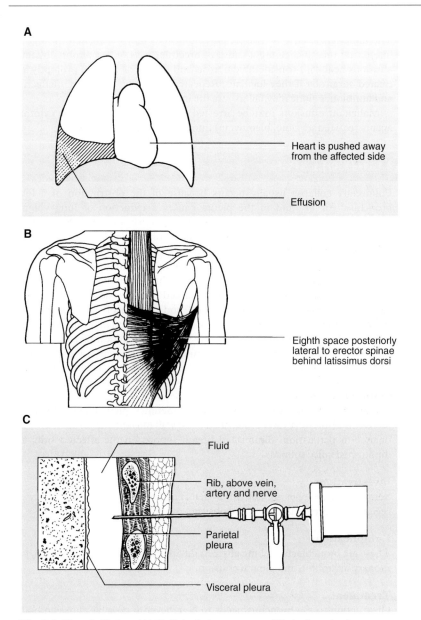

Fig. 2.9 Pleural effusion. **(A)** Radiological appearance; **(B)** the best site for aspiration of fluid; **(C)** aspiration. A plastic cannula may be used.

cells may be diagnostic and specific organisms may be isolated. Lymphocytes and mesothelial cells are non-specific.

Pleural biopsy is best performed using a special needle at the time of the first chest aspiration. It is valuable in cases of suspected malignancy and tuberculosis.

Treatment

The underlying cause is treated. Large effusions may be drained through an intercostal tube if they are a cause of breathlessness or discomfort. Infected effusions heal with considerable fibrosis and should be drained promptly and treated surgically if they loculate. Repeated aspiration is usually ineffective, and antibiotics alone may fail to cure the infection.

Malignant effusions may be arrested by instilling sclerosant or cytotoxic agents (e.g. tetracycline, bleomycin) into the drained pleural cavity.

LUNG COLLAPSE

Pulmonary collapse usually occurs because of the obstruction of a lobar bronchus. Air or fluid in the pleura causes a reduction of lung volume. Absorption collapse then occurs as alveolar oxygen is absorbed. Nitrogen follows more slowly. Shrinkage of the lung volume leads to a rise in the diaphragm on the affected side, overdistension of the rest of the lung, mediastinal shift towards the affected side and flattening and diminished movement of the affected side. The main causes are bronchial carcinoma, inhaled foreign body, compression of a bronchus by enlarged lymph nodes (e.g. lymphoma, primary tuberculosis), aspergillosis (p. 69) and viscid inspissated mucus which is not expectorated. The latter occurs postoperatively and in bronchial asthma.

Air or fluid in the pleural cavity also causes a reduction of volume of the lungs which resolves when they are drained. This is discussed elsewhere (p. 100-101).

Symptoms and signs

Symptoms include breathlessness and sometimes pleural pain. Signs are increased respiratory rate, diminished chest wall movement, partial loss of resonance to percussion, diminished breath sounds on the affected side, and diminished voice sounds.

Investigations

Some collapsed lobes are difficult to detect on chest X-ray. Bronchoscopy will reveal the nature of the bronchial obstruction.

Complications

These are bronchiectasis, lung abscess, differential diagnosis, pneumonia, pulmonary infarction, and pleural effusion.

Treatment

Obstruction to the bronchus needs to be relieved if possible. Foreign bodies are removed at bronchoscopy. Physiotherapy may aid expectoration of mucus plugs. Corticosteroids are given in asthma and allergic aspergillosis.

OBSTRUCTIVE SLEEP APNOEA SYNDROME

The pharyngeal and laryngeal muscles normally maintain the patency of the upper airway during inspiration. A number of factors may combine to narrow the upper airway, including enlargement of the adenoids, tonsils, the tongue and the cervical soft tissues. Such individuals snore easily. When this is accompanied by failure of the pharyngeal muscles to maintain the patency of the upper airway during inspiration, there is intermittent obstruction of breathing during sleep with multiple episodes of transient hypoxaemia, multiple arousals from sleep and reduction of sleep quality.

Symptoms and signs

The major symptom is daytime hypersomnolence, resulting in interference with work and driving or poor school performance.

There are no specific signs, but most subjects without obvious upper airway disease are obese, and many have thickening of the tissues of the enlarged tonsils and adenoids and neck, with a large collar size. Predisposing causes include hypothyroidism, acromegaly and macroglossia.

Investigation

Sleep apnoea syndrome is confirmed by the use of instruments to record transcutaneous oxygen saturation, oronasal airflow and respiratory movement during sleep. These demonstrate transient hypoxaemia and the cessation of ventilation.

Differential diagnosis

Central neurogenic hypoventilation may coexist. Other causes of insomnia and nocturnal waking include abnormal leg movements, 'restless legs', anxiety and narcolepsy.

Treatment

Weight reduction may help, as may avoidance of alcohol, sedation and sleeping in a slightly tilted position. Most patients will respond to the application of positive pressure to the upper airway via a nasal mask at night, though this has to be continued long term.

VENTILATORY FAILURE

Ventilatory failure is defined as the failure of the lungs to oxygenate the blood to a normal level and to maintain the arterial CO_2 pressure at or below the normal level when breathing air at normal PO_2.

Ventilatory failure may be acute (such as drowning, laryngeal obstruction or acute bronchial asthma in a previously healthy patient), neurogenic respiratory failure, or acute-on-chronic (e.g. acute exacerbations of chronic bronchitis).

Acute ventilatory failure

Progressive hypoxaemia and CO_2 retention may result in bradycardia and cardiac arrest within 4–8 minutes. Whatever the cause, treatment involves clearing the airway and administering artificial ventilation with the highest possible concentration of oxygen by the most efficient route available (endotracheal intubation, mask ventilation, an airway or mouth-to-mouth respiration). False teeth should be removed and obstructing material such as regurgitated food hooked out from the back of the tongue before positive pressure ventilation begins. Cardiopulmonary resuscitation is given if the carotid pulse is absent.

Sudden death in restaurants is usually caused by the inhalation of large pieces of food, usually meat. Talking while eating, coupled with impaired co-ordination of swallowing are responsible. Supraglottic obstruction may be relieved manually. Food in the trachea cannot be coughed up; away from equipment, emergency treatment consists of a vigorous upward push on the upper abdomen in the hope of displacing the diaphragm upwards and dislodging the wedged material (Heimlich manoeuvre).

Causes of laryngeal obstruction include angio-oedema, epiglottitis, diphtheria (rare), inhaled foreign body (e.g. child's dummy) and also croup or pertussis (see p. 401).

Laryngoscopy and intubation are performed when available. Needle tracheostomy or, in adults, cricothyroid puncture, may be life saving.

The treatment of severe acute bronchial asthma or bronchiolitis is described on pages 59 and 80. Severe pneumonia can also cause respiratory failure in previously healthy people (see p. 59).

Neurogenic respiratory failure

Neuromuscular weakness. Acute paralytic disorders such as myasthenia, polyneuritis and poliomyelitis may cause respiratory insufficiency. In the early stages, breathlessness results in a low PCO_2 but when VC falls below 1.0 litre, there is a risk of hypoventilation. Artificial ventilation is used.

Loss of respiratory drive. Several rare syndromes have in common periodic apnoea during sleep, causing transient hypoxaemia and its consequences. In the presence of lung disease, hypoxaemia may be profound and result in polycythaemia, pulmonary hypertension and heart failure. Sudden infant death may occur. Morning headache, daytime somnolence and intellectual deterioration are minor manifestations.

Ondine's curse. Complete loss of automatic periodicity and metabolic control of breathing occurs in some children. Treatment is by artificial ventilation via a nasal mask at night.

Pulmonary insufficiency: chronic and acute-on-chronic respiratory failure

Severe lung disease is accompanied by an increased work of breathing and disturbance of the pulmonary gas exchange mechanism. These result in hypoxaemia, with or without CO_2 retention and patients may acclimatise to quite severe abnormalities of blood gases. When such patients develop acute bronchial infections or fluid retention, they suffer severe rises of PCO_2 and deterioration of PO_2. Relief of hypoxaemia and sedation further reduce respiratory drive without improving the underlying condition and cause progressive under-ventilation and acute respiratory acidosis.

There are no consistent physical signs of CO_2 retention and hypoxaemia. All patients with such exacerbations of pre-existing respiratory disease need blood gas analysis. However, mood disturbance, confusion or aggression, coma or flapping tremor of the hands may occur.

With severe CO_2 retention there may be a reduction of respiratory movement, warm hands, dilated veins, papilloedema and raised intracranial pressure mimicking cerebral tumour.

Artificial ventilation is indicated for worsening blood gases and respiratory muscle fatigue. The following measures may postpone the need for this:

1. controlled oxygen therapy (not more than 24–28%)
2. regular arousal
3. assisted coughing
4. measures to improve lung function, e.g. bronchodilators, diuretic and corticosteroids
5. infusion of respiratory stimulants may help if respiratory depression is reversible, e.g. after injudicious administration of oxygen or sedation.

Artificial ventilation is used if the patient becomes unconscious, uncooperative, unable to cough or exhausted.

Oxygen therapy

Hypoxaemia caused by ventilation/perfusion imbalance may be relieved wholly or in part by increasing the inspired concentration of O_2.

Previously healthy patients, not acclimatised to hypoxaemia, urgently require restoration of PO_2 to normal levels to maintain cerebral and renal function. This can generally be achieved by means of a suitable mask except in the presence of very severe diffuse lung or pulmonary vascular impairment, hypotension or an anatomical shunt.

High concentrations of oxygen, approaching 100%, can be administered only by systems which include a valve. Generous oxygen therapy is used for acute severe dyspnoea with hyperventilation, e.g. left ventricular failure, bronchial asthma, pulmonary embolism. A firm plastic mask with holes capable of taking 12 l/min of oxygen flow is used. Oxygen concentration delivered to the patient depends on flow rate and the rate and depth of breathing.

Patients acclimatised to chronic hypoxaemia with or without CO_2 retention may develop severe respiratory failure during acute cardiorespiratory illnesses or after trauma, surgery or sedation. Rapid relief of hypoxaemia in these patients may lead to CO_2 retention, respiratory acidosis and narcosis by reducing hypoxic respiratory drive and acidifying haemoglobin (Bohr effect). Controlled oxygen therapy aims to increase PO_2 to around 60 mmHg (8 kPa), using masks employing the Venturi principle. The inflowing oxygen entrains large volumes of air, delivering a draught of fixed oxygen concentration. There is no CO_2 retention.

Nasal cannulae are used when continuous oxygen therapy is required but exact concentration is not critical. The patient can eat and talk. This is well tolerated by convalescent subjects and those with chronic lung disease.

Home oxygen. Chronic respiratory insufficiency may be improved in selected patients by prolonged inhalation (15 hours or more daily) of oxygen at 2–4 l/min via a nasal cannula to achieve 95% saturation in the arterial blood: longevity is increased, polycythaemia is reduced and there are fewer episodes of oedema, fluid retention and infective exacerbations requiring admission to hospital. Long-term oxygen therapy is known to benefit patients with chronic airflow obstruction (FEV1 below 1.0 litre) who have a resting arterial PO_2 below 55 mmHg (7.2 kPa), and documented episodes of heart failure. Patients must give up smoking, and must be assessed to verify improvement, but can avoid a progressive rise in PCO_2 with this form of treatment.

Home oxygen can be delivered by means of a concentrator which extracts nitrogen from room air.

Palliative oxygen therapy relieves hypoxaemia in end stage fibrotic obstruction and malignant lung disorders and may relieve Cheyne-Stokes respiration in heart failure. Life expectancy is not improved. Some patients who develop arterial desaturation during exercise benefit from portable oxygen therapy which prolongs effort tolerance.

3

INTENSIVE CARE

John Vann Jones, David P. Coates

Most hospitals have a high dependency unit (HDU) or an intensive therapy unit (ITU) for the management of particularly ill patients. Although some units care specifically for patients with renal and liver failure, most are concerned with maintaining the circulation and respiration in patients with potentially reversible illnesses like acute asthma, sepsis, severe metabolic acidosis, drug overdosage, trauma etc.

SHOCK

Acute circulatory failure with inadequate cellular oxygenation is commonly referred to as shock. This can have a wide variety of causes (Table 3.1).

The body responds to shock in a number of different ways.
1. Increased sympathetic nervous system activity releases catecholamines from the adrenal medulla.
2. Renin release from the underperfused kidneys leads to an increase in angiotensin II levels. Angiotensin II is a very potent vasoconstrictor which also causes the adrenal cortex to release aldosterone, thereby retaining salt and water.
3. A variety of pituitary hormones (e.g. adrenocorticotrophic hormone, growth hormone, antidiuretic hormone) cortisol, glucagon, and beta-endorphin are released into the circulation.

All of these measures are intended to restore tissue perfusion. Where shock is caused by infection (septic shock) or tissue damage (e.g. crush injury) other changes occur. These include:

Table 3.1. Common causes of shock

Blood loss, e.g. gastrointestinal haemorrhage	Allergic (anaphylaxis)
	Cardiogenic (primary cardiac damage)
Fluid loss, e.g. severe burns	Cardiac tamponade (pericardial effusion)
Acute infection	Pulmonary embolus

4. increased prostaglandin activity, especially prostacyclin, thromboxane, and PGF_2,
5. complement cascade activation,
6. cytokine release,
7. platelet activating factor release,
8. release of lysosomal enzymes.

These mediators have a wide range of different, often opposing, activities, for example prostacyclin is a vasodilator that inhibits platelet aggregation while thromboxane is a vasoconstrictor and promotes platelet adhesion.

MICROCIRCULATORY CHANGES

The initial changes at the small arteriolar and capillary level depend on the type and degree of shock. Eventually local accumulation of metabolites (e.g. lactic acid) leads to vasodilation with fluid loss into the interstitial spaces. This in turn makes the blood more coaguable and viscous, increasing the potential for intravascular coagulation. Paradoxically, because clotting factors are consumed so heavily within the microcirculation, the patient is often effectively anticoagulated. This condition is known as disseminated intravascular coagulopathy (DIC) or consumption coagulopathy (see p. 358).

Poor tissue perfusion leads to metabolic changes and anaerobic metabolism supervenes. All of the changes outlined eventually lead to multiple organ failure which has a poor prognosis.

CLINICAL PRESENTATION AND TREATMENT

These depend on the cause. For example severe blood loss presents an entirely different picture from cardiac tamponade (pericardial effusion). Therefore it is important to establish a cause for shock although some general principles can be applied.

1. Adequate haemodynamic monitoring to ensure correct fluid balance, e.g. central venous pressure, direct arterial pressure (most frequently using the radial artery). Sometimes cardiac output and pulmonary artery occlusion (wedge) pressure, an indirect measurement of left atrial filling pressure, are also monitored.
Correct volume restoration is very important in managing most forms of shock (Table 3.2).
2. Adequate oxygenation which may require the patient to be ventilated. The balance between oxygen demand and delivery is critical. The oxygen requirements of the ventilatory muscles, including the diaphragm, for example, may be increased several fold in shock.
3. Analgesia and sedation.
4. Inotropic support and the use of vasoactive drugs to redistribute cardiac output.

In most forms of shock even where the heart was previously healthy, the myocardium is depressed. It is therefore important to monitor closely and adjust cardiac work by manipulating the factors affecting cardiac filling (pre-

Table 3.2. Fluids used to replace circulating volume in shock

Whole blood

SAGM blood*

Colloid solutions:
    Gelatin solutions, e.g. Gelofusine, Haemaccel
    Dextrans, e.g. Dextran 70 in Saline 0.9%
    Hetastarch, e.g. Hespan, Elohes
    Human albumin solution 4% (HAS)
    Fresh frozen plasma (FFP)

Crystalloid solutions:
    Saline 0.9%
    Hartmann's solution

* SAGM blood = red cells suspended in an optimal preservative Saline, Adenine, Glucose, Mannitol.

Table 3.3. Inotropes and vasoactive drugs

Dobutamine	Vasodilating inotrope. Direct myocardial stimulant. Ensure adequate circulating volume
Dopamine	At low doses: dopaminergic renal and splanchnic vasodilation. At high doses: beta-1 adrenergic stimulation and increasing alpha adrenergic vasoconstriction
Dopexamine	Dopamine analogue: 1/3 peripheral dopaminergic but 60 times more beta-2 and only 1/6 beta-1 stimulation. Significant vasodilator
Phosphodiesterase inhibitors, e.g. Amrinone, Milrinone	Increased myocardial and smooth muscle cAMP resulting in increased contractility and vasodilation: 'inodilation'
Noradrenaline	Alpha stimulant: vasoconstrictor redirecting cardiac output. Particularly useful in septic shock
Adrenaline	Beta stimulant. Used in reversible myocardial depression, e.g. cardiac surgery

load) and impedance to ejection (afterload). In septic shock in particular, it has recently been appreciated that it is sometimes necessary to redirect the increased cardiac output from the vasodilated peripheral circulation to the major organs. In addition it may be necessary to stimulate cardiac output pharmacologically by using inotropic drugs (Table 3.3).

RESPIRATORY FAILURE

(see also p. 103)

Type I. Occurs with damage to the lungs itself. This may be acute (e.g. pulmonary oedema) or chronic (e.g. pulmonary fibrosis). The PaO_2 is low and the $PaCO_2$ is low or normal.

Type II. Occurs with poor ventilation, as in chronic bronchitis and emphysema or neuromuscular disease. The PaO_2 is low but the $PaCO_2$ is high.

In patients suspected of developing ventilatory failure, blood gases and acid–base status need to be carefully monitored. These results and the clinical picture will determine the need for admission to an ITU and indicate the need for controlled ventilation. Sometimes specific ventilatory function tests are required.

Management

1. Seek the cause, e.g. acute exacerbation of chronic bronchitis, sepsis.
2. Achieve adequate oxygen delivery by supplementary oxygen administration with or without controlled ventilation (Table 3.4)

ADULT RESPIRATORY DISTRESS SYNDROME (ARDS)

ARDS is sometimes referred to as shock lung. The pulmonary capillaries leak and result in hypoxia, reduced lung compliance and diffuse pulmonary infiltration radiographically. ARDS occurs as a non-specific reaction to a variety of

---

Table 3.4. Forms of ventilatory support

1. Controlled mandatory ventilation (CMV) by intermittent positive pressure ventilation (IPPV) through an endotracheal tube (ETT). A variety of functions may be adjustable, e.g. frequency, tidal volume, peak inflation pressure. This can be undertaken for several weeks.

2. CMV + positive end expiratory pressure (PEEP). During expiration a resistance of up to 20 cm H_2O is maintained which tends to increase functional residual capacity (FRC) enhancing oxygenation. There may be detrimental cardiovascular effects.

3. Synchronised intermittent mandatory ventilation (SIMV). The ventilator is programmed to deliver a predetermined number of mechanical breaths of specified tidal volume after a suitable pause in the patient's spontaneous ventilatory efforts. May help weaning from CMV.

4. Pressure support ventilation. Breaths initiated by the patient, sensed as a predetermined reduction in the ambient airway pressure, are assisted by a preset positive pressure supplement. This may assist weaning from CMV or SIMV.

5. Continuous positive airway pressure (CPAP). The patient breathes spontaneously through either an ETT or a tightly fitting face mask. There is a persistently positive airway pressure during both inspiration and expiration which increases FRC and reduces the work of breathing. It requires a large flow of gas to achieve the continuous positive pressure, especially during inspiration. It assists weaning from CMV or SIMV.

NB. Inspired oxygen concentration can always be independently adjusted.

problems that have a final common pathway of capillary cellular functional deficit. Common causes include sepsis, burns, blunt chest trauma, fat embolism and aspiration.

Cellular respiration can usually be maintained (see Table 3.4) in the short term with increased inspired oxygen concentrations, controlled mandatory ventilation (CMV) using minimised inflation pressures and adjusted inspiration : expiration ratios, and PEEP.

The poor prognosis usually relates to the development of multiple organ failure rather than to the inability to maintain ventilation.

4

NEUROLOGY

Iain Ferguson

Faced with the neurological patient, the student may elicit physical signs which are unequivocal but hard to interpret. This leads to the view that neurology is a difficult specialty. There is no doubt that a good grounding in anatomical and physiological principles is essential to the understanding of how pathology disrupts normal function of thought, movement and sensation. Once this academic hurdle has been overcome, however, it must be realised that the essence of neurology is a detailed clinical history complemented by physical examination.

Certain factors are important in the history.

1. The age of the patient. A progressive, spastic paraparesis in a child is more likely to be caused by a tumour, whereas in the young adult multiple sclerosis is the more likely diagnosis.

2. Mode of onset. The dramatic onset of focal neurological symptoms may suggest a localised epileptic attack or ischaemic episode.

3. Duration of symptoms. A migraine rarely persists for longer than 48 hours, yet tension headache may last days or even weeks.

4. Family history. A tentative diagnosis of Huntington's chorea may be reinforced by establishing this disease in another relative.

5. Previous medical history. A subarachnoid haemorrhage in early life may predispose to hydrocephalus or syringomyelia.

Physical signs may range from a gross disturbance of gait, as in cerebellar ataxia, to a subtle, dissociated sensory impairment seen in spinal cord lesions. Such signs, and a detailed history, allow definition of the disease and its situation. Appropriate tests may then be applied to specific regions. Images of great clarity may be obtained using computerised tomography (CT), magnetic resonance scanning (MRI) and Doppler ultrasound. Neurophysiological tests include electroencephalography (EEG) and nerve conduction studies with electromyography (EMG).

DISEASES OF THE CRANIAL NERVES

OLFACTORY (I) NERVE

Anosmia, or loss of the sense of smell, is commonly caused by nasal or sinus disease. Head injury may also cause anosmia. A subfrontal meningioma can cause anosmia although this is usually overlooked if visual failure and intellectual impairment are prominent features. Episodic disturbances of smell may be a feature of temporal lobe epileptic attacks (uncal fits).

OPTIC (II) NERVE

Disease here may affect colour vision, visual acuity, visual fields (Fig. 4.1) and optic disc appearance. Papilloedema, or swelling of the optic nerve head, has an identical appearance to papillitis but the latter is associated with a marked reduction of visual acuity. If left untreated, papilloedema will eventually result in reduction of acuity, concentric diminution of visual fields and finally blindness (Table 4.1).

Optic neuritis

Painful eye movements caused by traction on the inflamed nerve, poor visual acuity, impaired colour vision, afferent pupillary defect and central scotoma are features of this condition. Optic neuritis can occur with multiple sclerosis, syphilis, giant cell arteritis, tobacco and alcohol amblyopia, and methanol poisoning. Severe neuritis usually results in optic atrophy.

Optic atrophy

1. Primary. Leber's sex-linked recessive disease affecting males, Devic's disease (optico-myelopathy), multiple sclerosis and optic neuritis.

2. Secondary. Compression of the nerve by tumour or aneurysm, glaucoma, papilloedema, central retinal artery thrombosis, trauma, drugs and toxins, e.g. chloroquine, tobacco, quinine, and methyl alcohol.

The optic disc may appear pale in normal patients with myopia. Glaucoma causes enlargement of the optic cup.

Pupillary abnormalities

Large pupils occur in the young and smaller pupils in older healthy individuals. Irregular pupils may complicate chronic uveitis or follow iridectomy.

An Argyll Robertson pupil is small irregular and unequal, unreactive to bright light, and reacts normally to accommodation. It occurs in neurosyphilis, diabetes mellitus and some autonomic neuropathies.

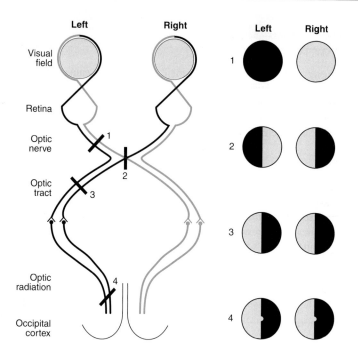

Fig. 4.1 Visual field defects and their causes. Common causes of lesion at site 1 = optic neuritis (MS), tumour, trauma, aneurysm; 2 = pituitary tumour, craniopharyngioma, aneurysm; 3 = tumour, stroke; 4 = stroke, tumour. The shaded area shows the visual defect. NB: Macular sparing at site 4.

Table 4.1. Causes of papilloedema

Raised intracranial pressure by tumour, abscess and meningitis due to failure of retinal venous drainage

Thrombosis of cerebral venous sinuses

Orbital tumour or pseudo-tumour

Malignant hypertension

Chronic hypercapnia and hypoxia

Benign intracranial hypertension

In papilloedema the blind spot is enlarged and this can be used as a sign to monitor treatment

The myotonic or Holmes Adie pupil

This is benign and usually unilateral. Patients complain only of a mild blurring of vision. The pupil is dilated, and reacts sluggishly to light and accommodation. A brisk reaction may be obtained from dilute (2.5%) metacholine. Absent deep tendon reflexes may be present in the full syndrome.

Table 4.2. Site and causes of Horner's syndrome

Site of lesion in sympathetic pathway	Causes
Hypothalamus	Tumour
Brainstem	Stroke, trauma, tumour
Cervical cord	Syringomyelia, glioma, trauma
Cervical root–stellate ganglion	Pancoast tumour, cervical rib surgery, trauma
Carotid artery in neck	Trauma, carotid dissection or angiography
Cavernous sinus	Migrainous neuralgia
Retrorbital	Aneurysm or tumour

Horner's syndrome

This is the result of a unilateral, rarely bilateral, sympathetic nerve lesion. The pupil is small (miosis) because of the unopposed action of the parasympathetic nerve. There is also a mild ptosis from weakness of Müller's muscle, and an apparent enophthalmus and lack of sweating in the upper and sometimes lower half of the face. The causes of Horner's syndrome are summarised in Table 4.2.

OCULO-MOTOR (III) TROCHLEAR (IV) ABDUCENS (VI) NERVES

Good ocular motility is essential to bring the full field system to bear on any new object. Horizontal eye movements are controlled by the pons. Failure of conjugate horizontal gaze may arise from a lesion in the medial longitudinal bundle, a fibre pathway which co-ordinates sixth and third nerve function. Nystagmus of the lateral rectus in the direction of gaze, and weakness of the adducting eye (medial rectus) gives a clinical picture known as internuclear ophthalmoplegia. This is commonly caused by multiple sclerosis. Failure of vertical eye movement is seen in progressive supranuclear palsy and tumours of the midbrain periaqueductal region.

In a third nerve lesion there is weakness of all extra-ocular muscles except the lateral rectus and superior oblique. The nerve also supplies levator palpebrae superioris and the pupillo constrictor fibres.

Features of a complete third nerve palsy are dilated pupil, marked ptosis and a downward and outward deviated eye.

Lesions of the third nerve nucleus in the midbrain are commonly vascular or tumour. In diabetes mellitus where there is microvascular damage, there is sparing of the peripherally lying pupillomotor fibres and so the pupil is unaffected. This is often called a 'medical' third nerve palsy. 'Surgical' third nerve palsy is commonly caused by a posterior communicating aneurysm or pituitary tumour and the pupil is affected. As the nerve leaves the dura it may be involved in an invasive basal process, such as tumour or sarcoid or tubercular granulomata.

A lone sixth nerve palsy is more common than isolated trochlear nerve lesions. More often, it occurs in association with third and sixth nerve palsy, when the lesion of the cavernous sinus is a tumour, granuloma or giant internal carotid aneurysm. Myasthenia gravis may present with ophthalmoplegia and a variable diplopia which is worse towards the end of the day. Thyroid eye disease causes ophthalmoplegia and proptosis.

TRIGEMINAL (V) NERVE

Facial sensation is appreciated via the three divisions (ophthalmic, maxillary and mandibular), supplying the skin of the face, cornea, sinuses, mucous membranes of nose, teeth, tympanic membranes, and sensation but not taste, to the anterior two-thirds of tongue. The motor division supplies the temporalis, masseter and pterygoid muscles. A brainstem lesion of the pons and medulla may cause numbness and tingling of the face. The pattern of sensory loss is sometimes in an 'onion skin' or concentric distribution. This is seen in syringobulbia, brainstem glioma or vascular disease. Trigeminal nerve trunk lesions occur from compression by an aneurysm of the internal carotid in the cavernous sinus or an acoustic neuroma in the cerebello-pontine angle. Intrinsic nerve trunk disease may be caused by herpes zoster.

FACIAL (VII) NERVE

This nerve innervates muscles of facial expression and the chorda tympani with taste to the anterior two-thirds of the tongue. The nerve to stapedius muscle dampens bony ossicle movement which, if damaged, results in hyperacusis. Parasympathetic fibres to the lacrimal gland may cause a dry eye when disturbed.

Upper motor neurone facial palsy occurs with damage to the anterior frontal fibres controlling facial movements. It spares voluntary movements but affects emotional ones. The other type of upper motor neurone lesion damaging suprapontine fibres results in a lower half facial weakness with sparing of the upper half because of bilateral cortical innervation of the forehead muscles.

A lower motor neurone lesion will cause complete paralysis of half of the face because the final motor pathway is affected.

Bell's palsy is caused by swelling of the facial nerve into the facial canal (Fig. 4.2).

Retroaural pain precedes palsy in 50% of patients. The facial muscles are stiff and weak; food collects in the mouth. Other features are loss of taste and excessive tears (crocodile).

Early steroid therapy will aid recovery; however, 90% of patients recover spontaneously.

Causes of bilateral facial weakness include Guillain–Barré syndrome, myotonic and facioscapulohumeral dystrophy and myasthenia gravis.

Brainstem lesions more commonly cause unilateral facial weakness and are the result of cerebrovascular accident, multiple sclerosis, tumour, motor neurone disease or syringobulbia.

Blepharospasm (intermittent involuntary forceful closure of the eye) may also occur in Parkinson's disease, or as a more widespread oromandibular

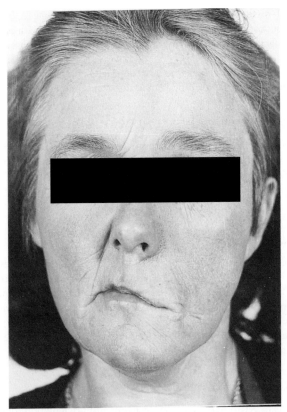

Fig. 4.2 The facial appearance in Bell's palsy (left side).

dyskinesia known as Meige's syndrome. Treatment is by intramuscular injection of small amounts of botulinus toxin.

Hemifacial spasm (clonic spasm of facial muscles involving the eye and mouth) is frequently distressing and also treated with botulinus toxin.

Facial myokymia, if restricted to the eyelids, is usually benign. When it involves facial muscles, producing a fine, rippling, 'bag of worms' appearance, it suggests pontine multiple sclerosis or glioma.

AUDITORY (VIII) NERVE

Sudden-onset lesions

1. Geniculate herpes zoster (Ramsay Hunt syndrome) causes vertigo, deafness, unilateral facial palsy and a vesicular rash in the external aural canal and hard palate.
2. Occlusion of the anterior inferior cerebellar artery will precipitate sudden unilateral deafness, more commonly in the elderly.
3. Mumps.
4. Head injury is a common cause of sudden deafness.

Gradual-onset lesions

1. An acoustic neuroma causes progressive deafness, with trigeminal and mild facial nerve involvement. There may also be unilateral cerebellar signs.
2. Other causes of deafness include bacterial meningitis, syphilis, sarcoidosis, Meniere's disease, streptomycin toxicity and brainstem multiple sclerosis.

GLOSSOPHARYNGEAL (IX) AND VAGUS (X) NERVES

The gag reflex, and palatal and pharyngeal movement are affected, as are sensation and movement of the vocal cords. Other features are bilateral vocal paralysis and a bovine cough, stridor and loss of explosive cough. These symptoms are collectively known as either a bulbar or pseudobulbar palsy (Table 4.3).

SPINAL ACCESSORY (XI) NERVE

This nerve supplies the trapezius and sternomastoid muscles. Unilateral lesions are rare. Causes of XIth nerve palsy include glomus tumour of the jugular foramen, and surgical dissection of lymph glands in the neck and may result in weakness of shrugging of the shoulder with slight winging of the scapula.

Upper motor neurone lesion such as a stroke will cause weakness of the sternomastoid contralateral to the side of the hemiparesis.

HYPOGLOSSAL (XII) NERVE

The signs of XIIth nerve palsy are wasting and fasciculation, deviation of the tongue to the weak side, with difficulty in manipulating food. The causes are tumour and malignant meningitis, glomus tumour, and skull base fracture. The lesion is unilateral.

Table 4.3. Bulbar and pseudobulbar palsy

Site of lesion	Clinical signs	Causes

Bulbar
  Lower motor
  neurone
	Dysarthria — nasal,
	slow voice, dysphagia
		Myasthenia gravis
		Motor neurone disease
		Muscular dystrophy (rare)
		Guillain–Barré syndrome

Pseudobulbar
  Upper motor
  neurone
  corticobulbar fibres
  —a supranuclear
  and nerve lesion
	Dysarthria—jerky type,
	dysphagia, spastic rapid
	tongue movements,
	brisk jaw jerk,
	emotional lability
		Stroke
		Multiple sclerosis
		Motor neurone disease

DISORDERS OF CONSCIOUSNESS

EPILEPSY

Epilepsy is defined as a continuing tendency to have seizures caused by a sudden excessive electrical discharge of cerebral neurones. Synchronous paroxysmal bursts of large numbers of neurones correlate with the EEG sharp and spike waves. These occur often in the inter-ictal period in patients with epilepsy and are extremely helpful in the diagnosis. Approximately 0.5% of the population will have a seizure. The highest incidence is in the first year of life, slowly declining between 10 and 50 years with another peak in the over 50s, usually caused by tumours, and vascular and degenerative diseases.

10 to 20% of patients may not have epilepsy but rather syncope or pseudo-seizures. A witness account is invaluable.

Aetiology

1. A birth history may suggest trauma, hypoxia, or metabolic insult.
2. A positive family history of epilepsy may be obtained.
3. Symptomatic disease may affect the cortex diffusely.
4. Medical conditions include alcohol excess, barbiturate withdrawal, uraemia, hypoparathyroidism, hypoxic encephalopathy, post–cardiac arrest, bacterial meningitis, viral encephalitis, subacute sclerosing pan encephalitis and Creutzfeldt–Jakob disease.
5. Focal seizures are almost always an expression of intracranial localised pathology, such as trauma, tumours, abscess or stroke.
6. Trigger factors for seizure include, alcohol, late nights, hypoglycaemia, drugs and flashing lights.

Classification of epilepsy

1. Generalised
a. tonic and/or clonic = 'grand mal'
b. absence = 'petit mal'
c. myoclonic
d. atonic
2. Partial (focal)
a. simple motor
b. simple sensory
c. complex partial with or without secondary generalisation (also known as psychomotor or temporal lobe epilepsy).

Symptoms and signs

Generalised seizures

These are characterised by clinical symptoms and EEG discharges which are bilaterally symmetrical with no focal onset.

Tonic/clonic or generalised attacks have an initial phase of widespread tonic muscular contractions, followed by rhythmical clonic jerks. Duration is 1–2 minutes with no aura. Consciousness is lost at onset and not recovered until minutes after the clonic phase. Lip or tongue biting, and urinary incontinence occur frequently. The post-ictal confusion may last minutes or hours.

Absence and petit mal attacks are short-lived episodes of loss of consciousness (5–15 seconds) with only minimal motor manifestations. True petit mal appears only in childhood and is associated with an EEG pattern of 3 per second spike and wave abnormality.

Absence attacks must be differentiated from petit mal. They often occur in adults, with complex partial epilepsy. Such patients may also have myoclonic jerking—brief sudden muscular contractions either affecting the whole body, or localised to the hand or leg.

Tonic or akinetic seizures occur predominantly in childhood with repetitive short bursts (5–10 seconds) of tonic posturing or loss of tone, where the patient suddenly falls to the ground. This is often associated with mental retardation and is difficult to treat.

Partial or focal seizures

These are characterised by clinical symptoms and EEG changes localised to one region of the brain. The focus may move to other areas of the motor cortex resulting in a spreading movement or sensory disorder (Jacksonian seizure).

Sensory seizures may be simple from the primary sensory cortex, or more complex visual, auditory or even olfactory illusions or hallucinations. This often takes place at the aura or prodrome of an attack. Déja vu or entendu feelings of familiarity, or an epigastric sensation rising to the head may also occur.

Complex partial seizures arise from the temporal lobe, sometimes with automatisms such as lip smacking, grimacing and fugue like states. Violent behaviour occasionally occurs but flailing of the arms is usually haphazard and poorly directed.

Investigations

The EEG may provide supportive evidence of the diagnosis (Fig. 4.3) but it can be normal in epilepsy and abnormal in non-epileptic individuals. A resting EEG or 24-hour ambulatory monitoring is useful in differentiating psychogenic from true seizures. The type and localisation of the epileptic discharge may be shown on EEG. MRI and/or CT are useful in determining the cause of epilepsy. Table 4.4 shows the differential diagnosis of epilepsy.

Treatment

Most types of recurrent seizure will improve with an appropriate anticonvulsant. Monotherapy is the aim. Certain types of epilepsy respond to specific groups of anticonvulsants.

1. Phenytoin and carbamazepine are most effective in partial and secondary generalised tonic/clonic epilepsy.

    The side-effects of phenytoin tend to be overemphasised but include hirsutism and gingival hyperplasia. Many patients are well controlled with a

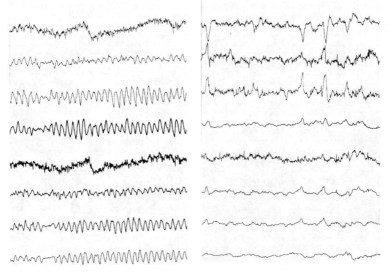

A   B

Fig. 4.3 EEG from a normal subject (A). Left hemisphere leads show normal alpha rhythm. (B) a subject with spike focus and phase reversal in temporal leads from left hemisphere. Note the fast paper speed of 3 cm/sec in both records.

low therapeutic blood level. Drug interactions occur. Phenytoin is a potent enzyme inducer and can reduce the efficacy of the oral contraceptive pill .

The side-effects of carbamazepine include blurred vision, drowsiness, skin rash, ataxia and diplopia. Benign leukopenia in 30% of cases will settle with cessation of the drug. Aplastic anaemia and hepatitis are rare.

2. Sodium valproate is the drug of choice for primary generalised tonic/clonic seizures, myoclonic or absence seizures.

Side-effects are nausea, vomiting and abdominal pain, which will improve if the dose is lowered. Tremor, hair loss and weightgain may occur. Hepatotoxicity is rare and occurs exclusively in children.

3. Ethosuximide is only of value for petit mal attacks.

4. Young patients with partial and secondary generalised fits often respond well to carbamazepine.

Patients should be seen regularly initially, in order to encourage good compliance. Changing anticonvulsants must be done slowly, and poly-pharmacy should be avoided if possible.

Surgical excision of an epileptic focus is rarely required.

Special problems relating to epilepsy

Pregnancy. All drugs can be teratogenic. Carbamazepine is the preferred drug.

Driving. If the patient has had even one witnessed seizure, and has an abnormal EEG, then the licencing authorities state that patients cannot drive until

Table 4.4. Diagnostic features of loss of consciousness in epilepsy, vasovagal syncope and hypoglycaemia

	Fit	Vasovagal syncope	Hypoglycaemia
Early warning	Uncommon Sometimes vague epigastric sensation in partial complex seizures	Blurred vision, lightheadedness	Pallor or bradycardia before and during attack
Onset	Dramatic	Gradual Helped or prevented by lying flat	Slow
Signs	Eyes roll up, often open Limbs rigid Tonic muscle contractions, pallor normal heart rate or tachycardia	Eyes closed Hypnotic, pale, bradycardia	Variety of involuntary movements, pale, bradycardia
Plantar reflexes	Plantars extensor	Plantars flexor	Reflexes lost
Corneal reflex	Absent	Present	Lost
Sphincter control	Lost	Preserved	Lost
Recovery	Disorientated, unreal, feeling sleepy Headaches lasting for hours	Drained, cold, sweaty Rapid recovery within 5 minutes	May be slow if glucose is not given

they have been free of fits for 2 years. Heavy Goods and Public Service Vehicle licences cannot be held if the patient has had even a single seizure after the age of 5 years.

Social implications. Most patients lead a normal life, but some care has to be taken with certain activities such as swimming and climbing.

Status epilepticus. This is defined as the failure to recover consciousness between serial seizures. Permanent brain damage will occur if patients are allowed to continue fitting for more than 1 hour. Mortality is 12%. Principles of treatment include maintaining an airway and inserting an intravenous line with glucose, vitamin B complex and specific anticonvulsant therapy.

NARCOLEPSY

This is a rare disorder of the reticular activating system, characterised by excessive daytime sleepiness often associated with cataplexy (sudden loss of muscular tone with collapse precipitated by emotion such as laughing or crying). Hypnagogic hallucinations and sleep paralysis may also occur.

COMA

There is relative or total absence of cerebral activity caused by disturbance of metabolism, blood supply or by direct injury.

Coma of sudden onset

Cardiac arrest is associated with apnoea and absence of pulse. The patient is limp, with moist, cool skin because of peripheral shut down. Eyes are slightly open, pupils in midposition and there is no eye movement on passive head rotation. Rapid return of cerebral perfusion will result in complete recovery without any neurological damage.

There are many syndromes of cerebral damage resulting from inadequate brain perfusion, varying from cortical blindness and language difficulties to the persistence of coma and limb paralysis. Sudden rupture of blood into the sub-arachnoid space from an intracranial aneurysm is suggested by a cry, headache and vomiting before loss of consciousness. Subhyaloid haemorrhages in the optic fundus may appear.

The diagnosis is made by CT scan of the brain and a lumbar puncture. Other cerebral insults which can result in sudden coma include occlusion of the basilar artery and pontine haemorrhage.

Coma occurring over minutes or hours

This is often of the metabolic type caused by hyperglycaemia with or without ketosis, hypoglycaemia, drug overdose or hypoxia. Ruptured arteriovenous malformation, meningitis, encephalitis, cerebellar haemorrhage, hypertensive encephalopathy, metabolic, renal and hepatic failure are other causes.

Slow evolution of coma with lateralising signs

This is often associated with head injury. If there is a rapid rise in pressure from swelling or blood clot, then the temporal lobe will herniate downwards and compress the brainstem (Fig. 4.4).

Cerebellar infarction with swelling, may produce a brainstem compression syndrome with coma. There is little chance of recovery from a coma with pupillary and eye movement changes.

Investigations and treatment (See Tables 4.5 and 4.6)

Some patients fail to recover after a general anaesthetic. This may be from anoxia. A dramatic rise in temperature, pulse and respiration rate, and meta-bolic acidosis during anaesthesia, suggest malignant hyperpyrexia which is an inherited autosomal dominant trait. Sensitivity to succinylcholine or halothane in patients with muscle disease may be a problem. This is treated with intravenous dantrolene.

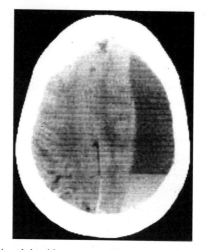

Fig. 4.4 Chronic subdural haematoma. Unenhanced CT scan shows a collection of altered blood with a fluid level from sedimentation of blood breakdown products.

Table 4.5. Assessment of the comatose patient

1. Inspect for signs of trauma to scalp and body
2. Endotracheal intubation if cyanosed
3. Smell for alcohol and acetone on the breath
4. Remove vomitus from throat
5. Suction and maintain clear airway
6. Insert intravenous line, check calcium, sugar and creatinine levels, osmolality, prothrombin time, APTT, drug screen, haemoglobin, white cell count
7. Infusion of intravenous glucose 50% and 50 mg thiamine to treat possible Wernicke's encephalopathy
8. Look for signs of drug abuse
9. Assess level of coma on Glasgow Coma Scale (see Table 4.6)
10. Observe the eye position and movement—horizontal roving eyes suggest intact brainstem, therefore a bihemisphere problem; check oculocephalic reflex only if a neck fracture has been excluded
11. Insert urinary catheter
12. If brain CT scan is negative then perform lumbar puncture providing there is no evidence of papilloedema: look for features of meningitis, encephalitis and haemorrhage. Centrifuge sample of cerebrospinal fluid and look for xanthochromia
13. If brain CT scan shows mass lesion, refer to neurosurgeons.

Special coma syndromes

The locked-in syndrome is caused by damage to the ventral pons, resulting in paralysis of all four limbs and lower cranial nerves. The patient is awake and

Table 4.6. Glasgow coma scale

1.	*Eye opening*	*Score*
	Spontaneous	4
	To speech	3
	To pain	2
	Nil	1
2.	*Verbal response*	
	Orientated	5
	Confused conversation	4
	Inappropriate words	3
	Incomprehensible sounds	2
	Nil	1
3.	*Best motor response*	
	Obeys command	6
	Localises to pain	5
	Withdraws to pain	4
	Abnormal flexion to pain	3
	Extension response	2
	Nil	1

15 = fully conscious   3 = Severe brain damage

This scale is widely accepted as a method for quantifying level of coma.

fully aware. Communication may be possible only with vertical eye movements.

A chronic vegetative state occurs where there is no higher function. The patient is totally dependent on support staff. He has a normal sleep–wake cycle and eyes are often open. There is extensive damage to the cortex and forebrain.

Brainstem death occurs where there is artificial ventilatory support in a patient whose heart continues to beat, yet the brain is irreversibly damaged. The cause of death must be known and hypothermia, metabolic disturbance such as hypoglycaemia, or drug effect, e.g. barbiturate or muscle relaxant, must be excluded.

In order to establish brainstem death, apnoea should persist when there has been prior ventilation with oxygen, when the patient is taken off the ventilator. Oxygen is given at 6 l/min via a tracheal cannula to prevent further brain damage. The $PaCO_2$ must rise to act as a stimulant to the brainstem. The patient should be unresponsive except for spinal reflexes. All brainstem reflexes should be absent, including pupil response to light, oculo-cephalic, oculo-vestibular, corneal and gag reflexes. Only after discussion with the family and full documentation by two experienced doctors giving independent assessments can the ventilator be switched off.

MOVEMENT DISORDERS

PARKINSON'S DISEASE (PARALYSIS AGITANS)

The cause of the most common disorder affecting the extra-pyramidal system is unknown. 1% of the population over 60 is affected. Parkinson's disease (PD) results from degeneration, with neuronal loss, of the pigmented nuclei of the brainstem. Intracytoplasmic hyaline inclusions (Lewy bodies) in the remaining neurones is the histological hallmark of the disease. The chemical changes in the region known as the nigro-striatal system are responsible for the clinical features of PD which emerges when 80% of the total dopaminergic cells are lost.

Symptoms and signs

The cardinal features are tremor, rigidity and akinesia. Other signs include disturbance of posture and abnormal autonomic function. Subtle early symptoms are often put down to advancing years. There is slow loss of agility, lack of facial expression, increased blinking, tilted trunk posture and hesitant rise from a chair. Generalised poverty of movement and problems with fine movements such as dressing occur. The tremor is present at rest.

Rigidity is of the cogwheel type and often unilateral. The general body posture is flexed, with the centre of gravity thrown forward. The gait is small and shuffling, described as festinant.

As the disease progresses, freezing occurs. Other problems include dysarthria, dysphagia and drooling of saliva. Autonomic features include thermal paraesthesiae, increased sweating and flushing, postural hypotension with inadequate bladder emptying. The skin is often greasy and eczematous. 60% of patients will eventually develop dementia.

Differential diagnosis

A Parkinsonian syndrome occurs in patients on dopamine blocking drugs such as chlorpromazine.

The arteriosclerotic extrapyramidal syndrome is characterised by a 'marche a petit pas' and pyramidal signs often with a pseudobulbar palsy.

Benign essential postural tremor is of a faster frequency and does not have the other associated features.

Treatment

Drug treatment may not be required early on.

Benzhexol and orphenadrine suppress excess cholinergic activity in the striatal neurones. These drugs tend to help tremor but are often limited by the side-effects of dry mouth, constipation, prostatism and difficulty focusing. They are not well tolerated in the elderly.

Leva-dopa (L-dopa) with a dopa decarboxylase inhibitor, e.g. sinemet plus or madopar, represent the most effective medication. The duration of action of leva-dopa may be up to 8–10 hours initially, but tends to diminish with time.

Dopamine agonists such as bromocriptine, lysuride and pergolide can be useful supplementary treatment.

Subcutaneous apomorphine is only used in selected patients with severe unpredictable swings in motor performance.

Selegeline the monamine oxidase type B inhibitor, has been shown to slow the progression of PD and is therefore recommended in most patients.

The central nervous system side-effects of L-dopa and the dopamine agonists include abnormal movements of various types with 'on–off' effects and psychiatric problems. As the disease progresses, an increasing dosage of L-dopa is often required. After many years, a range of involuntary movements may emerge: tics, chorea, dystonia and even ballismus. Treatment is by reducing the dose of L-dopa and adding a small amount of a dopamine agonist.

Psychiatric effects occur in 50% of patients who have had the disease for 5 years or more. These may take the form of vivid dreams, progressing to frank hallucinations. The psychosis may have a strong paranoid element. Treatment consists of reducing the dose of L-dopa or dopamine agonist. Drugs such as phenothiazines may exacerbate PD. Sudden cessation of anti-Parkinsonian drugs should be avoided because this can precipitate an acute confusional state and rigidity. Postural instability with frequent falls, freezing and swallowing problems are very difficult to manage.

Brain implantation with human fetal mesencephalic cells is still at the experimental stage.

Prognosis

PD patients are living longer—15 to 20 years from the time of diagnosis is not unusual—but the degree of disability by then is marked.

CHOREA

Chorea is characterised by non-rhythmical involuntary jerking movements affecting different areas of the body in an irregular, unpredictable fashion. It may affect the distal limbs, the face, swallowing, articulation or breathing.

Causes

1. In the young. Sydenham's chorea (St Vitus dance or rheumatic chorea) from *Streptococcus* group A infection, pregnancy and the contraceptive pill.

2. In the elderly. Huntington's disease, benign hereditary and senile chorea.

3. Systemic diseases. Systemic lupus erythematosus (SLE), thyrotoxicosis, hypoparathyroidism, patients with Parkinson's disease on L-dopa.

Vascular hemichorea, or hemiballismus, is caused by infarction in the basal ganglia subthalamic nucleus and is treated with small doses of haloperidol or tetrabenazine.

Huntington's chorea is an autosomal dominant condition with complete penetrance and a very low mutation rate. Prevalence is 5–10 per 100 000. The onset of chorea, behavioural abnormality and dementia in the fourth and fifth decade is followed by a progressive course and death within 15–20 years. The pathological features are thinning of the head of the caudate nucleus from neuronal loss and gliosis. This is seen on MRI or CT scan as a flattening of the frontal horns of the lateral ventricles. The gene for Huntington's chorea is related to a DNA segment mapped to the short arm of chromosome 4 (see p. 467).

Treatment is with dopamine blockers, such as tetrabenazine, haloperidol or pimozide, to control movements.

ESSENTIAL TREMOR

There is regular rhythmical oscillation of segments of the limb and trunk whilst maintaining posture or moving parts of the body. It is a type of action tremor most noticeable when the arms are outstretched. It is often familial and is helped by alcohol. The commonest cause of tremor is anxiety, but it is also seen with alcohol abuse and thyrotoxicosis. The incidence of Parkinson's disease is increased in patients with essential tremor. Treatment is with propranolol, clonazepam and sometimes prednisolone.

MYOCLONUS

Sudden involuntary contraction of muscle groups results in movement of the corresponding joint. Nocturnal myoclonus is a normal phenomenon associated with sudden jerking of the whole body during the hypnagogic state. Epileptic myoclonus, or epilepsia partialis continua, is often precipitated by sensory stimuli and occurs with a spike focus on the EEG. It is commonly the result of stroke, tumour or cerebral abscess. Other causes of myoclonus include post-cardiac arrest cerebral hypoxia, Creutzfeldt–Jakob disease, benign essential myoclonus and subacute sclerosing panencephalitis (SSPE). It also occurs as a complication of hepatic, renal and respiratory failure. Treatment is with clonazepam or sodium valproate.

DYSTONIA

Dystonia can be either focal or segmental and consists of muscle agonist and antagonist contracting in a slow fashion to distort limb posture. A common example is spasmodic torticollis. Patients with Parkinson's disease on L-dopa or dopamine agonist treatment will often develop dystonia affecting one foot or one arm.

The rare primary idiopathic dystonia musculorum deformans is a progressive disease requiring large doses of anticholinergics, phenothiazines, L-dopa and benzodiazepines.

Wilson's disease, an inherited disorder of copper metabolism, is characterised by stiff dystonic posturing and a fixed smile. If treated early it will respond to penicillamine.

Spasmodic torticollis and other dystonias may be treated with local injections of botulinus toxin into the affected muscles.

Writer's cramp is believed to be a form of focal dystonia.

ATHETOSIS

Slow, sinuous writhing movement occurs along the long axis of the limbs, again most commonly seen as an L-dopa side-effect, but also in patients with cerebral palsy.

TICS OR HABIT SPASMS

These are common, repetitive semi-purposive movements, which patients can suppress, and are often associated with stress. They can take the form of some purposeful action, such as winking or shrugging of the shoulder. An extreme form occurs in the Gilles de la Tourette syndrome which is associated with extreme vocalisation and treated with clonidine.

PAIN SYNDROMES

At a peripheral level, unmyelinated C fibres are responsible for diffuse, long-lasting slow pain. A-delta fibre discharges result in well localised, brief, fast pain. Pain may be distributed to the dermatomes, in which case it is well localised and often associated with paraesthesiae. Pain may also radiate to the myotomes or sclerotomes (skeletal or ligamentous structures) where it tends to be less well localised. Dermatome pain is of a pricking, burning, well-localised nature. Deep pain is a diffuse dull ache and bears no relationship to skeletal or visceral structures, making diagnosis problematical. Disease of visceral or skeletal structures is referred to the skin supplied by the same spinal segments, e.g. cardiac pain. Central nervous system sources of pain are exemplified by so-called thalamic pain after a stroke. This is characterised by dysaesthesiae or pain on touching skin.

MIGRAINE

50% of men and 30% of women will suffer such headaches at some time in their lives. Pain is caused by dilatation of the arteries in the distribution of the external carotid arteries. During the prodrome the blood flow is reduced by vasoconstriction and increased during the headache phase. This dilatation has been linked to increased levels of 5-hydroxytryptamine and other vasoactive substances in the serum. Migraine usually begins in the second to third decade, sometimes the fifth, and a positive family history is common.

Symptoms

Headaches begin suddenly, reaching a peak in minutes or hours. The pain is described as throbbing, pulsing or pounding. A typical migraine begins early in the day and often at weekends. Diuresis and euphoria are common. Common migraine is defined as unilateral headache with nausea and vomiting. Classical migraine has focal neurological features. The aura, e.g. a hemianopia, usually lasts 15 minutes. Flashing lights, shimmering, fortification spectra or teichopsia, bright moving lights, may be followed by a blind spot or hemianopia. Trigger factors include:

1. foods containing tyramine or other vasoactive substances, e.g. alcohol, cheese, caffeine, yoghurt
2. hormone fluctuations prior to and during menstruation, pregnancy and puerperium, and the contraceptive pill.
3. vasodilator drugs including nifedipine, and trinitrin
4. relaxing after a period of intense activity.

A variant of migraine is cluster headaches (migrainous neuralgia) and is characterised by localised pain around the eye, conjunctival injection, lacrimation and a Horner's syndrome.

Other types of migraine include facial, ophthalmoplegic and basilar syndromes.

Treatment

The acute attack usually only requires simple analgesics and an anti-emetic. If these fail then a combination of ergotamine and caffeine may be required. This is best limited to younger patients without vascular disease. Prophylaxis takes the form of cyclizine, beta-blockers, clonidine or pizotifen. The anti-serotonin drug methyserigde may be required in resistant cases. Sumatriptan, a selective 5-HT (hydroxytryptamine) agonist causes a selective vasoconstriction within the carotid arterial circulation in animals. It is an expensive new drug used to treat the acute migraine attack.

GIANT CELL (TEMPORAL) ARTERITIS

This is a very important condition which tends to affect those over 60 and is rare under the age of 55 years.

Diffuse steady headache, sometimes spreading from the temples over the face, is typical. The scalp is often tender when brushing hair because of the inflamed superficial temporal and occipital vessels. General symptoms of fatigue, malaise and proximal stiffness (from polymyalgia rheumatica) occur.

Although the erythrocyte sedimentation rate (ESR) is usually raised it may be normal in the early phase of the illness in 15% of cases. Patients may complain of a painful tongue which may develop ischaemic ulcers or even gangrene. Jaw claudication from masseter ischaemia is secondary to external carotid artery involvement.

The most important complication is sudden loss of vision caused by occlusion of the ophthalmic artery. Vertebrobasilar and, rarely, carotid arteries may be affected before they enter the dura resulting in focal ischaemic syndromes.

Diagnosis is confirmed by biopsy of the superficial temporal artery. Arteritic changes are often focal and segmental, so a negative biopsy does not exclude the diagnosis. The response to steroids is diagnostic.

The headache resolves within 24 hours of prednisolone 60 mg per 24 hours. This dose should then be slowly tapered using the ESR as a guide. Patients may have to remain on steroids for 12–18 months.

TENSION HEADACHES

These are experienced by everyone. The pain is characterised by a constant tight pressure and may radiate from the head into the neck and shoulders. It often builds up gradually during the day and may continue for days. Headache lasting longer than 6 months is unlikely to be caused by serious intracranial disease. Alcohol and exercise alleviate tension headache whereas they exacerbate migraine. Cervical headache may be associated with spondylosis. Emotional factors can influence tension headaches. Physiotherapy, soft collar, muscle relaxants and antidepressants may alleviate the pain.

TRIGEMINAL NEURALGIA OR TIC DOULOUREUX

An important disease of the elderly, the pain is usually in the distribution of the maxillary and/or mandibular divisions. In idiopathic tic, degenerative or fibrotic changes in the Gasserian ganglia have been reported. Secondary causes of neuralgia include multiple sclerosis and compression of the nerve by tumour or anomalous blood vessel.

The onset of idiopathic trigeminal neuralgia is usually in mid to late life and is unusual under the age of 35.

Symptoms and signs

The symptom is a paroxysmal pain (like electric shock) from a trigger zone, radiating out into the trigeminal divisions. It is often precipitated by cold wind, washing the face, shaving or eating. Paroxysms last for 1–2 minutes. There is no objective loss of sensation during or after an attack, although the patient may complain of hyperaesthesia. The frequency of attacks vary from many times a day to several times a month. The patient may be undernourished from a lack of eating or from fear of precipitating an attack.

Differential diagnosis

Facial pain involves disease of the temperomandibular joint, maxillary sinusitis, teeth glaucoma, or nasopharyngeal disease. Atypical facial pain where no organic cause is found can be difficult to treat. Antidepressants and carbamazepine are usually employed.

Treatment

Simple analgesics are ineffective. Opiates will work but are addictive. Intravenous phenytoin will abort an attack. Oral carbamazepine is usually effective, but may cause sedation in the elderly. Surgery, including alcohol injection of the infra-orbital nerve, can be effective. Radiofrequency thermocoagulation of trigeminal nerve rootlets is often used, as is decompression by separating anomalous vessels from nerve roots via a small posterior fossa approach.

Prognosis

Remission in trigeminal neuralgia is very common. Months or years may go by before the next attack.

LIMB PAIN

Causalgia. Severe limb pain and intense burning secondary to partial injury is often associated with varying degrees of sympathetic nervous system disturbance. It is similar to reflex sympathetic dystrophy secondary to minor limb trauma, also known as Sudeck's atrophy, where there are skin changes and reduced sweating.

Phantom limb pain as seen in amputees and caused by central mechanisms.

Radicular pain may be caused by herpes zoster, a tumour or irradiation.

Plexus pain is seen in brachial neuralgia, tumour and trauma.

Peripheral nerve pain is seen in amyloidosis, diabetes and entrapment mononeuropathy.

CERVICAL RADICULAR PAIN SYNDROMES

C5/6 level disease involving the C6 root produces pain in the trapezius ridge, shoulder, anterior arm, radial forearm and thumb.

C6/7 disc level involving the C7 root causes pain in the shoulder blade, pectoral region, posterolateral upper arm, dorsal forearm, elbow, index and middle finger.

Other causes of upper limb pain include polymyalgia rheumatica, fibromyalgia, viral myalgia, cellulitis, ischaemia, superficial venous thrombosis, collagen vascular disease and paraproteinaemia from vasospastic disease.

LOW BACK PAIN

Lumbar disc disease may cause pain through a number of mechanisms. These include a torn tendon at muscle attachment to vertebrae, stretching of the periosteum, a bulging disc against annulus fibrosis, inflammation around the disc (discitis), compression of nerve roots from bulging of the annulus or frank herniation of disc material, and a root compressed by osteophytes, intervertebral joints and facets. Abdominal or pelvic disease may also be referred to the back. Chronic low back pain is a major cause of loss of work. 95% of lumbosacral disc lesions occur at L4/5 and L5/S1 level.

Symptoms

The clinical features of lumbar root lesions are shown in Table 4.7. The mode of onset and type of pain may give a clue to the aetiology of back pain.

Table 4.7. Clinical features of lumbar root lesions

Root	Site of pain	Sensory loss	Weakness	Tendon reflex affected
L3	Anterior thigh	Anterior thigh	Hip flexion adduction Quadriceps	Knee jerk
L4*	Anterior thigh	Anterior thigh	Quadriceps Tibialis anterior	Knee jerk
L5*	Lateral thigh	Lateral lower leg and dorsum of foot	Hip abduction Hamstrings Foot eversion	—
S1*	Posterior thigh	Lateral foot	Eversion of foot	Ankle jerk
S2	Posterior thigh	Rear calf	Small foot muscles	—

* = Most commonly affected roots

1. Pain of gradual onset suggests tumour.
2. Pain of sudden onset suggests mechanical stress.
3. Intermittent pain associated with walking suggests spondylitic radiculopathy with narrow spinal canal.
3. Discomfort at rest with continuous irritation suggests inflammation of the pain-sensitive periosteum.

The quality of bone pain is a referred discomfort, often a deep aching, whereas root pain is often very intense and sharp, and distally distributed to the dermatomes.

Differential diagnosis

Other causes of low back pain include lumbosacral or sacroiliac sprain, fractured lumbar vertebra, metastatic bone disease, infection of bone, spondylolisthesis (slip forward of vertebra), spondylosis and ankylosing spondylitis.

Investigations

These include plain x-ray of the lumbosacral spine. Spinal CT and MRI are very helpful, showing the soft tissue and bone. Contrast myelography shows indentation of the thecal sack by a mass lesion.

Treatment

Narcotics may be necessary for acute pain relief. Anti-inflammatory and anti-depressant drugs are used for chronic pain, as are physiotherapy, massage and traction, and enforced bedrest. Surgery is considered if medical treatment fails.

STROKE

Cerebrovascular disease is the third most common cause of death in Western society and a major cause of disability. Stroke is defined as the rapid onset of neurological deficit which may build up over minutes, hours or even days. The incidence of stroke in the community is 2 per 1000 population per year.

Pathology

1. reversible ischaemia
2. infarction—major vessel occlusion, either embolism or thrombosis
3. infarction with secondary haemorrhage
4. haemorrhage (15% of cases).

Aetiology of infarction

1. local thrombosis
2. emboli from the great vessels or heart
3. poor perfusion pressure
4. abnormal platelets or coagulation
5. vasospasm
6. arteritis.

The overall incidence of stroke is falling in the Western world, possibly because of attention to treatable risk factors.

Risk factors

1. Hypertension—persistently raised blood pressure, diastolic greater than 100 mmHg.
2. A family history of stroke, hypertension and coronary artery disease.
3. Cardiac disease, particularly valvular, with or without artrial fibrillation.
4. Transient cerebral ischaemic attacks.
5. Raised haematocrit, greater than 0.5.
6. Smoking, lack of exercise, high serum cholesterol levels, excess alcohol intake.
7. Oral contraceptive pill.

Symptoms and signs

The temporal syndrome

1. Transient cerebral ischaemic attack (TIA) lasts less than 24 hours.
2. Minor stroke lasts longer than 24 hours but less than 1 week.
3. Major stroke lasts longer than 1 week.

The anatomical syndrome

Carotid territory features include amaurosis fugax and language problems.

Vertebrobasilar territory features include dizziness, dysarthria, double vision, dysphagia, hemianopia, clumsiness and loss of consciousness.

Specific arterial occlusive syndromes

Common carotid. Occlusion often fails to produce a deficit because of the good anastomosis between the two carotids, and between the carotid and vertebrobasilar systems.

Internal carotid. Stenosis with eventual thrombosis leads to a gradual stuttering onset with transient ischaemic attacks preceding the major event in a number of cases. Embolism is usually dramatic and calamitous. Features are those of unilateral hemisphere dysfunction:

1. contralateral hemiparesis
2. contralateral sensory loss
3. aphasia (dominant hemisphere)
4. homonymous hemianopia is infrequent and usually takes the form of temporary neglect of opposite visual fields.

Middle cerebral artery. This is the artery most likely to be affected by embolism. Damage is to the ipsilateral internal capsule and basal ganglia. Features include:

1. contralateral hemiplegia
2. contralateral hemianaesthesia
3. contralateral hemianopia
4. aphasia if dominant hemisphere is affected.

Anterior cerebral artery (Fig. 4.5)
Features include:

1. contralateral numb weak leg
2. akinetic mutism and abulia (reduced rate and complexity of language and motor response) in bilateral disease.

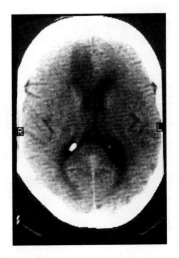

Fig. 4.5 Infarction in territory of right anterior cerebral artery—a low-density area in front of the right frontal horn involving grey and white matter. There is no compression of the ventricle.

Posterior cerebral artery. Signs are of contralateral homonymous hemianopia.

Vertebrobasilar arteries. Occlusion produces a wide spectrum of syndromes that depend on the site of thrombosis. If of sudden onset, usually embolic, occlusion results in quadraplegia and ocular dysfunctions. The lateral medullary syndrome is from occlusion of the basilar or posterior inferior cerebellar artery. Findings include:
1. vertigo, vomiting, nystagmus
3. dysphagia
3. hoarseness
4. ipsilateral loss of pain and temperature in the face, palate and vocal cord paralysis, Horner's syndrome and limb ataxia
5. contralateral pain and temperature loss in the limbs and trunk (there are *no* motor limb signs)
6. crossed hemiplegias occur with brainstem lesions when a cranial nerve nucleus and pyramidal tract are affected.

Investigations

These include haemoglobin, packed cell volume, ESR or viscosity, blood sugar, serum cholesterol, lipids (controversial because it is not known whether lowering blood cholesterol will reduce incidence of stroke), Venereal Disease Research Laboratory (VDRL). In a patient with stroke a CT brain scan:
1. may be normal
2. may show a low-density large lesion caused by a major vessel occlusion, or small lacunar infarctions (lacunes are 3–5 mm cystic lesions)
3. may show patchy enhancing lesions thought to be caused by luxury perfusion
4. may show evidence of haemorrhage.

Doppler carotid artery studies represent a non-invasive technique to show stenotic lesions (Fig. 4.6). Carotid arteriography may be necessary to define stenotic lesions more accurately.

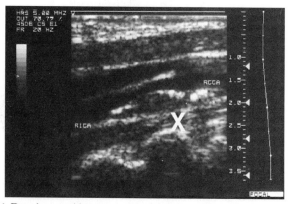

Fig. 4.6 Doppler carotid artery studies show stenotic lesions.

Treatment

Transient cerebral ischaemic attacks, if untreated, lead to stroke in 22–50% of cases within 5 years. Treatment is with aspirin 300 mg per 24 hours. If this fails then anticoagulants should be considered. Carotid endarterectomy may be effective when there is 70% or greater carotid artery stenosis.

Anticoagulants may be of value for stroke in evolution and as prophylaxis in valvular heart disease, especially where there is atrial fibrillation. Surgery to evacuate a cerebellar haemorrhage may be beneficial.

Rehabilitation involves the physiotherapist, and the occupational and speech therapist.

Prognosis

40 to 50% of patients die within 3 weeks. The highest mortality occurs in cerebral haemorrhage (70–80%). Mortality is lower in infarction—20%. Adverse factors for long-term outlook include aphasia and incontinence. 50% of patients will be left with a substantial neurological deficit.

SUBARACHNOID HAEMORRHAGE

Bleeding into the subarachnoid space is usually from a ruptured berry aneurysm (Fig. 4.7) or arteriovenous malformation. Saccular berry aneurysms are caused by a congenital defect in the supporting tissue resulting in a bulge in the arterial wall. Aneurysms are usually located at the division of a major intracranial artery.

A transient sudden increase in blood pressure is often the stimulus for rupture. The aneurysm is more likely to rupture if it is between 10 and 20 mm in diameter. An aneurysm of less than 3 mm in diameter has a low risk of rupture.

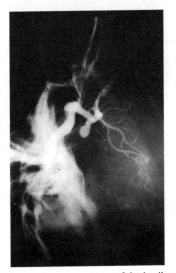

Fig. 4.7 Angiogram shows a berry aneurysm of the basilar artery.

The volume of blood released varies from a few millilitres to a massive haemorrhage which can be fatal in seconds. The consequences of rupture are

1. direct brain injury
2. susceptibility to re-rupture
3. secondary hydrocephalus from blockage of CSF circulation
4. vasospasm.

Symptoms and signs

Symptoms include sudden onset of severe occipital headache, unconsciousness in 50% of patients, vomiting, epileptic fits and lumbar pain in the case of spinal subarachnoid haemorrhage.

The signs are neck stiffness, positive Kernig's sign, papilloedema, subhyaloid retinal haemorrhages, focal neurological signs, and cranial nerve palsies.

Investigations

A CT scan may show subarachnoid blood in sylvian and interhemispheric fissures and occasionally in the ventricular system. If the CT scan is negative then lumbar puncture may be necessary. This should show a uniformly blood-stained CSF, not a bloody traumatic tap (Fig. 4.8). Xanthochromia in the supernatant of the centrifuged sample may persist for up to 14–20 days. Lymphocytes may be present in small numbers in the late phase.

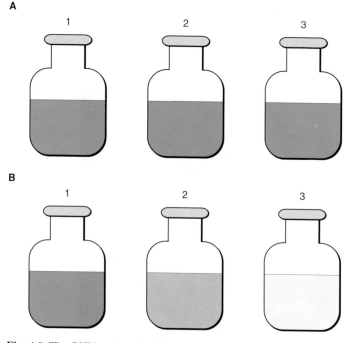

Fig. 4.8 The CSF in subarachnoid haemorrhage (**A**) and in a bloody tap (**B**).

Differential diagnosis

Other causes are encephalitis, meningitis, migraine and cervical spondylosis.

Treatment

The risk of re-rupture remains high at 1–2% per day for the first 3–4 weeks. Blood pressure should be well controlled. Intravenous nimodipine reduces the morbidity from vasospasm.

Surgery involves clipping the neck of the aneurysm and the best results are obtained in middle cerebral and posterior communicating aneurysms.

Prognosis

1. 30% of patients will die in the first 24 hours.
2. 30% will survive 8 weeks and 20% of these will re-bleed, usually within the first 3 weeks.
3. 50% of the survivors at 1 year will go back to work.
4. Persistent disability results from hemiplegia, cranial nerve palsies and epilepsy.

Arteriovenous malformations (AVM) comprise arteries and veins of mixed size but not capillaries. There is usually an arteriovenous (AV) fistula. The AVM may rupture, or cause epilepsy or headache. It is often detected incidentally on a CT brain scan. A proportion of patients will have a skull bruit. Treatment takes the form of catheter embolisation, surgery or radiotherapy.

DISEASES OF THE SPINAL CORD

The spinal cord in utero approximates to the bony levels, but after growth the lower cord is several segments above the bony level. The cord terminates at the Ll vertebra but lower lumbar sacral roots continue in the canal until they reach their point of exit.

In lesions of the spinal cord, the level of damage should be assessed so that appropriate radiology can be accurately directed. However, it is not always possible to determine the exact site of the cord lesion from symptoms and signs. It is often necessary during myelography to run the contrast medium the full length of the cord from conus to foramen magnum.

ACUTE SPINAL CORD LESION (MYELOPATHY)

Compressive lesions must be looked for immediately. Failure to do this and to treat surgically may result in permanent cord damage. Causes include:

1. trauma.

2. extradural compression from
a. disc herniation, cervical and thoracic spine
b. metastatic tumour from primary prostate, lung, breast and also myeloma

c. osteomyelitis, tuberculosis.

Less common causes such as epidural abscess, haematoma and tumour may be not associated with bony X-ray changes.

Damage to the cord occurs by means of compression of its blood supply with subsequent ischaemia.

Other causes of acute myelopathy include:

1. transverse myelitis caused by viral infections, syphilis and HIV
2. multiple sclerosis
3. Devic's disease (neuromyelitis optica)
4. systemic cancer-necrotising non-metastatic myelopathy
5. vascular disease, haematomyelia or anterior spinal artery thrombosis.

Symptoms and signs

Symptoms include painful back from bone disease, segmental root pain, progressive difficulty in walking, a numb tingling sensation in the legs, and difficulty in passing urine.

The signs are sensory level below the point of lesion, enlarged bladder with overflow incontinence, and proximal hip flexion weakness leading to flaccid paralysis; spasticity emerges later with brisk reflexes and extensor plantars.

Investigations

1. Chest X-ray.
2. Rectal examination.
3. Lumbar puncture. CSF protein level may be very high, with xanthochromia, particularly if there is a complete block.
4. MRI and CT scanning.

Management of established complete paraplegia

1. Medical or surgical treatment of the cause.
2. Bladder function, with indwelling catheter using aseptic technique. Infections are treated with antibiotics.
3. Bowel care: enema, manual evacuation.
4. Regular turning to avoid pressure scores. A Ripple mattress should be used.
5. Avoidance of contractures with physiotherapy and regular passive exercises.
6. Later, transfer to a special paraplegic unit for rehabilitation.

CHRONIC SPINAL CORD DISEASE

This is slowly progressive, occurring over months or even years. Common causes include cervical spondylosis from osteoarthritic and degenerative changes in the neck, with osteophytes, disc protrusion posteriorly, resulting in local bony overgrowth. There may be progressive difficulty in walking, bilateral tingling, and numbness in the hands, and neck stiffness (absence of local pain is common). Bladder dysfunction is rare.

Spastic paraparesis, brisk deep tendon reflexes and extensor plantar responses are seen. The sensory level may involve the dorsal column, or spinothalamic function, and is not always an accurate guide to the level of the lesion.

Investigations

Plain neck X-ray, CT scan with myelogram, MRI scan.

MOTOR NEURONE DISEASE

This is a condition of unknown aetiology where there is degeneration of the corticospinal tracts, anterior horn cells and bulbar motor nuclei. It affects patients in the fourth to the sixth decades. Male to female preponderence ratio is 2.5 : 1.

The symptoms and signs of the disease are summarised in Table 4.8 and a combination of syndromes is common. Widespread fasciculations beyond the focal weak muscles is a common picture.

Investigations

Investigations are directed to exclude other diseases. Nerve conduction studies and concentric needle electromyography may show features of denervation in a widespread distribution.

Differential diagnosis

1. cervical spondylitic myelopathy
2. pure motor neuropathy as in paraproteinaemia
3. foramen magnum or cord tumour
4. a pseudobulbar palsy may be secondary to vascular disease.

Management

There is no cure. Dysphagia may be treated by sucking ice or taking neostigmine 15 mg before meals. Feeding is by gastrotomy in cachectic patients using an endoscopic technique. Physiotherapy, speech and swallowing therapy, suction machines, foot drop orthotic splints are needed. Motor Neurone Disease Association care assistants will provide support.

Death almost invariably occurs within 3 years. Inhalation pneumonia is common because of the weak cough reflex.

SPINAL CORD TUMOURS

These may be caused by lesions arising from the nerve roots, the covering of the spinal cord, extradural fat, vascular networks and sympathetic chain of the vertebral column itself.

Benign encapsulated tumours (meningiomas and neurofibromas) account for the majority of all spinal cord primary tumours. Intramedullary tumours are more common in children and extramedullary tumours in adults. Tumours of the spinal cord are much less frequent than intracranial tumours, with a ratio of 1 : 4. Extramedullary tumours can cause symptoms by involving nerve roots and compression of the spinal cord, including occlusion of spinal blood vessels. Intramedullary tumours such as a glioma may extend the whole length of the spinal cord early in the disease (Fig. 4.9).

SUBACUTE COMBINED DEGENERATION OF THE CORD

Deficiency of vitamin B_{12} (cyanocobalomin) is the cause. Neurological lesions may result from inactivity of the B_{12} dependent enzyme methionine synthetase. This occurs in pernicious anaemia (PA), post-gastrectomy and some malabsorption syndromes. PA is often seen in association with other autoimmune diseases. The pathology is in the white more than the grey matter, although peripheral nerves are involved. There is loss of the myelin sheath and, to a lesser extent, the axons.

Neurological symptoms may appear early in the disease and even antedate the onset of anaemia (see Ch. 11).

Folic acid if given prematurely, before vitamin B_{12}, may exacerbate the neurological symptoms.

FRIEDREICH'S ATAXIA

This most common of the spinocerebellar degenerations is an inherited disorder (autosomal recessive) causing degeneration of cells in the posterior root ganglia, with secondary change in the peripheral nerves and posterior column of the spinal cord and cerebellum.

Development is in childhood, although the disease can present for the first time in adults. The signs are difficulty in walking, cerebellar dysarthria, ataxic weak limbs, absent deep tendon reflexes and extensor plantar responses. Posterior column function is affected with Rhombergism. There may also be club foot, scoliosis and cardiac involvement.

The ECG is usually abnormal with widespread T wave inversion. There is no treatment and the mean age of death is 35 years, from heart failure.

SYRINGOMYELIA

Syringomyelia is caused by an irregular cavitation in the central grey part of the spinal cord and brainstem. In the early stage of what is mainly a slowly progressive disease there is disruption of the central decussating pain and temperature fibres. The process then extends to the anterior horn cells, and eventually disrupts the corticospinal fibres. Dorsal column function abnormality is a late feature.

The disorder is occasionally associated with craniocervical junction anomalies. These include cerebellar tonsilar herniation and adhesions at the foramen magnum. They cause interruption of the free flow of CSF in and out

Table 4.8. Symptoms and signs of motor neurone disease

Clinical syndrome (location of pathology)	Symptoms	Signs
Progressive muscular atrophy (PMA) (anterior horn cell)	Weakness, wasting fasciculations	Often asymmetrical proximal or distal wasting Preservation of deep tendon reflexes
Amytrophic lateral sclerosis (ALS) (Corticospinal tracts)	Spastic gait, weak legs, cramps	No sensory signs Spastic quadraparesis Brisk reflexes, plantars extensor Bladder function preserved until very late
Bulbar palsy (motor lower cranial nerve nuclei)	Dysphagia, dysarthria, dysphonia, weak cough, risk of inhalation	Nasal speech, nasal regurgitation, and a wasted fasciculating tongue
Pseudobulbar palsy (bilateral corticobulbar tracts)	Dysarthria, spastic tongue, dysphagia, emotional lability	Spastic tongue, increased jaw jerk

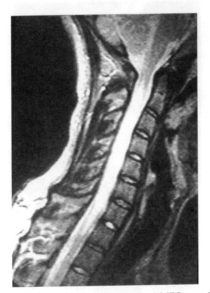

Fig. 4.9 Astrocytoma of the spinal cord. A sagittal MRI scan (T2 weighted) of the cervical spine showing a high signal from within the cord extending from C2 to C7.

of the fourth ventricle to the subarachnoid space. CSF is then forced downwards into the central cord.

Symptoms and signs

In the early stages patients may experience painless burns and sudden-onset pain in the back, chest or arms. The sensory signs are often dissociated anaesthesia with pain and temperature being affected, and sparing of dorsal column function. The hands may be weak and the reflexes are usually depressed or absent in the upper limbs. A Horner's syndrome and nystagmus may be present and some patients have a short neck with kyphosis.

Late in the disease, patients exhibit severe wasting of the hands, with difficulty in walking from spastic paraparesis. There is increasing sensory loss, and the skin of the hands takes on a red, shiny, dry trophic appearance. Charcot joints may develop, particularly involving the shoulders and elbows. Patients may develop a bulbar palsy (syringobulbia).

Differential diagnosis

Tumour of the cord, haematomyelia and cervical spondylitic myelopathy.

The diagnosis is made on an MRI scan (Fig. 4.10) of the cord, or CT myelogram.

Treatment is by craniocervical junction decompression. Most patients will do moderately well, although a small number of patients will experience slow progression despite surgery.

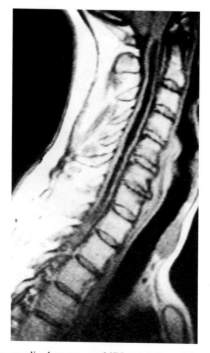

Fig. 4.10 Syringomyelia shown on an MRI scan (T1 weighted) showing cystic dilatation of the cervical cord.

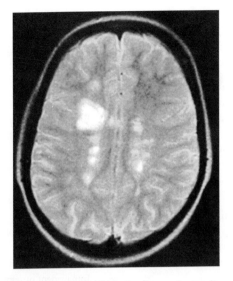

Fig. 4.11 Multiple sclerosis. Several high signal areas in a periventricular distribution within the white matter of the cerebral hemispheres are shown on the MRI scan (T2 weighted).

MULTIPLE SCLEROSIS (MS)

MS is the commonest disorder of the central nervous system to affect the young in the Western World. Lesions are confined to the central nervous system white matter, with preservation of axons compared with loss of myelin. The multiplicity of lesions and their sclerotic appearance (plaques) are evident on gross pathological specimens. The MRI scan (Fig. 4.11) shows well-established periventricular high signal abnormalities. Lesions also occur in the brainstem, cerebellum and spinal cord.

A susceptibility to the disease may be acquired during childhood. Disease prevalence is 5 : 100 000 in Africa and Asia, whereas in northern Europe it is 80 : 100 000. If migration from one zone to another takes place before the age of 10 then individual susceptibility is determined by the new region. If migration takes place later in life, the patient takes with him the susceptibility of the home country. Altered host reaction to an agent (?virus) not yet identified is a possible factor, set against a background of genetic and immune abnormality. MS is more frequent in identical twins and amongst members of the immediate family.

An immunological basis for the disease is supported by the finding of a raised CSF IgG with oligoclonal banding. Immunological studies have shown collection of T cells and macrophages in the perivenous white matter near the plaques.

The course of the disease is more severe in women with onset in the mid-thirties. Those patients whose disease begins with pure optic neuritis or pure sensory symptoms have a better prognosis than those with other syndromes. The average onset is between the second and fourth decades.

Table 4.9. Symptoms and signs in multiple sclerosis (in order of frequency)

Symptoms	Signs
Muscle weakness	Spasticity
Ocular disturbance	Hyperreflexia
Urinary disturbance	Extensor plantars
Gait ataxia	Absent abdominal reflexes
Paraesthesiae	Intention tremor
Dysarthria	Optic atrophy
Mental disturbance	Nystagmus
Pain	Impaired vibration sense
Vertigo	Impaired position sense
Dysphagia	Impaired pain appreciation
Convulsions	Facial weakness
Hearing loss	Impairment of touch
Tinnitus	Impairment of temperature

Symptoms and signs

These are listed in Table 4.9.

Relapses and remissions are very common in MS. The acute episodes may develop over several hours or days and resolve gradually over weeks.

The diagnosis of MS depends on demonstrating scattered lesions throughout the central nervous system. In a proportion of patients the disease runs a chronic progressive course, with no remission. In such cases, most commonly in the elderly, it is essential to exclude other disease such as spinal cord compression.

Although there is considerable individual variation, the majority of patients will experience progressive deterioration, often punctuated with acute relapses. This results in a progressively increasing difficulty in walking, a spastic ataxic gait, failing vision and urinary difficulty.

Investigations

Although the diagnosis is commonly made on clinical grounds, laboratory support, particularly in the early stages, can be invaluable.

The CSF lymphocyte count is usually less than 20 cells per mm^3. The IgG total protein ratio is raised at greater than 15% which is taken along with a serum IgG sample to compensate for any leakage of blood into the CSF at the time of lumbar puncture. Oligoclonal banding in the CSF is the most sensitive test.

Electrophysiology—visual evoked potentials (VERs) are used to check the integrity of the visual pathway. This test is abnormal in all patients with a previous attack of optic neuritis, even if the visual acuity has returned to normal.

Myelography—may be necessary to exclude a mass lesion in patients who present with a spinal cord syndrome.

MRI *scanning* (Fig. 4.11) is the most sensitive method of providing evidence of multiple lesions within the central nervous system. T2 weighted images will show established pathology, and gadallinium enhances areas thought to relate to an acute breakdown in the blood–brain barrier associated with a new lesion.

Differential diagnosis

1. Visual loss—consider optic nerve compression, vascular or toxic disease.
2. Paraplegia—think of other causes of cord compression.
3. Ataxia—consider tumour and vascular disease.

Treatment

There is no cure for multiple sclerosis.
1. An acute relapse may be shortened by an intensive course of i.v. methyl-prednisolone 500 mg per 24 hours for 5 days.
2. Dietary regimens have been studied, but appear to confer no long-term benefit. Nevertheless many patients claim benefit from linoleic acid or sun-flower seed oil, and take a low animal fat or gluten-free diet.
3. Immunopressive drugs such as azathioprine and cyclophosphamide confer no long-term benefit.

Symptomatic management

1. Infections are controlled with antibiotics.
2. For bladder dysfunction anticholinergic drugs (probanthine and terodi-line) may reduce urinary urgency and frequency but can precipitate acute retention. A Conveen sheath may help incontinence but there is no ade-quate apparatus for females. Intermittent self-catheterisation in the early stages is usually followed by a permanent indwelling catheter or a suprapu-bic catheter. A small number of patients are managed with an ileal bladder, with the ureters transplanted into an ileal loop.
3. Baclofen, diazepam and dantrolene may reduce muscular spasms but, in the higher doses, the limbs may become excessively hypotonic. This can result in patients collapsing if they use their spasticity to maintain the upright posture. Some patients use a self-administered intrathecal baclofen pump.
4. If the immobile patient is left for periods without passive exercises, then tendon contractures appear which may have to be treated surgically.
5. Special attention is paid to support services, including physiotherapy, occu-pational therapy and adaptation of the house.

Most patients remain active, working normally in the early stages of the dis-ease. Thereafter they are managed at home and occasionally admitted to hos-pital or a special young disabled unit for respite care. The average duration of the disease is 20 years from time of diagnosis. Some patients are still ambulant 20 years or more after onset.

CEREBRAL INFECTIONS

BACTERIAL MENINGITIS

Bacterial meningitis is due to inflammation of the meninges, but not primarily brain parenchyma. Any cerebral cortex changes occur as the result of vascular occlusion. Meningitis in children is usually caused by blood-borne organisms spreading from paranasal sinuses, middle ear, mastoid or respiratory infections. Organisms may enter the skull from a fracture. Neonates are often infected with *Haemophilus influenzae* which is rare after the age of 6 years. Adults are usually affected by the meningococcus, with its haemorrhagic skin rash, or *Streptococcus pneumoniae*.

Symptoms and signs

These comprise fever, headache, fits, confusion and alteration of conscious level. There is a rapid onset over 24 hours. The patient is sick, irritable, with neck stiffness, photophobia and limited straight leg raising.

Diagnosis

Confirmed by CSF cell count and culture. If there are papilloedema and focal neurological signs, a CT brain scan is required to exclude an abscess. CSF usually contains 1000 white cells per ml and most are polymorphs. There is increased protein and a low glucose. Organisms may be hard to find in the partially antibiotic-treated patient.

Chronic meningitis with cranial nerve signs, hydrocephalus and a moderate CSF lymphocytic pleocytosis raises the possibility of tuberculous meningitis. Confirmation of this diagnosis may be difficult but is aided by a positive history of tuberculosis contact, TB on the chest X-ray, or a positive Heaf test. If in doubt, the patient should be treated.

Treatment

In bacterial meningitis, intravenous antibiotics are given as soon as possible, eg ampicillin, chloramphenicol, benzyl penicillin, cefatoxime. When sensitivity of the organism is known, a specific antibiotic is used and continued for 14–21 days. Serial CSF examinations may help to monitor difficult cases.

Prognosis

The mortality is 8–10%. Outlook is best in meningococcal meningitis. Long-term complications include deafness, epilepsy and mental retardation.

NEUROSYPHILIS

This is a rare condition. The majority of deaths occur from cardiovascular or neurological complications caused by the spirochaete *Treponema pallidum*. The early stages of primary infection may be followed years later by meningovascular involvement. Gummata in the brain occasionally occur and will mimic a space-occupying lesion. Tabes dorsalis and general paralysis of the insane may develop years later.

Tabes dorsalis

Tabes is due to degeneration of posterior roots of spinal nerves and posterior column of the spinal cord.

Symptoms and signs

These include lightning pain (rectal and bladder 'crises'), painless urinary retention, impotence, falling in the dark because of the loss of proprioception, Argyll Robertson pupils, bilateral ptosis, optic atrophy, high stepping, stamping gait, Romberg's test positive and patchy sensory loss to face in a cuirasse distribution. Charcot joints develop with absent deep pain and joint position sense.

General paralysis of the insane (GPI)

GPI is caused by progressive inflammation of the brain parenchyma by the spirochaete.

Symptoms and signs

Lack of judgement, personality deterioration, grandiose ideas. Cognitive impairment, Argyll Robertson pupils, tremor of tongue (rare), limb tremor, increased reflexes with extensor plantars are also present.

Investigations

CSF and blood, VDRL, *Treponema pallidum* haemaglutination assay (TPHA), Fluorescent treporemal antibody test (FTA). Lymphocytic pleocytosis is seen in most cases. The IgG/total protein ratio is raised.

Treatment

3 weeks of intramuscular penicillin. Response to treatment is measured by the number of cells in the protein CSF. When treated early, improvement may occur.

INTRACRANIAL ABSCESS

CT brain scanning has improved early diagnosis of this disease but the mortality is still 30%. Local spread of infection occurs from middle ear, mastoid, sinuses or local bone infection. Blood spread is often from a remote site such as chronic pulmonary or cyanotic congenital heart disease. Abscesses tend to develop in areas of focal ischaemia or necrosis in grey or white matter, cerebral cortex and cerebellum. Beginning as a cerebritis with a necrotic centre, it then slowly enlarges with capsule formation. If untreated, the abscess slowly expands or ruptures into a ventricle or subarachnoid space with resultant pressure on the brainstem.

Symptoms and signs

The local infection site may be apparent, e.g. mastoid. Focal neurological symptoms may be seen. Headaches and papilloedema point to raised intracranial pressure.

Focal signs are:

1. Dominant hemisphere—dysphagia, hemiparesis
2. Temporal lobe—dysphasia, quadrantanopia and epilepsy
3. Frontal lobe—disinhibition, epilepsy
4. Cerebellum—nystagmus and ataxia.

Investigations

CT and MRI scans are useful. EEG will show a focal abnormality. Lumbar puncture should be avoided because of the risk of coning.

Blood cultures, especially in haematogenous spread, are required, as are chest and skull X-rays, middle ear and mastoid films.

Complications

Pus may rupture into a ventricle. Epilepsy is often difficult to control.

Differential diagnosis

Other intracranial masses and meningitis.

Treatment

Surgical drainage with instillation of antibiotics, and intravenous antibiotics, usually broad spectrum with cover for gram-negative bacteria and anaerobes.

INTRACRANIAL THROMBOPHLEBITIS

This may occur in the presence of infection but is now more common in a non-infective form. It is also seen in women on the contraceptive pill and in patients with protein S or C deficiency, or in those with a general increase in clotting tendency.

1. Cavernous sinus thrombosis may result from spread of infection from the face or nose. It is characterised by orbital oedema and proptosis, leading to cheimosis and ophthalmoplegia.
2. Thrombosis of the lateral sinus may be caused by spread of infection from the middle ear and lead to raised intracranial pressure.
3. Superior sagittal sinus thrombosis is characterised by headaches, monoparesis or hemiparesis and fits.

Investigations

1. CT brain scans may show a contrast enhancing venous sinus.
2. MRI scans may show a venous filling failure.
3. Intravenous digital subtraction angiography shows a failure to fill affected venous sinuses.
4. CSF may show raised pressure and protein, but no cells.

Treatment is with antibiotics. Anticoagulants may be indicated in certain cases. Although many patients make a good recovery morbidity and mortality are significant.

VIRAL DISEASE OF THE CENTRAL NERVOUS SYSTEM

1. Neurotropic viruses attack certain nerve cells, e.g. poliomyelitis affects the anterior horn cell and herpes zoster the dorsal root ganglion.
2. Viruses cause inflammation of the meninges.
3. Viruses cause acute demyelinating disease with inflammation. This affects the white matter, causing an encephalitis and myelitis.
4. 'Slow' viruses are unconventional agents or 'prions'. They cause a spongiform encephalopathy, the rare Creutzfeldt–Jakob disease. This condition is transmitted in a specific way, either by the use of contaminated instrumentation or by injection or implantation of affected tissue, e.g. corneal transplant. The disease usually presents after a very long incubation period.

Acute aseptic viral meningitis

This is a self-limiting illness with meningeal irritation and CSF pleocytosis, with no evidence of bacteria or fungi. The majority of cases are viral but *Leptospira* and *Mycoplasma pneumoniae* have been reported. Non-infectious agents, such as contrast dye and fluid from CSF cysts, can cause a similar picture. The commonest viruses involved are enteroviruses, coxsackie, Epstein–Barr, herpes simplex, polio, HIV and lymphocytic choriomeningitis. This is a condition usually seen in children and young adults and is uncommon over the age of 50.

Symptoms and signs

These include fever, neck stiffness and headache. The CSF is clear, with a raised lymphocyte count, raised protein and sterile culture.

The duration of the illness is 1–2 weeks. The vast majority of patients make a complete recovery. The prognosis is excellent.

Differential diagnosis

Partially treated bacterial meningitis, with a low CSF cell count, epidural or subdural abscess, tuberculous meningitis, neurosyphilis, fungal (cryptococcal) infection, neurosarcoidosis, carcinomatous meningitis and leukaemia.

ENCEPHALITIS

Encephalitis is defined as inflammation of the surface of the brain. Encephalitis must be distinguished from metabolic or toxic causes of stupor fits and confusional states. Common viruses causing encephalitis include mumps, measles, varicella and influenza. Herpes simplex encephalitis is often a fatal condition characterised by haemorrhagic necrosis of the temporal lobe.

Symptoms and signs

These include headache, drowsiness, confusion, odd behaviour, focal neurological signs, coma, fits and papilloedema.

Investigations

A CT brain scan often shows a swollen low-density temporal lobe in herpes simplex encephalitis. The EEG is very helpful, showing focal slow wave abnormality.

Specific features of herpes simplex encephalitis (HSE)

1. It is of abrupt onset.
2. There is a rapid progression but great variability in the clinical picture.
3. 75% have fever, personality change, headache or dysphasia.
4. 30% have fits, autonomic dysfunction, ataxia, hemiparesis.
5. The EEG is abnormal in 80%, characterised by high-voltage complexes of a periodic nature over the temporal lobe.
6. A brain biopsy of the temporal lobe is diagnostic.

Treatment

Intravenous acyclovir, if given rapidly, can improve the survival rate to 80%. If untreated, the mortality from HSE is 70%. Intravenous dexamethasone may reduce cerebral oedema.

Acute disseminated post-infectious encephalomyelitis

Characterised by perivascular cerebral infiltration and patchy demyelination of the white matter of brain and spinal cord, this differs from acute viral encephalitis in which there is grey matter involvement and no demyelination. There are 100 cases per 100 000 population. It may complicate acute childhood illnesses, such as measles, influenza, rubella, Epstein–Barr virus infection and rarely may follow vaccination for influenza, rubella, smallpox and rabies. There are encephalitic and myelitic forms and the CSF findings are the same as those in acute viral encephalitis. Early vaccination reduces the risk of this condition. Steroids may help to reduce complications, but efficacy is not proven. In mild cases recovery is complete. Morbidity and mortality are significant.

HERPES ZOSTER (shingles)

Infection is characterised by acute inflammation of the dorsal root ganglia, with a painful vesicular eruption in the involved dermatome. Motor root involvement occurs in 15% of cases. The disease may emerge at any age, but the risk increases with advancing years. The condition may complicate trauma, surgery or deep X-ray therapy, and there is an increased incidence in patients with systemic illness such as pneumonia.

Symptoms and signs

1. The skin is hypersensitive and associated with painful paraesthesiae.
2. When it affects the ophthalmic division, it may produce corneal ulceration, scarring and blindness.
3. Geniculate herpes (Ramsay Hunt syndrome) is characterised by vertigo, pain in the ear, and facial palsy with a ventricular rash on the tongue, palate and external auditory canal.

Treatment

1. Herpes zoster infection is treated with acyclovir.
2. Topical preparations are available.

3. Hydroxyuridine in solution can also be applied to the skin. The pain of post-herpetic neuralgia may be severe enough to warrant pethidine.

OTHER INFECTIOUS DISEASES AFFECTING THE NERVOUS SYSTEM

Poliomyelitis

Though effective vaccination has made this disease rare, it still occurs in the Third World and sporadically elsewhere. There are three types of polio virus and the incubation period is 3–21 days.

Symptoms and signs

An initial febrile illness with sore throat and headache that may be so mild it is not noticed. The major illness is accompanied by signs of meningism with muscle pains and flaccid paralysis of the limbs. Bulbar involvement causes dysphagia, dysphonia and instability of the blood pressure. Respiratory paralysis may be a result of diaphragmatic, intercostal or bulbar involvement.

The paralysed limbs are hypotonic, areflexic and quite characteristic of an anterior horn (lower motor neurone) lesion. There is no sensory involvement. Paralysis, though rare, is more likely if vigorous exercise has been taken at the time of the initial illness.

Investigations

1. The diagnosis is principally a clinical one.
2. Lumbar puncture shows a CSF with increased numbers of cells (early on polymorphs, then lymphocytes) together with increased protein levels.
3. The virus can be isolated from throat swabs but more successfully from the stools.

Treatment

Treatment includes analgesia for muscle pain and respiratory support if there is a reduction in regular measurements of vital capacity. Recovery from paralysis is variable but may take up to 6 months—and the patient may be left with one or more wasted, weak and hypotonic limbs, as well as possibly needing long-term respiratory support. Intensive physiotherapy is required for muscle weakness.

Prophylaxis is with three doses of oral live polio vaccine. In children it is given in a sugar lump with a 6–8 week interval between the doses. A reinforcing dose is given at school entry. HIV positive subjects may excrete the virus for longer than normal subjects, and household contact should be warned of this.

Tetanus

Tetanus results from infection of a wound with *Clostridium tetani*, a commensal in the human gastrointestinal tract and also found commonly in soil. Farm and agricultural workers are especially at risk and the wound is often trivial, e.g. a splinter. The tetanus spores can remain dormant for years at the site of a previous wound and only germinate when conditions are correct, i.e. anaerobic. Tetanus neonatorum occurs in neonates when the umbilical stump is infected.

Pathology
The organism stays locally at the site of infection but produces a neurotoxin which attacks motor nerve endings and the anterior horn cells of the spinal cord. It also attacks sympathetic nerve fibres.

Symptoms and signs
After a variable incubation period there is:

Trismus. Spasm of the masseter muscles (lockjaw) spreads to affect other facial and neck muscles (risus sardonicus). Eventually muscle spasm may affect the trunk and back, which is arched.

Violent spasms. In severe cases there may be generalised spasms occurring every few minutes. These can be provoked by extraneous stimuli such as noise or by disturbing the ill patient in any way.

Exhaustion. The severe spasms or convulsions may exhaust the patient.

Pneumonia. Involvement of the respiratory muscles together with the convulsions leads to inhalation pneumonia.

Local tetanus. Sometimes tetanus remains localised to the area around the wound site.

Treatment
Local. An obviously infected wound should be opened and drained. Surgery should be delayed for at least 1 hour following the administration of antitoxin.

Antitoxin. Either human or equine antitoxin should be given as soon as the diagnosis is suspected (diagnosis is usually made on clinical grounds alone).

Antibiotics. Large doses of intravenous penicillin are required and should be started immediately.

Supportive. Minor spasms may be relieved by diazepam. In more severe cases curarisation and artificial ventilation are required (the latter is often unavailable in Third World countries).

Prevention. Tetanus is a preventable disease. Everyone should be immunised by means of toxoid vaccines. The initial course should be maintained by booster injections at 5 yearly intervals. Boosters should also be given following at-risk wounds when a long-acting penicillin is also given.

Prognosis
The neonatal form of tetanus is almost always fatal, while the local form has a good prognosis. The rate of onset and severity of convulsions determines the outcome in others, as do the medical facilities available. Overall mortality is still 40–50%.

Botulism

This is caused by poisoning with an enterotoxin derived from *Clostridium botulinum* found in contaminated and often tinned meat or fish.

Symptoms and signs

After nausea, vomiting and diarrhoea which develop 10–40 hours after ingestion of the contaminated food, the hallmark of the disease is the presence of severe autonomic (hypotension and dryness of the mouth and throat) and bulbar (diplopia, dysphagia and nasal regurgitation) palsy. Respiratory and limb weaknesses also occur.

Treatment

This is supportive only, and the mortality, once there is bulbar involvement, is high.

INTRACRANIAL TUMOURS

Tumours of the brain may cause symptoms of a focal nature depending on their location. Raised intracranial pressure is another mode of presentation. Because the skull is a rigid box, any rise in pressure will force the brain downwards. Herniation of the medial temporal lobe occurs through the tentorium, and so the brainstem becomes compressed against the opposite free edge of the tentorium. The cerebellar tonsils are forced downwards between the foramen magnum and the medulla. Vital brainstem functions such as respiration, conscious level, blood pressure, heart rate and circulation are then impaired. Patients are treated by acute medical and surgical decompression.

The behaviour of a tumour depends on a number of factors:

1. histology, speed of growth and tendency to bleed
2. local invasion
3. oedema surrounding the tumour mass
4. obstruction to CSF flow leading to hydrocephalus in the posterior fossa fourth ventricular tumour
5. location: tumour on the parasagittal cortex on one side will produce weakness of the opposite leg
6. raised intracranial pressure.

PRIMARY BRAIN TUMOURS

Most primary brain tumours are malignant and do not respond to treatment. Death for most patients occurs within 2 years. In adults the primary brain tumour arises from supporting tissues not from neurones. Of primary tumours, 50% are glial in origin, 30% arise from the meninges and the remainder from pituitary or ependymal tissue. Glial tumours include astrocytoma and oligodendroglioma. A glioblastoma is a poorly differentiated, highly malignant tumour (Fig. 4.12). Assessing the degree of malignancy is important. This depends on the number of mitotic figures and amount of vascular

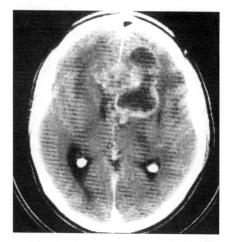

Fig. 4.12 Malignant glioma. Contrast enhanced CT scan shows irregular enhancement with surrounding oedema involving the left frontal lobe and extending into the right hemisphere across genu of the corpus callosum.

hyperplasia, necrosis, cellularity and haemorrhage. The pilocytic astrocytoma and the radiosensitive reticulum sarcoma are relatively benign tumours. Glioblastoma and oligodendrogliomas are prone to haemorrhage and may therefore be mistaken for a stroke.

Ependymomas represent 5% of primary brain tumours and develop at any site along the ependymal lining of the walls of the ventricles, even in the aqueduct and spinal cord. They spread via the ventricles and subarachnoid space in 20% of cases.

Investigations
The diagnosis is usually confirmed by CT or MRI. Biopsy is recommended in most cases of single tumour to determine histology.

Differential diagnosis
This includes brain abscess, infarction and encephalitis.

Treatment
Treatment may be surgical or by irradiation, or both. Chemotherapy is controversial and the results disappointing. Dexamethasone reduces brain oedema. Primary brain lymphoma is rare but is increasing with HIV and the use of immunosuppressives. This type of tumour metastasises to the dura and is treated by deep X-ray therapy (DXT).

CNS METASTASES

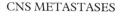

1. These represent 20% of all brain tumours (Fig. 4.13).
2. 80% are solitary with an identifiable primary; 15% are late manifestations after the primary has been successfully treated and 5% are solitary lesions with no known source.

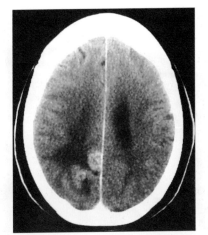

Fig. 4.13 Malignant deposits. Two enhancing lesions in the upper hemisphere and a cystic lesion with an enhancing ring in the right thalamus.

3. The mode of spread is often haematogenous via microtumour emboli.
4. Deposits occur in proportion to the size and blood flow of various regions of the brain.
5. Lung and breast adenocarcinomas and malignant melanoma have a high micro-embolic release rate, and are prone to vascular endothelial penetration into brain tissue.
6. A biopsy may be necessary for a single lesion, and often yields an adenocarcinoma but no indication of the primary site.

Treatment
1. DXT and steroids.
2. Intrathecal radio-labelled monoclonal antibodies for targeting radiotherapy to the tumour tissue represents an important development. This is useful in carcinomatous meningitis but less successful with solid tumours.
3. Methotrexate and cytarabin are usually of value in meningeal metastases.

MENINGIOMAS

15% of intracranial tumours arising from arachnoid cells are meningiomas. Common sites include cerebral convexity, sphenoid wing, parasagittal regions, olfactory groove, posterior fossa tentorium, cerebellopontine angle, and occasionally the sellar region.

Symptoms and signs
Patients may present with seizures from the indentation of healthy cerebral cortex. Focal sensory hallucinations are often mistaken for transient cerebral ischaemic attacks. Focal motor or dysphasic episodes are often a presenting feature in a slow growing benign tumour.

Sometimes there are no symptoms until the tumour is very large, when it presents with raised intracranial pressure or a progressive hemiparesis.

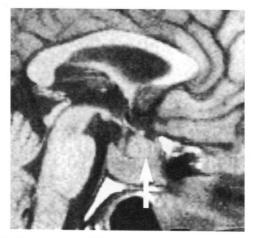

Fig. 4.14 Pituitary adenoma. Mid sagittal MRI scan (T1 weighted) showing normal midline structures. The pituitary gland is grossly expanded up into the suprasellar cistern.

Investigations
A CT brain scan shows a dense mass with a uniform pattern of enhancement after contrast.

Treatment
Treatment is by surgical removal if possible (sometimes the tumour is too large to remove). Recurrence is common but slow growth is measured in years. In the elderly surgery may be unnecessary.

TUMOURS IN THE SELLAR REGION (Fig. 4.14)

Acidophilic adenomas present with acromegaly, and basophilic adenomas with Cushing's disease. Microadenomas and prolactinomas are prolactin-secreting tumours which cause less obvious physical changes.

Infertility, galactorrhoea and amenorrhoea may be present. A tiny lesion, it is sometimes difficult to detect on a CT scan even with high resolution and contrast. MRI scanning is more accurate. Serum prolactin levels are helpful.

Treatment
Treatment is with either oral bromocriptine 2.5 mg twice daily or surgical removal, particularly if there are signs of compression of optic nerves. DXT may be necessary.

Chromophobe adenoma

This tumour may present as large mass with no endocrinopathy or with hypopituitarism and diabetes insipidus. CT appearances are of a high-density lesion with contrast enhancement. 50% of cases are referred because of visual

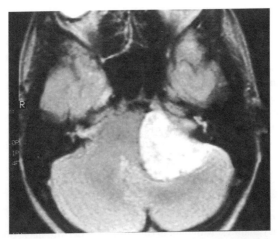

Fig. 4.15 Acoustic neuroma. An MRI scan (T2 weighted) through level of the internal auditory meati. The large high signal area in the cerebellopontine angle is a tumour.

failure. This is often of very gradual onset and patients are unaware of the deficit. Routine skull X-ray may show a large sellar turcica.

Treatment is by surgical removal.

ACOUSTIC NEUROMAS (Fig. 4.15)

Representing 8% of all intracranial tumours, acoustic neuromas are generally unilateral but bilateral in 5%. Tumours arise from Schwann cells that envelop axons of the vestibular branch of the eighth nerve.

Symptoms and signs

Presentation is often of very gradual onset. There is progressive unilateral deafness, numbness of the ipsilateral face and an absent corneal reflex.

Mild seventh nerve weakness occurs as does brainstem compression with ataxia, weak legs and upper motor neurone signs. Papilloedema is a late feature.

Investigations and treatment

Brainstem auditory evoked potential monitoring is sensitive. MRI scanning is more sensitive than CT, especially for intracanalicular tumours.

Treatment is by surgical removal. Intraoperative brainstem auditory evoked potential monitoring is used to detect excessive traction on the brainstem. This has reduced morbidity to less than 3%. Care must be taken to preserve facial nerve function.

NERVE ROOT AND PLEXUS DISEASE

The peripheral nervous system is that part of the nervous system lying outside or distal to the pia arachnoid membrane. Disease of these fibres is characterised by weakness, wasting, pain, and sensory and reflex loss. Anterior horn cell diseases, including syringomyelia and motor neurone disease, also produce lower motor neurone signs. A knowledge of the anatomy of the nerve supply to myotomes, dermatomes and deep tendon reflexes is essential in order to make an accurate assessment of the localisation of pathology. Motor and sensory nerve conduction velocities may distinguish between segmental demyelination and axonal disease. Identification of slowing of nerve conduction across two points of the nerve may point to a source of entrapment, for example in the carpal tunnel syndrome. Concentric needle electromyography is of value in nerve and muscle disease. Nerve biopsy, usually sural or superficial radial, may be of value in identifying some causes of peripheral nerve disease.

CERVICAL ROOT LESIONS

Symptoms and signs (Table 4.10)

These may manifest with pain in the arm, shoulder and neck, often in a radicular distribution or in the myotomes, with numbness and paraesthesiae in the dermatomes. Wasting and weakness occurs in a radicular distribution.

Causes are most commonly cervical spondylosis, but also the Pancoast lung tumour affecting the T1 root, herpes zoster and Guillain–Barré syndrome.

BRACHIAL PLEXUS DISEASE

The brachial plexus consists of three trunks—upper, middle and lower—comprising C5/6/7/8 T1 nerve roots. The plexus is liable to damage by trauma, tumour invasion and compression by a fibrous band or cervical rib.

1. Lower plexus. C8/T1 (medial cord) may be damaged by hyperextension of the arm, with or without traction. A birth injury is called Klumpke's paralysis. Acquired lesions include dislocation of the shoulder, thoracic outlet syndrome (cervical rib or fibrous band) and tumour invasion. These result in paralysis of the small muscles of the hand, and painful paraesthesiae of the medial part of the forearm and hand.

2. Middle plexus. C5/6/7/8 (lateral cord) is often damaged in a motorcycle accident, with violent downward pulling on the arm which may result in paralysis of biceps, flexors of the wrist and fingers, together with sensory loss to the lateral aspects of the forearm and hand.

3. Upper plexus. C5/6/7 (posterior cord) damage may result in a Duchenne-Erb's paralysis, an unusual paralysis of deltoid, triceps, brachioradialis and extensor muscles of wrist and fingers. The patient adopts the 'waiter tip' posture.

NEURALGIC AMYOTROPHY

This is an acute syndrome of excruciating pain in the shoulder or arm, which when resolved is followed by rapid-onset focal weakness and wasting not always of a specific root or peripheral nerve type.

It often follows infection, inoculation, trauma or surgery and is the result of acute inflammation of the nerve roots, plexus or its branches. Patients slowly

Table 4.10. Clinical features of cervical root lesions

Pain	Segmental root
Shoulder	C5
Lateral forearm, thumb and index finger	C6
Posterior arm, scapulamedial border	C7
Medial forearm	C8
Medial arm and hand	T1
Weak muscles	
Spinati, deltoid, rhomboid, biceps	C5
Biceps, brachioradialis, pronator, supernator, extensor carpi radialis	C6
Sternal head of pectoralis major, triceps, wrist extensors	C7
Finger flexors	C8
Intrinsic hand muscles	T1
Sensory loss to lateral upper arm	
Lateral forearm, thumb and index finger	C5 and C6
Middle finger, posterior forearm	C6 and C7
Medial forearm, little finger	C8
Inner aspect of upper arm	T1
Deep tendon reflexes affected	
Biceps	C5
Brachioradialis	C6
Triceps	C7
—	C8
—	T1

recover, and prognosis is generally good, but weakness may persist for months despite active physiotherapy.

THORACIC OUTLET SYNDROME

This is produced by pressure on the medial cord of the brachial plexus, often by a cervical rib or fibrous band. Features include pain in the inner aspect of the arm, after carrying heavy weights, and weakness of the small muscles of the hand and sensory loss in a C8/T1 distribution. There may be a supraclavicular bruit with or without a thrill and obliteration of the radial pulse on arm hyperabduction.

A chest X-ray may show a cervical rib. A fibrous band or thickened scalenus anticus muscle will not show on plain X-ray. This will only be evident at operation. A subclavian arteriogram may show kinking or compression of the subclavian artery. Differential diagnosis includes carpal tunnel syndrome and cervical spondylitic radiculopathy.

Treatment is surgical.

CAUDA EQUINA LESIONS

Common causes of cauda equina syndrome include fracture dislocation of the vertebra, tumour, arteriovenous malformation and prolapsed intervertebral disc. Posterolateral protrusion affects one root only; central disc lesions may affect several roots.

Symptoms and signs
The cauda equina syndrome is characterised by neurogenic claudication, i.e. pain and foot drop worsening on walking.

Reduction in straight leg raising, weak muscles, depressed deep tendon reflexes and sensory impairment depend on which roots are involved. There is urinary retention with bladder distension and incontinence, loss of anal reflex, impotence, and numb legs and buttocks.

Investigations and treatment
Plain X-rays of lumbar sacral spine, CT radiculogram and an MRI scan are useful.

Surgical decompression is mandatory if bladder function is involved. Delay may produce permanent damage. Single nerve root disease with pain and paraesthesiae may respond to traction. Bedrest on hard boards may help. Surgery may be required if there is wasting and weakness, or central disc protrusion.

PERIPHERAL NEUROPATHY

There are a number of conditions where there is non-acute traumatic degeneration of the nerves of the limbs. The clinical picture is variable. It may be of rapid onset as in post-infective polyneuritis, or the slow-onset hereditary sensorimotor neuropathy (HSMN), sometimes called Charcot-Marie-Tooth disease. The following types are recognised:
1. acute Guillain–Barré syndrome
2. subacute or chronic distal neuropathy, which can be motor, sensory, autonomic or mixed
3. mononeuropathies
   a. entrapment type
   b. non-compressive mononeuritis multiplex as seen in diabetes mellitus, polyarteritis nodosa, carcinoma and amyloidosis.

Pathology
1. Acute infective allergic process e.g. Guillain-Barré syndrome.
2. Occlusion of the vasa nervorum with focal infarction of the nerve, e.g. polyarteritis nodosa.
3. Amyloid infiltration.
4. Segmental demyelination, such as in diabetes and diphtheria.
5. Peripheral dying back phenomenon, as in hereditary neuropathy.

ACUTE GUILLAIN-BARRÉ SYNDROME (GBS)

This is an acute demyelinating neuropathy which accounts for 40% of all adult neuropathies. It is multifocal and proximal, and appears to be caused by an immune response directed against a component of myelin in the peripheral nerve. The decreased suppressive T cell response in GBS is consistent with a cell-mediated immune response. There may also be humoral antigen, although the basis for this is unknown. It is the rationale behind plasma exchange treatment. A non-specific viral infection precedes the onset of neurological symptoms by 2–4 weeks in 50% of cases.

Symptoms and signs

Weakness spreads upwards from the legs. Involvement is diffuse, symmetrical, and usually reaches maximal effect within 4 weeks. There is mild distal paraesthesiae, back muscular pain in 50% of cases and dysphagia.

Areflexia, proximal weakness, and later total paralysis are seen. Asymmetrical facial weakness occurs in 50% of cases. Other cranial nerve motor weakness gives rise to dysphagia, dysarthria and a weak cough.

Respiratory weakness is an important sign, and may not be immediately apparent because of the lack of distress on the face. Serial lung function measurements are therefore essential.

Autonomic signs appear in 70% of cases. Sympathetic features include orthostatic hypotension even when sitting, transient bladder paralysis and tachycardia. Parasympathetic features are generalised warmth, bradycardia and the inappropriate ADH syndrome.

Investigations

There is a raised CSF protein yet no increase in the number of white cells. Nerve conduction studies may be normal or show slow conduction velocity and block with increase in distal latency.

Treatment and prognosis

All patients should be admitted to hospital because respiratory failure may occur at any stage during the illness. Some patients need artificial ventilation.

The major causes of a 13% mortality are pulmonary embolism, autonomic dysfunction and overwhelming infection.

The illness is usually complete within 3–6 months but plasmaphaeresis within the first 2 weeks of neurological symptoms may accelerate recovery. The role of steroids is still unresolved.

Most patients make a good recovery but 5% will be left with a mild or severe disability and 10% will experience relapses.

SUBACUTE AND CHRONIC NEUROPATHIES

The picture is motor, sensory, autonomic or mixed. In most cases the feet are more severely affected than the hands. Although in 50–60% no cause can be identified, it does occur with diabetes mellitus, toxins (N-hexane), drugs (amiodarone) and alcohol, carcinoma (often occult) or vasculitis (SLE or polyarteritis), vitamin deficiency, e.g. B_{12}, and hereditary Charcot-Marie-Tooth disease.

Symptoms and signs

There is slowly progressive sensory loss, with numbness and tingling in the feet and hands. The fingers are clumsy and the feet often catch the ground, wearing the tips of shoes.

Wasting of distal muscles occurs with areflexia (sensory neuropathies may have intact deep tendon reflexes). A glove and stocking distribution of sensory loss is found.

Perforating skin ulcers, neuropathic joints and foot deformities (particularly in hereditary neuropathy) occur.

Investigations

1. Drug, occupational, social and family history together with details of alcohol intake.
2. Blood sugar, vitamin B_{12} level, porphyrins, paraproteins.
3. Chest X-ray.
4. Nerve conduction studies, EMGs.
5. CSF. If CSF protein is high, there may be inflammatory demyelinating neuropathy which can respond to steroids or plasma exchange.

Treatment

1. Depends on underlying cause.
2. Vitamin B_{12} injections, tight control of diabetes, removal of tumour.
3. Symptomatic treatment: below the knee orthotic splints.
4. Practical aids to daily living.

Prognosis

Toxic neuropathies will improve when the cause is removed. Hereditary neuropathies will slowly progress with increasing disability which rarely shortens life span.

ENTRAPMENT MONONEUROPATHY

Incomplete injury to the peripheral nerve where the nerve is macroscopically intact is common in compressive neuropathy. The nerve may be compressed against bone or tendon. In the early stages the patient may only complain of numbness and paraesthesia, but when the syndrome is well developed a fixed sensory loss and muscle atrophy may be present. By this stage any treatment is unlikely to result in complete recovery. It is therefore important to diagnose entrapment syndromes early.

Features of upper and lower limb peripheral nerve lesions are shown in Tables 4.11 and 4.12.

CARPAL TUNNEL SYNDROME

This is caused by compression of the median nerve at the wrist. Features include tingling, numbness and pain in the tips of the fingers, thumb, index and middle finger which may waken the patient at night. Less commonly there will be weakness of the abductor pollicis brevis.

Table 4.11. Peripheral nerve lesions—arm

Nerve	Weakness	Sensory loss
Axillary/circumflex	Deltoid	Patchy over deltoid
Long thoracic	Serratus anterior—winged scapula	None
Musculocutaneous	Biceps (and absent jerk)	Lateral forearm
Radial spiral groove of humerus (upper arm)	Brachio radialis (and absent tendon jerk) wrist extensors, finger extensors, supinator and forearm plus triceps muscle (and absent tendon jerk) for a high lesion	Back of hand at base of thumb
Median at wrist	Thenar eminence, (abductor pollicis brevis)	Radial 3½ fingers
Ulnar at elbow	Flexor digitorum profundus (4/5, fingers) lumbricals (4/5), interossei, and hypothenar eminence.	Ulnar 1½ fingers

Table 4.12. Peripheral nerve lesions—leg

Nerve	Weakness	Sensory loss	Affected tendon reflex
Femoral	Quadriceps—iliopsoas (in a proximal lesion)	Anterior thigh medial shin	Knee jerk
Lateral cutaneous nerve of thigh	None	Anterior and lateral thigh	None
Obturator (rare)	Adductors of hip	Medial thigh	—
Common peroneal (lateral popliteal)	Dorsiflexors and eversion of foot = foot drop	Lateral shin dorsum of foot	None
Posterior tibial	Plantar flexion of foot	Sole of foot	Ankle jerk
Sciatic	Hip extensor abduction and knee flexion	Lateral shin sole rear of calf	Ankle jerk

The syndrome is commonest in females in their 50s. There is an increased frequency of the syndrome with hypothyroidism, acromegaly, the contraceptive pill, pregnancy and rheumatoid arthritis.

Reduced pinprick and light touch in the tips of the radial 2½ fingers and thumb are seen. Later features include wasting and weakness of the thenar muscles.

Treatment

Immediate relief of pain may be achieved by injecting steroids into the carpal tunnel and by wearing a night splint. Definitive treatment is section of the transverse carpal ligament.

ULNAR NERVE COMPRESSION

Repetitive minor injuries (often not reported by the patient) to the medial epicondyl region may result in localised slowing of ulnar nerve conduction across the elbow. This will ultimately result in progressive wasting of all small muscles of the hand except the thenar group. Sensory loss involves the fifth and ulnar half of the fourth finger.

Treatment consists of transposition of the ulnar nerve from the cubital tunnel to the anterior aspect of the arm.

LATERAL CUTANEOUS NERVE OF THE THIGH

This may be compressed by the inguinal ligament, usually in overweight people, producing the syndrome of meralgia paraesthetica. There is burning pain experienced over the anterolateral aspect of the thigh.

Weightloss is required and, sometimes, local steroid injection or, rarely, section of the nerve.

COMMON PERONEAL NERVE

It may be compressed at the head of the fibula from too tight a plaster cast. Sitting cross legged for long periods may also result in weakness of dorsiflexion and eversion of the foot. The pattern of sensory loss involves the lateral aspect of the leg, dorsum, and lateral aspect of the foot.

POSTERIOR TIBIAL NERVE

Entrapment at the transverse intertarsal ligament in the ankle, produces pain and paraesthesiae in the toes and ball of the foot. These symptoms are often worse on walking. Treatment is by avoiding the precipitating cause and weightloss. Sometimes, surgical release of the transverse intertarsal ligament is required.

DISEASE OF THE NEUROMUSCULAR JUNCTION

MYASTHENIA GRAVIS

Myasthenia gravis (MG) is an autoimmune disease characterised by fluctuating fatigueable weakness caused by a defect in neuromuscular transmission. It is often associated with other autoimmune diseases, such as pernicious anaemia, hypothyroidism and rheumatoid arthritis. Although the cause is unknown, an autoimmune response may be centred on the thymus with production of antibodies directed against striated muscle acetylcholine receptors.

The antiacetylcholine antibody is positive in 95% of patients. The condition is associated with thymic hyperplasia in 70% of cases, thymic tumour in 15% and atrophy in the remainder.

Penicillamine may induce a temporary autoimmune myasthenia, with high antibody titres.

Symptoms and signs

The disease affects mainly adults. The purely ocular form is seen in 20% of patients and is more benign, with a lower titre of antiacetylcholine receptor antibodies than in the generalised form. Transient neonatal MG affects the offspring in 11% of affected mothers. It is a temporary condition, disappearing within 4–6 weeks.

There is diplopia, dysarthria, dysphagia, weakness of mastication and of the facial and proximal limb muscles.

Diagnosis is confirmed by a positive intravenous edrophonium chloride 'tensilon' test. Further confirmation may be obtained from repetitive nerve stimulation studies which demonstrate a decrimental muscle response.

Treatment

Treatment is with the long-acting anticholinesterase drug, pyridostigmine. The shorter acting neostigmine can aid swallowing. Alternate day prednisolone and immunosuppressive drugs such as azathioprine and cyclophosphamide may be required in severely affected patients.

Thymectomy is of benefit, particularly in young females, and is mandatory in all patients with thymoma.

Plasmaphoresis may be particularly helpful.

MUSCLE DISEASES

Rapid advances have been made in recent years in the understanding of the genetics of inherited myopathies, particularly Duchenne muscular dystrophy (DMD). Features of the inherited dystrophies are shown in Table 4.13.

Muscle diseases are often classified by the affected muscle group, e.g. facioscapulohumeral dystrophy. Metabolic disorders of muscles are rare and include McArdle's disease (myophosphorylase deficiency), periodic paralysis (hypo-normo-or hyperkalaemic), glycogen storage disorders, lipid myopathies and mitochondrial defects. Myotonia or a failure of muscle relaxation may accompany certain disorders, such as dystrophia myotonica.

DUCHENNE MUSCULAR DYSTROPHY (DMD)

This is an inherited sex-linked recessive disorder affecting males. The female offspring are carriers. There is a milder variant (Becker's muscular dystrophy). Prenatal diagnosis has been greatly improved by the availability of DNA markers for the DMD gene. The disease has the following features:

1. The onset of DMD is often before 4 and always under 10 years.
2. Walking is delayed in half the patients, and they present with clumsiness and frequent falls.

Table 4.13. Inherited muscular dystrophy

Type	Inheritance	Onset	Progress	Muscles affected	Serum CPK level
Duchenne (DMD) and the milder Becker's form	Sex-linked recessive males affected30% spontaneous mutation rate	Early childhood < 4 years	Rapid In wheelchair by age 10 Dead by age 20	Pelvic, pectoral girdle, myocardium	Very high, 10–20 000 iu/l
Limb girdle	Autosomal recessive	Variable Age 20–30 years	Variable slow progression	Pelvic, pectoral girdle	Slightly elevated, may be high
Facioscapulohumeral	Autosomal dominant	Variable Age 10–20 years	Variable, be severe within 20 years of onset	FSH, pelvic girdle	Elevated or normal
Dystrophia myotonica (myotonia congenita, rare, no wasting)	Autosomal dominant	Variable Age 20–60	Most patients unable to walk 20 years after onset	Facial, sternomastoid distal limbs	Normal

3. Signs include a waddling gait, and positive Gower's sign, characterised by the patient climbing up his own legs from a seated position on the floor.
4. Proximal limb weakness and pseudohypertrophy of the calves are common signs.
5. Cranial nerve muscles and bladder function are spared.
6. When confined to a wheelchair, these boys often develop kyphoscoliosis and hip and knee contractures. Reduced lung function then follows.
7. Most patients die before the age of 20.
8. Although the ECG is abnormal in 60% of cases, clinical cardiac involvement is rare.

Investigations

The serum creatine phosphokinase (CPK) is very high. Concentric needle EMGs show a myopathic pattern. Muscle biopsy shows a typical pattern with increased internal nuclei and variation of fibre size in the early stages, leading to fibrosis and fat replacement in severely affected muscles.

Treatment

There is no cure for this disease. Patients are treated with passive muscle stretching and spinal supports. It is important to keep weight down. Genetic counselling is essential.

5

ENDOCRINOLOGY

Martin Hartog

THE PITUITARY

ANTERIOR PITUITARY

Control of anterior pituitary function is via hypothalamic factors/hormones released into the hypophyseal portal system. The synthetic activity of hypothalamic cells is affected by circulating levels of the relevant hormone by negative and sometimes positive feedback.

Many of the hypothalamic hormones, or their synthetic analogues, are used in clinical practice either as agonists or, via downregulation of receptors on prolonged exposure to the hormone analogue, as antagonists (Table 5.1).

POSTERIOR PITUITARY

The posterior pituitary is made up of nerve cell tissue and it is controlled via neurological pathways.

Table 5.1. Clinical applications of hypothalamic factors/hormones or analogues

Hypothalamic factor/hormone	Clinical application
TRH	Diagnosis hyper/hypothyroidism Treatment thyroid carcinomas
LHRH (gonadorelin)	Via agonist effect: Treatment infertility Via antagonist effect: Treatment hormone dependent carcinomas, sexual precocity
Somatostatin	Treatment acromegaly, **GI** endocrine tumours
GHRH	Treatment shortness
CRH	Diagnosis Cushing's syndrome
Dopamine	Dopamine agonists: Treatment hyperprolactinaemia

PITUITARY TUMOURS

Tumours of the anterior pituitary may be derived from any of the hormone-secreting cells and are thus classified according to the hormone(s) they secrete.

Effects of pituitary tumours

Pituitary tumours may cause endocrine and/or pressure effects. The commonest pressure effects are headaches and visual field defects, the latter from upward extension of the tumour affecting the optic nerve(s), chiasma or tract, classically causing a bitemporal hemianopia.

The bony margin of the pituitary fossa can be seen on skull radiology but this gives no indication of pituitary anatomy. This can be demonstrated by either CT or, better, MRI scan which shows suprasellar extensions and may outline microadenomas too small to be seen otherwise.

HYPERSECRETION

Prolactin: Hyperprolactinaemia

Hyperprolactinaemia is common. It is much more frequent in women than in men and causes 10–15% of all secondary amenorrhoea in gynaecological clinics. The main causes are pregnancy, prolactinomas, hypothalamus/pituitary stalk lesions, primary hypothyroidism, chronic renal failure and the use of dopamine antagonists such as phenothiazines.

Symptoms and signs

Amenorrhoea, infertility, oestrogen deficiency and galactorrhoea are seen in women. Rarely, impotence is seen in men, and men and women may present with pressure effects of a prolactinoma.

Investigations

Diagnosis is based upon the detection of a raised serum prolactin on at least two occasions. Pregnancy must be excluded, a drug history taken and serum thyroid function tests performed. Many prolactinomas are too small to be seen on plain X-ray of the skull (microadenoma) but may be detected on CT or MRI scan.

Differential diagnosis

The normal level of serum prolactin is up to approximately 700 mU/l. Even higher levels in normally menstruating women are unlikely to be significant. Levels above 5000 mU/l usually indicate a prolactinoma. In women with a lesser degree of hyperprolactinaemia, a prolactinoma must be distinguished from a lesion affecting the hypothalamus or pituitary stalk, such as a non-functioning tumour.

Treatment
Dopamine agonist treatment, usually with the ergot alkaloid derivative bromocriptine, is very effective, reduces prolactin levels to normal and relieves symptoms. During a subsequent pregnancy there is a risk of tumour enlargement, rarely causing a visual field defect. A major long-term indication for treatment is the prevention of osteoporosis, by restoration of ovarian function, although this incurs the need for contraception. Because dopamine agonist-treatment also reduces the size of prolactinomas, they can usually be treated medically with long-term bromocriptine, and surgery or pituitary irradiation is not often needed.

Growth hormone (GH): Acromegaly/gigantism

This is an uncommon condition in which there are a number of physical and biochemical changes arising from excessive GH secretion, almost always from an anterior pituitary tumour.

Symptoms and signs (See Table 5.2, Figure 5.1)
Investigations
Diagnosis is predominantly clinical and is confirmed biochemically by measuring serum GH levels during an oral glucose tolerance test when, because of the suppressive effect of hyperglycaemia, the level normally falls to <5 mU/l. In acromegaly, owing to autonomous secretion of GH by the underlying tumour, normal suppression is not seen and GH levels may even rise paradoxically. In addition, a CT or MRI scan of the pituitary should be performed to demonstrate the tumour.

Differential diagnosis
The classical syndrome is readily recognised, but may be overlooked because of its slow progression; comparison with old photographs is invaluable.

Treatment
This is usually surgical, using the trans-sphenoidal route, when relatively small tumours may be excised, leaving normal pituitary function intact. Otherwise,

Table 5.2. Symptoms and signs of acromegaly

Symptoms	Signs
Change in appearance	Acromegalic facies
Enlargement of hands and feet	Large extremities
Paraesthesia of hands	Carpal tunnel syndrome
Sweating	Greasy, sweaty skin
Headaches	Prognathism (protrusion lower jaw)
Joint pains	Osteoarthrosis
Diabetes mellitus	Hypertension
In children (before fusion of epiphyses)	Excessive growth (gigantism)

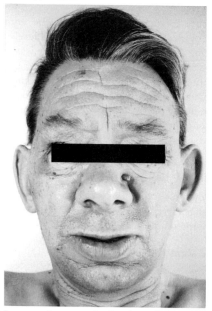

Fig. 5.1 Facial features of acromegaly showing soft tissue enlargement and coarse skin.

ablative treatment with pituitary irradiation may be required. Medical treatment with bromocriptine can also be used in a minority sensitive to dopamine agonists. This is a paradoxical response since L-dopa normally stimulates GH secretion. In addition there is now an analogue of somatostatin available, given by subcutaneous injection, which reduces GH levels.

Adrenocorticotrophic hormone (ACTH): Cushing's syndrome. (See p. 184)

Follicle stimulating hormone/luteinising hormone (FSH/LH): Sexual precocity

Sexual precocity occurs when changes of puberty are seen in girls and boys before the ages of 8 and 9 respectively. It may arise from an organic lesion, such as a pinealoma affecting the hypothalamus, or, more often in girls than boys, as a functional disorder.

Symptoms and signs

The precocious puberty commonly causes associated psychological problems.

The signs are those of precocious puberty and disordered growth. The premature secretion of gonadal steroids results in early excessive growth but ultimate shortness from fusion of the epiphyses.

Investigations

Serum gonadotrophin levels are raised and a CT or MRI scan of the hypothalamus/pituitary will detect an underlying tumour.

Differential diagnosis

The condition must be distinguished from sexual precocity caused by congenital adrenal hyperplasia and gonadal hormone secreting tumours.

Treatment

Treatment is of the underlying conditions, if possible, or, otherwise, by subcutaneous injection of an LHRH analogue which inhibits FSH and LH secretion. Resolution of the endocrine syndrome and reduction in the excessive rate of growth results.

Vasopressin: Water intoxication

Although tumours of the posterior pituitary do not occur, inappropriate secretion of vasopressin is common and found in many conditions such as primary hypothyroidism, pneumonia and head injury. In addition, some malignant tumours, in particular small cell carcinomas of the bronchus, secrete vasopressin ectopically. Inappropriate secretion of vasopressin results in water retention and, eventually, the syndrome of water intoxication, the clinical features of which depend upon the severity and rapidity of onset.

Symptoms and signs

The patient may have headaches and progress to fits, drowsiness and, ultimately, coma and death.

Peripheral oedema is not seen as the excess water is distributed both intra- and extracellularly and the patient would die from intracellular oedema before pitting oedema was detected.

Investigations

Diagnosis is based on finding dilutional hyponatraemia in which low levels of serum sodium, and normal or low levels of serum urea and/or creatinine are found. Urine osmolality is inappropriately high compared with plasma.

Differential diagnosis

The serum biochemical findings must be distinguished from those of depletional hyponatraemia, resulting from sodium deficiency, in which hyponatraemia is associated with impairment of renal function because of the depletion of extracellular fluid volume.

Treatment

Treatment is usually with fluid restriction to 500–100 ml per 24 hours when the serum sodium level gradually rises. Rarely, emergency treatment is needed, for instance because of fits, in which case hypertonic saline (3 or 5%) is given. This may precipitate heart failure, and too rapid correction can also cause the rare, but fatal, neurological condition of central pontine myelinolysis.

HYPOSECRETION

Non-selective

Non-selective hypopituitarism is usually caused by a pituitary tumour or its treatment. Other causes include pituitary infarction, which occurs particularly post-partum (Sheehan's syndrome), and granulomas.

Symptoms and signs

Symptoms and signs depend on the extent of pituitary hormone deficiency. Thus, deficiency of GH in a child results in shortness, that of gonadotrophins in hypogonadism, that of ACTH in glucocorticoid deficiency, that of thyroid stimulating hormone (TSH) in (secondary) hypothyroidism and that of vasopressin in diabetes insipidus.

Investigations

Serum GH levels during a stimulation test, serum gonadotrophins, thyroid function tests and serum cortisol, usually also during a stimulation test, may need to be measured. A CT or MRI scan of the pituitary is usually indicated.

Differential diagnosis

Secretion of gonadotrophins and GH are practically always impaired before those of TSH and ACTH. Thus, preservation of normal gonadotrophin secretion as indicated by persistent menstruation or the normal postmenopausal elevation of gonadotrophins in a woman, and normal potency and serum testosterone in a man, virtually excludes a clinically significant degree of hypopituitarism.

Treatment

Treatment depends upon the age of the patient and extent of hypopituitarism. Patients with panhypopituitarism require full replacement therapy with thyroxine, glucocorticoids, GH (for children) and desmopressin for diabetes insipidus. Thyroxine should not usually be given without glucocorticoid as TSH and ACTH deficiency commonly occur together and thyroxine treatment alone may precipitate an adrenal crisis. Men are treated with androgens and women, at least until the age of 50, with oestrogens, both for their immediate effects and the long-term prevention of osteoporosis. Infertility can be treated with injections of gonadotrophins.

Growth hormone: Shortness

This may occur as an isolated idiopathic defect or from an organic lesion such as a craniopharyngioma.

Symptoms and signs

The child is markedly short, usually more than 2.5 standard deviations below the mean, and is usually chubby as GH has a lipolytic effect.

Investigations

Subnormal GH levels are found during one or more stimulation tests, of which the most definitive is insulin-induced hypoglycaemia.

Differential diagnosis

See section on Growth (p. 195)

Treatment

Growth can be restored with subcutaneous injections of human growth hormone which is manufactured by recombinant DNA technology. This has replaced material extracted from human pituitaries, which has been responsible for instances of Creutzfeld-Jacob disease.

ACTH

ACTH deficiency is rare as an isolated defect, except from long-term treatment with glucocorticoids or ACTH.

FSH/LH: HYPOGONADOTROPHIC HYPOGONADISM

Gonadotrophin deficiency occurs as a manifestation of hypopituitarism, for instance secondary to craniopharyngioma, or as an isolated hypothalamic defect. The latter is more common in boys than in girls and may be associated with other congenital disorders (e.g. Kallmann's syndrome).

Symptoms and signs

In Kallmann's syndrome, in addition to the lack of pubertal development, other abnormalities such as absence (anosmia) or deficiency (hyposmia) of sense of smell, cleft palate, harelip and dental anomalies are present.

Investigations

Serum gonadotrophin levels are measured and a skull X-ray and CT or MRI scan may be performed.

Differential diagnosis

Isolated gonadotrophin deficiency must, in particular, be distinguished from constitutional delayed puberty; this may only be possible after a period of follow-up.

Treatment

Treatment is with androgens or oestrogens but, when inducing puberty, it is very important that the dosage is kept low to avoid premature maturation and fusion of the epiphyses and shortening of ultimate height.

Vasopressin: Diabetes insipidus

Diabetes insipidus is caused either by a lesion of the posterior pituitary and pituitary stalk leading to vasopressin deficiency (cranial diabetes insipidus), or by resistance to the action of vasopressin on the renal tubules (nephrogenic diabetes insipidus) as in hypercalcaemia, hypokalaemia, the action of certain drugs such as lithium, and in a rare sex-linked congenital abnormality. The deficiency of or resistance to vasopressin results in failure of urine concentration.

Symptoms and signs

Thirst is the predominant symptom, with polyuria of >3 litres per 24 hours. If, for whatever reason, the subject is unable to maintain an adequate fluid intake (e.g. after a head injury) there is the risk of rapid and profound water depletion.

There are usually no signs unless the patient becomes fluid depleted.

Investigations

Urine volume should be measured and plasma electrolytes and serum calcium levels determined. If there is doubt as to the diagnosis, a fluid deprivation test should be performed in which fluid intake is stopped, usually for up to 8 hours, and bodyweight, plasma and urine osmolality serially measured.

Differential diagnosis

Polyuria needs to be distinguished from frequency of micturition. The most difficult differential diagnosis is from compulsive water drinking which is not uncommon and does not necessarily indicate a serious underlying psychiatric disorder.

Treatment

Treatment is with desmopressin, a synthetic long-acting analogue of vasopressin. It is given intranasally, usually twice daily.

THE THYROID

The thyroid gland synthesises thyroxine (T4) and tri-iodothyronine (T3), and also calcitonin in the C cells. Control of the thyroid is by TSH, the secretion of which is stimulated by TRH from the hypothalamus. Circulating levels of thyroid hormones exert a negative feedback effect upon the hypothalamus and anterior pituitary.

Manufacture of the thyroid hormones begins with the trapping of iodide from blood and ends with the release of T4 and T3 into thyroid capillaries from their loose association with thyroglobulin in colloid. Over 99% of T4 and T3 circulate bound to plasma proteins, particularly thyroxine binding globulin (TBG), and it is the free fractions that determine the thyroid state of the individual.

HYPERFUNCTION: THYROTOXICOSIS, HYPERTHYROIDISM

Thyrotoxicosis occurs with a prevalence in the UK of 1.1% for established cases and 1.6% with the inclusion of possible cases. It is commonly due to Graves' disease, an autoimmune condition in which thyroid overactivity is caused by a number of circulating thyroid-stimulating immunoglobulins that bind to the TSH receptor. Graves' disease occurs in association with other organ-specific autoimmune diseases such as Addison's disease, diabetes mellitus and pernicious anaemia.

Autonomous oversecretion by one or more thyroid nodules, associated with suppression of the activity of the rest of the gland, underlies thyrotoxicosis of

Table 5.3. Symptoms and signs of excessive thyroid hormone secretion

	Symptoms	Signs
General	Loss of weight (despite good appetite) Heat intolerance Increased sweating	Evidence of weightloss Warm, moist skin
Cardiovascular system	Shortness of breath Palpitations	Tachycardia Peripheral vasodilation Increased pulse pressure Atrial fibrillation ⎫ Particularly in Cardiac failure ⎭ the elderly
Muscles	Weakness	Muscle weakness and wasting (thyrotoxic myopathy)
Nervous system	Anxiety state Irritability	Fine tremor Brisk tendon jerks
Gastrointestinal system	Diarrhoea	
Eyes	Staring appearance	Lid retraction, lid lag

the elderly. Transient thyrotoxicosis occurs in thyroiditis—either autoimmune or subacute (de Quervain's)—caused by the release of preformed thyroid hormone from the inflamed gland.

Symptoms and signs
The effects of excessive thyroid hormone secretion are listed in Table 5.3 Usually, but not always, a goitre which is diffuse in Graves' disease and nodular in the elderly is present.

Ophthalmopathy (Fig. 5.2). This is clinically present in about 50% of patients with Graves' disease and is also autoimmune in origin. It is not necessarily associated with thyrotoxicosis and can occur in patients who are euthyroid and, rarely, hypothyroid. The external ocular muscles are grossly hypertrophied and the orbital contents increased from oedema, fat, connective tissue, inflammatory cells and mucopolysaccharide deposition.

It comprises one or more of the following features:
Exophthalmos (protrusion). This is occasionally unilateral and thus may be confused with an intra-orbital tumour.
Impaired eye movement (ophthalmoplegia). Upward gaze is affected most often from tethering of the inferior recti.
Lid bulge.
Oedema of the conjunctiva (chemosis).
Rarely, the eye involvement causes visual impairment from corneal ulceration (with severe exophthalmos) or from pressure on the optic nerve.

Pretibial myxoedema. This occurs in up to 5% of patients with Graves' disease. It is an infiltration with a mucopolysaccharide which characteristically

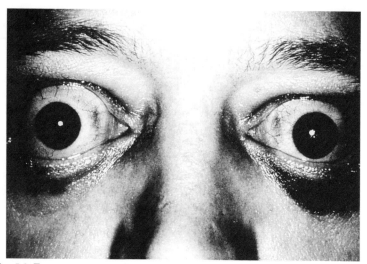

Fig. 5.2 Eye appearances in Graves' disease showing marked exophthalmos and lid retraction.

affects the front of the shins, sometimes asymmetrically, causing redness, thickening, and puckering of the skin.

Investigations
The most sensitive laboratory tests are raised serum total or, preferably, free T3 levels and suppressed serum TSH.

Differential diagnosis
The diagnosis of thyrotoxicosis is essentially clinical. However, particularly in the elderly, the clinical features may be occult with non-specific symptoms such as weightloss and cardiac arrhythmias. The condition may be difficult to distinguish from an anxiety state and, indeed, the two conditions may coexist.

Treatment
Medical. Antithyroid drugs block the synthesis of thyroid hormone and will relieve the symptoms during the time they are taken. Persistent thyrotoxicosis is likely to be caused by inadequate dosage or lack of compliance of drug taking.

Carbimazole is the drug most commonly used in the UK. It is given in an initial dosage of 10–15 mg 8-hourly until the patient is euthyroid, which usually takes 4–8 weeks. The dosage is then reduced to a maintenance one of 5–15 mg per 24 hours and thyroxine, 100 µg per 24 hours, is often added to avoid hypothyroidism. The drug is usually well tolerated, but may cause rashes and/or scalp hair loss, in which case propylthiouracil can be given instead. Both drugs very rarely cause agranulocytosis which appears to be an idiosyncrasy. Treatment is maintained for 12–18 months, and longer in children. However, relapse occurs in 50% and cannot be predicted. The best results are seen in young women with small goitres.

Non-selective beta-blockers are sometimes also used in the initial treatment of thyrotoxicosis as they relieve some of the symptoms, such as anxiety and palpitations, although they have no effect upon thyroid hormone secretion.

Radioiodine. Radioiodine treatment involves giving a drink of water containing the radioactive isotope ^{131}I. It is very effective and will cure the condition in approximately 75% of patients after a single dose. Those whose thyrotoxicosis persists after the first dose are given one or more further doses, as necessary, after an interval of at least 3 months. The treatment must not be given to pregnant mothers as ^{131}I crosses the placenta, and is best avoided in children. It use was formerly restricted in the UK to those over the age of 40 to avoid unnecessary radiation of the gonads in childbearing years, but it is now considered a potential first line treatment for all adults. The main disadvantage of ^{131}I therapy is the high incidence of subsequent hypothyroidism which is of the order of 15% in the first year and 3% per year thereafter. It is essential therefore that patients are aware of this risk.

Surgery. Surgery is by partial thyroidectomy which relieves the condition in more than 90% of patients and has a low incidence of relapse. There is a small risk of serious side-effects, such as damage to the recurrent laryngeal nerve and hypoparathyroidism. Hypothyroidism also occurs in the years following an operation, but the incidence is probably lower than that with radioiodine. It is essential that patients are euthyroid prior to surgery and so require initial treatment with antihyroid drugs.

The advantages and disadvantages of each form of treatment must be discussed with the patient. Radioiodine is being used more as first line treatment for adults, but it is common in young adults to use antithyroid drugs first, and then either radioiodine or surgery if there is subsequent relapse.

Ophthalmopathy

The symptoms and signs of ophthalmopathy are difficult to treat but, fortunately, gradual improvement may occur after months or years.

Associated thyrotoxicosis should be treated and hypothyroidism avoided as this can worsen the condition. Watering and discomfort may respond to hypromellose eyedrops, salt restriction and diuretics, and embarrassing lid retraction to guanethidine eye drops. More severe eye symptoms warrant the use of high-dose glucocorticoids. Tarsorrhaphy and prism lenses may be needed for marked exophthalmos and ophthalmoplegia respectively. Other forms of treatment for severe ophthalmopathy are immunosuppressants, plasma exchange and orbital decompression.

Thyrotoxic crisis

This is a medical emergency with a significant mortality. Urgent treatment is with beta-blockers, carbimazole and potassium iodide.

Rapid clinical deterioration of thyrotoxicosis occurs with florid clinical signs, e.g. marked tachycardia, tremor etc. There is usually some precipitating event such as infection, surgery or intercurrent illness.

Table 5.4. Causes of hypothyroidism

Primary*	Iodine deficiency
	Autoimmune thyroiditis (Hashimoto's disease)
	'Idiopathic atrophy' (often end stage of autoimmune thyroiditis)
	Iatrogenic: antithyroid drugs, radioiodine, surgery
	Drugs (e.g. lithium, amiodarone)
	Congenital enzyme defect
	Failure of development (cretinism)
Secondary (pituitary disease causing TSH deficiency)	
	Hypopituitarism
	Isolated TSH deficiency (rare)
Tertiary (hypothalamic disease causing TRH deficiency)	
	Craniopharyngioma

* The most common type, globally most often caused by iodine deficiency. In industrialised countries, the most common causes are autoimmune thyroiditis and treatment of thyrotoxicosis.

HYPOFUNCTION: HYPOTHYROIDISM, MYXOEDEMA

Hypothyroidism, as with thyrotoxicosis, is common with a prevalence in the UK of 0.8% of established cases with 1.1% with the inclusion of possible cases. Causes of the condition are shown in Table 5.4.

Primary hypothyroidism is much more common than the other types. Globally it is most often due to iodine deficiency, but in industrialized countries the commonest causes are autoimmune thyroiditis and secondary to the treatment of thyrotoxicosis.

Symptoms and signs

Hypothyroidism can cause a large number of different clinical features (Table 5.5) thus presenting in many different ways. In addition, there may be a goitre depending upon the cause. Hypothyroidism induces (secondary) hyperlipoproteinaemia and, thus an increased incidence of ischaemic heart disease.

Investigations

The biochemical hallmark of primary hypothyroidism is a raised serum TSH, absence of which excludes the diagnosis. A raised serum TSH together with a normal serum T4 indicates subclinical hypothyroidism and an increased risk of developing frank hypothyroidism.

Differential diagnosis

Hypothyroidism typically comes on gradually and so the changes may be missed by those who see the patient frequently. The diagnosis must be considered in patients presenting with such diverse symptoms as weightgain, angina and rheumatic pains.

Treatment

Treatment is with thyroxine which is cheap and stable. It has a half-life in euthyroid subjects of approximately 7 days, and so only needs to be given once

Table 5.5. Symptoms and signs of hypothyroidism

	Symptoms	Signs
General	Cold intolerance Weight gain	Dry, coarse skin and hair Pallor
From infiltration with myxoedematous tissue	Change in appearance Hoarseness of voice Paraesthesia of hands	Puffiness of face and extremities Involvement of larynx Carpal tunnel syndrome
Cardiovascular system	Angina of effort	Bradycardia Evidence of IHD Pericardial effusion
Muscles	Generalised aches	Stiff swollen muscles
Nervous system	'Slowing up' Poor memory Unsteadiness Sometimes frank psychosis	Slowness of speech and thought Delayed relaxation tendon jerks Cerebellar ataxia 'Myxoedema madness'
Gastrointestinal system	Constipation	Abdominal distension Paralytic ileus (rare) Ascites (rare)
Children	Retardation of growth	Shortness
Infants	Mental deficiency (if treatment delayed)	Cretinism

daily. In middle aged and elderly patients it is important to begin with a small dose of 25–50 μg per 24 hours to avoid exacerbating, or precipitating, underlying ischaemic heart disease. The usual maintenance dose varies within 50–200 μg per 24 hours and is determined not only clinically but by levels of serum TSH which should be neither suppressed, which indicates overtreatment, nor elevated, indicating undertreatment.

GOITRE

The term goitre is used for any swelling of the thyroid gland, the causes of which (Table 5.6) overlap those of primary hypothyroidism. A long-standing goitre, as seen in areas of iodine deficiency, commonly undergoes changes such as haemorrhage, infarction and fibrosis which cause it to become nodular.

Symptoms and signs

The patient usually becomes aware of a goitre because of the cosmetic appearance. True pressure effects, such as difficulty in swallowing and shortness of breath, are very unusual with benign goitres unless they are retrosternal.

Goitres vary in size, consistency and nature of their surface. Classically they are bilateral neck swellings which rise on swallowing.

Table 5.6. Causes of goitre

Autoimmune (Hashimoto's) thyroiditis	'Physiological', e.g. puberty, pregnancy
Congenital enzyme defect	Thyroiditis
Goitrogen induced	Reidel's
Dietary, (e.g. cassava contains thiocyanate)	Subacute (de Quervain's)
	Thyrotoxicosis
Drugs, e.g. amiodarone, antithyroid drugs, iodides, lithium	Tumours of the thyroid
Iodine deficiency	Adenoma
	Carcinoma

Investigations
Measurement of thyroid autoantibodies and thyroid ultrasound may be indicated in addition to thyroid function tests.

Differential diagnosis
The most important distinction to be made is between a benign goitre, for whatever reason, and thyroid carcinoma (see below).

Treatment
With small goitres, no treatment other than reassurance may be required. Thyroxine is usually successful in reducing the size of large diffuse (non-toxic) goitres but shrinks only a minority of nodular ones. Surgery may be required for goitres that do not respond to medical treatment.

THYROID CARCINOMA

Carcinomas of the thyroid are rare. In the young they are usually differentiated, either papillary (most often) or follicular, whereas in the elderly they are usually undifferentiated (anaplastic). Differentiated thyroid carcinomas may arise from exposure of the neck to ionising radiation, especially in childhood.

An additional type of malignant tumour is medullary thyroid carcinoma, arising from parafollicular (C) cells. This may occur sporadically or as part of the syndrome of multiple endocrine adenomatosis.

Symptoms and signs
The presentation is usually with a goitre. There may be pressure effects such as dysphagia, shortness of breath and hoarseness, the latter from involvement of the recurrent laryngeal nerve.

The goitre is typically a hard, apparently single, thyroid nodule of recent onset, or there may have been rapid increase in size of an existing goitre. There may be signs of pressure effects, such as stridor, and enlarged cervical lymph glands.

Investigations
Thyroid carcinomas characteristically do not take up radioisotope ('cold' nodule) and on ultrasound are either solid or, if cystic, are >4 cm in diameter.

Diagnosis is by fine-needle aspiration cytology, biopsy or surgical excision. Raised levels of serum calcitonin are found in medullary thyroid carcinomas.

Differential diagnosis

The possibility of a carcinoma has to be considered in anyone presenting with a goitre.

Treatment

Initial treatment for differentiated carcinomas is surgical. Subsequently thyroxine is given long term, as many are sensitive to TSH suppression, together with therapeutic doses of radioiodine as necessary for residual tumour and/or functioning metastases. Medullary thyroid carcinomas are also treated surgically. Anaplastic carcinomas are rapidly fatal but may respond temporarily to irradiation.

Prognosis

Papillary carcinomas tend to spread locally whilst follicular tumours spread distally. The prognosis for differentiated carcinomas is good, with a 10-year survival of papillary carcinomas of >80%.

ADRENALS

ADRENAL CORTEX

Three main groups of steroid hormones are secreted by the adrenal cortex: glucocorticoids and mineralocorticoids, the most important in man being cortisol (hydrocortisone) and aldosterone respectively, and androgens. All are derived from cholesterol by a series of enzyme steps (Fig. 5.3).

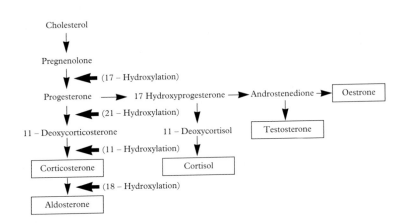

Fig. 5.3 Adrenal steroid biosynthesis.

Table 5.7. Causes of Cushing's syndrome

Type	Relative incidence (%)	Comments
Pituitary dependent	65	Underlying lesion usually a pituitary (micro) adenoma. Most common in young to middle aged women
Adrenal tumour		
Benign	10	
Malignant	10	
Ectopic ACTH secretion	15	Particularly small cell bronchial carcinoma, thymic and pancreatic tumours, bronchial carcinoid

Table 5.8. Symptoms and signs of Cushing's syndrome

Effect of glucocorticoid	Symptoms and signs
Protein catabolic	Muscle wasting, weakness, proximal myopathy Thinning of skin, easy bruising, striae (particularly abdominal) Osteoporosis In children: stunting of growth
Anti-insulin	Clinical features of diabetes mellitus
Others	Redistribution of body fat with central obesity, 'buffalo hump'. Round (moon), red face Hypertension Psychiatric disorders, especially depression Hirsutism, oligo/amenorrhoea Pigmentation (in types with increased ACTH secretion)

HYPERFUNCTION

Glucocorticoids: Cushing's syndrome

Cushing's syndrome is rare but of particular importance since it is part of the differential diagnosis of common conditions such as obesity and hypertension, and because high-dose glucocorticoid treatment causes the same clinical features. Causes of Cushing's syndrome are shown in Table 5.7.

Symptoms and signs (Table 5.8, Fig. 5.4)
The extent to which these develop depends upon the duration of the condition. Patients with ectopic ACTH secretion from a malignant tumour usually die before they can be detected, but their very high cortisol levels commonly cause mental confusion and weakness, the latter from potassium deficiency.

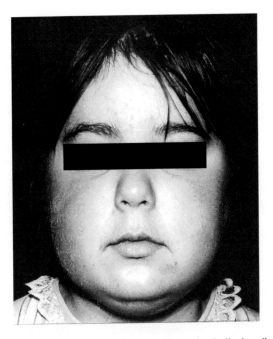

Fig. 5.4 Facial appearance in Cushing's syndrome classically described as a 'moon-face'.

Investigations

These are used initially to establish the diagnosis and then, if confirmed, to determine the cause (Table 5.9). The overnight dexamethasone suppression test is a particularly useful screening procedure, normal suppression of the serum cortisol virtually excluding the diagnosis.

Differential diagnosis

Patients with depression may have steroid abnormalities similar to those of Cushing's syndrome and alcoholics may develop a 'pseudo' Cushing's syndrome which remits on alcohol withdrawal. Slow-growing benign ACTH-secreting tumours, especially carcinoids, are often particularly difficult to diagnose.

Treatment

Treatment depends on the type of Cushing's syndrome. Patients with pituitary-dependent disease are usually treated by trans-sphenoidal pituitary surgery. If this fails, total adrenalectomy may be necessary but is a more serious surgical procedure and requires gluco- and mineralocorticoid replacement therapy. In addition, there is a risk of stimulating the growth of a pituitary adenoma, the patient commonly developing skin pigmentation (Nelson's syndrome) from the very high ACTH and lipotrophin levels.

Adrenal tumours are treated by surgery and ectopic ACTH-secreting tumours as appropriate. Preoperatively, or when it is not possible to relieve the

Table 5.9. Investigation of Cushing's syndrome

Test	Procedure	Typical findings
To establish diagnosis		
Overnight dexamethasone suppression	2300 h: 1 mg dexamethasone 0900 h: Serum cortisol	Failure to show normal suppression
Low-dose dexamethasone	0.5 mg dexamethasone 6-hourly for 2 days	Failure to show normal suppression serum/24 h urinary cortisol
Urinary free cortisol	24 h urine	Elevated levels
To determine cause		
Plasma ACTH	0900/h/2200 h— MN blood samples	Levels *high* in pituitary-dependent CS Levels *very high* with ectopic ACTH secretion Levels *suppressed* in adrenal tumour
High-dose dexamethasone	2.0 mg dexamethasone 6-hourly for 2 days	> 50% suppression serum/24 h urinary cortisol, in pituitary-dependent CS Other types show little or no suppression
Abdominal/skull CT scan		May show adrenal/pituitary tumour
Screening tests for non-adrenal tumour	e.g. chest X-ray. LFTs	May show site/evidence of source ectopic ACTH secretion

CS = Cushing's syndrome; LFTs = liver function tests; MN = Midnight

condition, medical treatment with drugs, such as metyrapone, that block cortisol synthesis are used.

Mineralocorticoids: Primary aldosteronism

Primary aldosteronism is caused by an adrenal tumour (almost always benign), or by bilateral hyperplasia. The excessive aldosterone secretion results in hypertension, from sodium retention, and hypokalemia, from potassium loss in urine. It accounts for <1% of patients with raised blood pressure.

Symptoms and signs

The main clinical feature is hypertension. In addition, the patient may have symptoms of potassium deficiency, such as polyuria, polydipsia and muscle weakness. Peripheral oedema does not occur because of an aldosterone escape mechanism.

Investigations

The levels of serum potassium are low, the serum bicarbonate elevated and the serum sodium either raised or in the upper half of the normal range. The diagnosis is established by finding an elevated plasma aldosterone level and suppressed plasma renin activity. CT scan may show an adrenal adenoma.

Differential diagnosis

The condition should be suspected in someone with hypertension and hypokalaemia, but the latter is more often the result of thiazide diuretic treatment of hypertension.

Treatment

Treatment is either by surgical excision of an adrenal tumour or, more commonly, with spironolactone which blocks the actions of aldosterone on the renal tubules.

Androgens: Congenital adrenal hyperplasia (CAH)

CAH is caused by a congenital, and sometimes familial, defect of one of the enzymes of cortisol synthesis, most commonly 21-hydroxylase. Although the main defect is in glucocorticoid secretion, there may be associated severe mineralocorticoid deficiency which results in a salt-losing state in newborn infants. Because of the glucocorticoid deficiency, there is stimulation of ACTH secretion which causes excessive adrenal androgen production.

Symptoms and signs

CAH may be recognised at birth because of masculinisation of the genitals of a female baby or, soon afterwards, from an acute salt-losing syndrome. The enzyme defect may be partial and the condition only recognised because of precocious puberty in boys and late onset hirsutism in women.

Investigations

Urinary and plasma steroid levels are abnormal with high levels of glucocorticoid precursors and adrenal androgens.

Differential diagnosis

The condition must be distinguished from other causes of masculinisation of a female infant and, later, from other causes of male precocious puberty and hirsutism in women.

Treatment

Treatment is with glucocorticoids together with fludrocortisone, an orally active mineralocorticoid in the salt-losing form. In infants and children the dose of glucocorticoid must be monitored with particular care to avoid stunting of growth.

HYPOFUNCTION

Non-selective: Addison's disease

Addison's disease is uncommon. The destruction of the adrenal cortices was formerly most often due to tuberculosis, but is now usually the result of autoimmune destruction. The condition may present acutely during a septicaemic illness, such as meningococcal infection, from bilateral adrenal infarction or haemorrhage.

Symptoms and signs

Acute adrenocortical deficiency causes a shock-like syndrome. Otherwise, the condition develops insidiously over several weeks or months with non-specific symptoms such as anorexia, weakness and weightloss.

The cardinal physical sign is brown pigmentation of the skin, particularly affecting exposed areas, scars and creases, and of the mucous membranes of the mouth and conjunctiva. This arises from excessive secretion of pituitary ACTH and lipotrophin. Hypotension, with further fall on standing, is also seen.

Investigations

The initial diagnosis is essentially clinical. In addition, serum biochemistry typically shows low serum sodium and raised serum potassium, urea and creatinine levels. If Addison's disease is strongly suspected, treatment should be started immediately to avoid an adrenal crisis and the diagnosis later confirmed by an adrenocortical stimulation test with tetracosactrin (Synacthen), a synthetic derivative of ACTH.

Treatment

Treatment of acute adrenocortical deficiency is with i.v. saline and cortisol 300–400 mg per 24 hours which, at this high dosage, has adequate mineralocorticoid effect as well. Chronic replacement therapy is with 20–30 mg cortisol per 24 hours in 2 divided doses, or an equivalent dose of an alternative glucocorticoid (see below), together with fludrocortisone, an orally active mineralocorticoid, 50–300 μg per 24 hours. The patient must double or treble the glucocorticoid dosage in the event of an intercurrent illness or accident.

Selective

Isolated glucocorticoid deficiency occurs from ACTH deficiency either because of long-term glucocorticoid or ACTH treatment, or as a manifestation of panhypopituitarism. Mineralocorticoid treatment is not necessary since aldosterone secretion is not under ACTH control.

Glucocorticoid therapy

Many glucocorticoids are available (e.g. cortisol, prednisolone, betamethasone, dexamethasone, triamcinolone). There is no clear superiority of one preparation over another and they incur similar side-effects. Replacement therapy for glucocorticoid deficiency, whether primary adrenocortical or secondary to ACTH deficiency, must be distinguished from pharmacological therapy when glucocorticoid is given for a variety of non-endocrine conditions such as rheumatoid arthritis, asthma and after transplantation. In the latter, every attempt must be made to keep the dosage as low as possible yet maintaining disease control. Occasionally ACTH rather than glucocorticoid is used. The higher the glucocorticoid/ACTH dose, and the longer it has to be given, the greater the risk of side-effects, which are the same as the clinical features of Cushing's syndrome (Table 5.8); in addition, there is a risk of adrenocortical suppression.

ADRENAL MEDULLA

Hyperfunction

Phaeochromocytoma

Tumours of the adrenal medulla, and similar tissue found around the aorta, are known as phaeochromocytomas. They are rare and may be unilateral or bilateral. The latter may be associated with conditions such as neurofibromatosis or medullary thyroid carcinoma. The tumours secrete adrenaline and noradrenaline sometimes intermittently. Hypertension is the major clinical feature (see p. 39).

THE GONADS

FEMALES

The ovaries contain oocytes and secrete oestrogens, progesterone and androgens (Fig. 5.5). The predominant circulating oestrogen during reproductive years is oestradiol whilst, after the menopause, it is oestrone. This is produced from androgens derived from both the adrenals and ovaries in adipose tissue.

Delayed puberty

Delayed puberty results from disorders of the hypothalamus, anterior pituitary and ovary (Table 5.10).

Symptoms and signs

Disorders of the hypothalamus or pituitary are not necessarily associated with failure of development of secondary sexual characteristics, as there may be

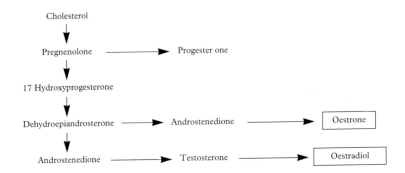

Fig. 5.5 Ovarian steroid biosynthesis.

Table 5.10. Causes of delayed puberty

Hypothalamic–pituitary disorders	Primary gonadal disorders
Constitutional	Chromosomal abnormalities
Isolated gonadotrophin deficiency (Kallmann's syndrome)	Gonadal dysgenesis (girls) Klinefelter's syndrome (boys)
Chronic disease, e.g. chronic renal disease, coeliac disease	Surgical excision Cytotoxic chemotherapy
Low bodyweight Anorexia nervosa (in extreme cases)	
Hypothalamic/pituitary disease, e.g. tumours, granulomas, post irradiation	
Primary hypothyroidism	
Hyperprolactinaemia (uncommon in children)	

adequate gonadotrophin secretion to achieve this but failure of normal cyclical secretion resulting in amenorrhoea.

Investigations

Detection of elevated serum gonadotrophin levels indicates a primary ovarian disorder, whilst the levels are normal or low with hypothalamic/pituitary disease. X-ray of the left hand for bone age indicates skeletal development.

Differential diagnosis

This is sometimes evident on clinical examination, e.g. gonadal dysgenesis.

Treatment

Treatment depends upon the cause. If it is not possible to restore ovarian function, replacement therapy with oestrogen is needed. Small doses of ethinyl oestradiol (up to 10 µg per 24 hours) are given initially to avoid disproportionate maturation of the epiphyses and stunting of growth. Later it is convenient to give a combined oral contraceptive.

Gonadal dysgenesis

Gonadal dysgenesis occurs in approximately 0.4 per 1000 female births. It is a disorder of sex chromosomes and a variety of different karyotypes are found, of which the most common is XO. The ovaries fail to develop and present as undifferentiated (streak) gonads.

Symptoms and signs

Clinical features are absent ovarian function, shortness and a variety of associated abnormalities which include webbing of the neck, increased carrying angle of the forearm, short fourth and fifth metacarpals and skin naevi. Diagnosis may be made at birth from (lymphoedema) of the hands and feet.

Investigations

Serum gonadotrophin levels are elevated and the karyotype is abnormal (sometimes a mosaic).

Differential diagnosis

The diagnosis is essentially clinical, but the condition needs to be distinguished from other causes of shortness and absent pubertal development.

Treatment

Severe stunting of growth is now treated with injections of an anabolic steroid, sometimes together with human GH. Subsequently, oestrogen replacement therapy is given (as above), which eventually induces withdrawal menstrual bleeds and prevents the development of osteoporosis.

Amenorrhoea

Failure of development of periods is known as primary amenorrhoea and its causes overlap with those of delayed puberty discussed above. Development of amenorrhoea at any time after periods have become established is known as secondary amenorrhoea of which there are a number of causes (Table 5.11).

Symptoms and signs

In addition to the absence of periods there may be features of oestrogen deficiency (see below).

Investigations

Serum prolactin is measured to detect hyperprolactinaemia and serum FSH/LH levels to distinguish between a disorder of the hypothalamus/pituitary (the levels are normal or low), and, less commonly, of the ovary (the levels are elevated).

Table 5.11. Causes of secondary amenorrhoea (after exclusion of pregnancy)

Hypothalamic–pituitary	Ovarian	Endometrial
Functional defect of gonadotrophin secretion	Polycystic ovarian disease	Fibrosis
Emotional upset	Primary ovarian failure	Tuberculosis
Excessive physical exertion	Autoimmune oophoritis	
Intercurrent illness	Cytotoxic chemotherapy	
Low bodyweight	Pelvic-irradiation	
Anorexia nervosa	Premature menopause	
Obesity	Surgical excision	
Hyperprolactinaemia		
Organic defect of gonadotrophin secretion		
Pituitary tumour		
Granuloma affecting the hypothalamus		

Treatment

Treatment is of the cause, if possible. Otherwise treatment may be indicated for absence of periods, associated infertility or oestrogen deficiency. Cyclical oestrogen therapy, most commonly with a preparation of the combined oral contraceptive, induces withdrawal bleeds unless there is a uterine disorder.

Oestrogen deficiency

This is inevitable at the time of the menopause but may also be an associated feature of amenorrhoea in younger women, depending upon the cause.

Symptoms and signs

Oestrogen deficiency causes hot flushes, sweats and dyspareunia, the latter from dryness of the vagina. It results in excessive loss of bone mineral content with a risk of osteoporosis.

Investigations

Serum oestradiol levels are low.

Treatment

Treatment is with oestrogen replacement therapy. However, this must be given in combination with a progestogen since unopposed oestrogen causes endometrial hyperplasia and a risk of carcinoma. In younger women it is convenient to use a preparation of the combined oral contraceptive.

Hirsutism

Excessive body hair is a common symptom among women and often causes great distress. It must be assessed in relation to the patient's country of origin since there are large racial variations. It is most often caused by polycystic ovarian disease, but is occasionally seen with other conditions such as adult congenital adrenal hyperplasia (CAH) and virilising syndromes, e.g. androgen-secreting tumours of the adrenals and ovaries.

Symptoms and signs

The excessive hair may affect the face, arms, legs, trunk and abdomen, the latter in the male type distribution. Disturbances of the menstrual cycle are common and, rarely, there is frank virilisation with amenorrhorea, increased muscularity, marked loss of scalp hair and enlargement of the clitoris.

Investigations

Serum testosterone and plasma/urinary adrenal androgen levels are measured. An ultrasound of the ovaries may show the typical changes of polycystic ovarian disease.

Differential diagnosis

Women with clinical virilisation require full investigation to detect the cause.

Treatment

Patients with CAH are treated with glucocorticoid. Adrenal or ovarian tumours require surgical excision. Otherwise, if various cosmetic measures are not effective, oestrogen treatment, with a preparation of the combined oral contraceptive, may be helpful. In women with severe hirsutism, the anti-androgen cyproterone acetate is often dramatically successful; however, because of the risk of failure of normal gonadal development of a male fetus, it must be given cyclically with ethinyl oestradiol to ensure contraception.

MALES

Spermatogenesis occurs within the seminiferous tubules of the testes, whilst testosterone is secreted by the interstitial (Leydig) cells. Testosterone is converted peripherally to dihydrotestosterone which, in some tissues, is the active form of the hormone.

Delayed puberty

Causes of delayed puberty are shown in Table 5.10. It is more often constitutional in boys than girls.

Symptoms and signs

Clinical features are those of lack of pubertal development of the genitalia and body hair, together with those of the underlying condition. Measurement of testicular size is particularly important, and enlargement is a clear sign that puberty is developing.

Investigations

Measurement of serum gonadotrophin levels and determination of the bone age and karyotype may be indicated.

Differential diagnosis

It is often difficult to distinguish functional delayed puberty from hypogonadotrophic hypogonadism except after a period of follow-up.

Treatment

Any treatment with androgens must be undertaken cautiously for fear of causing disproportionate maturation of the epiphyses and stunting of growth. It is given either by monthly low-dose intramuscular injection of testosterone ester or by human chorionic gonadotrophin (HCG), once or twice weekly, also by injection.

Klinefelter's syndrome

Klinefelter's syndrome is caused by a chromosomal abnormality which affects approximately 1 in 800 male births. Failure of normal development of the seminiferous tubules, which are hyalinised, and varying degrees of deficiency of interstitial cell function are seen. The most frequent chromosomal abnormality is an XXY karyotype.

Symptoms and signs

The condition commonly presents with delayed puberty and/or gynaecomastia associated with very small (pea sized) testes. However, if there is normal androgen secretion, it may not be recognised until adult life because of infertility.

Investigations

The serum testosterone level is measured and the karyotype determined. Semen examination shows azoospermia.

Differential diagnosis

Klinefelter's syndrome must be distinguished in children from other causes of delayed puberty and gynaecomastia and must be considered in the investigation of infertility in adults.

Treatment

Gynaecomastia, if embarrassing, may need surgery. Androgen deficiency requires replacement therapy. The infertility is, unfortunately, untreatable.

Adult hypogonadism

The onset of hypogonadism in men is relatively rare and may have a hypothalamic/pituitary cause, such as pituitary tumour, or a primary testicular cause, such as mumps orchitis.

Symptoms and signs

The testes are small and there may be clinical features of androgen deficiency with soft smooth skin, loss of body hair and impotence, as well as infertility. Osteoporosis is a complication of long-standing hypogonadism.

Investigations

Measurement of serum gonadotrophin levels distinguishes a hypothalamic/pituitary lesion, when the levels are normal or low, from a primary testicular one when they are elevated.

Treatment

Treatment is of the cause, if possible. There are a number of different preparations of testosterone. Some can be taken by mouth, but esters of testosterone, given intramuscularly 3–4 weekly, are often more effective.

Gynaecomastia

Gynaecomastia (enlargement of the breasts in males) occurs at puberty, probably from conversion of androgen to oestrogen, but usually resolves spontaneously over 1–2 years. In an adult it may signify serious disease (Table 5.12).

Table 5.12. Causes of gynaecomastia

Pubertal	Hormone-producing tumours
'Simple'	Adrenal cortex (oestrogens)
Klinefelter's syndrome	Carcinoma of bronchus (HCG)
Post pubertal	Germinal cell (HCG)
Chronic renal failure	Thyrotoxicosis
Cirrhosis of liver	
Drugs	
Androgens (transiently on starting treatment)	
Anti-androgens	
Cimetidine	
Spironolactone	
Digoxin	
Methyl dopa	
Oestrogens	

Symptoms and signs
Although fat deposition in the breasts is often found in overweight men, true gynaecomastia consists of glandular tissue which can be felt as a bud under the areolae and may cause marked breast enlargement.

Investigations
There is usually no need for any investigations in boys with apparently pubertal gynaecomastia, unless there is clinical evidence of Klinefelter's syndrome. Similarly, mild gynaecomastia in the elderly does not necessarily need investigation. Otherwise, chest X-ray, liver function tests, serum testosterone, oestradiol, LH and HCG levels may be helpful.

Differential diagnosis
In adolescent boys the main differential diagnosis is between simple pubertal gynaecomastia and Klinefelter's syndrome.

Treatment
Medical treatment of pubertal gynaecomastia with an anti-oestrogen, such as tamoxifen, is sometimes effective but, if the condition is marked and causing serious embarrassment, surgery is usually required. In adults, treatment is of the underlying condition.

GROWTH

The growth of an individual is determined by genetic and environmental factors, the latter including those in utero. Growth is assessed by comparison with growth charts derived from heights and weights of a large number of apparently normal girls and boys of different ages. In addition, parental height must

Table 5.13. Causes of shortness

Familial	Chromosomal disorders
Constitutional delayed puberty	Down's syndrome
'Light for dates' birthweight	Gonadal dysgenesis
Food deprivation	Endocrine disorders
Emotional deprivation	GH deficiency
Skeletal abnormalities	Hypothyroidism
Chronic disease	Glucocorticoid excess
bronchial asthma	Dysmorphic*
chronic renal failure	
coeliac disease	
diabetes mellitus	

* Includes a variety of conditions often associated with unusual facies, skeletal abnormalities and a low IQ.

be taken into account. Predictions of ultimate height can be made from bone age which is determined on an X-ray of the left hand and wrist.

SHORTNESS

Shortness is usually considered to exist if the height is less than the third centile (1.9 SD below the mean). Shortness may be familial or constitutional, or the result of 'light for dates' birthweight, nutritional or emotional deprivation, skeletal or chromosomal disorders or may result from chronic disease, such as bronchial asthma, diabetes mellitus, coeliac disease and chronic renal disease (Table 5.13).

Symptoms and signs
As well as shortness, there may be clinical features of the underlying condition. With food deprivation, comparison of weight and height centiles illustrates the thinness of the child.

Investigations
These include measurement of bone age, screening tests for chronic disease such as serum electrolytes, creatinine, ferritin and full blood count, thyroid function tests, stimulation tests of GH secretion, X-ray of the pituitary and determination of the karyotype.

Differential diagnosis
Although diagnosis may be apparent clinically, or made from results of initial investigations, the cause of shortness is sometimes difficult to establish, for instance with emotional deprivation or occult chronic disease such as coeliac disease.

Treatment
Treatment is of the underlying condition, if possible. When specific treatment is available, for instance with a gluten-free diet in coeliac disease, children

show 'catch up' growth to attain the height they would have achieved without the intercurrent disorder.

TALLNESS

Causes of excessive height are familial, Marfan's syndrome, homocystinuria and gigantism. Children with predicted excessive height from either of the two first causes are sometimes treated with large doses of gonadal steroid which, despite initial acceleration of growth, cause disproportionate maturation of the epiphyses and reduction in ultimate height.

HYPOGLYCAEMIA

Hypoglycaemia is defined as blood glucose level <2.2 mmol/l in subjects under 60 and <2.8 mmol/l in those over 60. There are a variety of causes (Table 5.14), insulin treatment being by far the most common.

Insulinomas are rare and may be part of the syndrome of multiple endocrine adenomatosis; they occur usually as a single adenoma and 10–20% are malignant. The mechanism(s) of hypoglycaemia with non-pancreatic tumours is uncertain but is not from ectopic secretion of insulin.

Symptoms and signs

Hypoglycaemia produces a variety of symptoms and signs that originate in the nervous system (neuroglycopenia) or are from stimulation of the sympathetic nervous system. These include hunger, shaking, anxiety, palpitations, sweating, poor concentration, slurred speech, fits, disorientation, drowsiness and ultimately unconsciousness, coma and death.

Table 5.14. Causes of hypoglycaemia

Fasting hypoglycaemia	Hypoglycaemia in response to a stimulus
Endocrine disease	Drugs
Addison's disease	Alcohol
Hypopituitarism	Insulin
Hepatic disease	Sulphonylureas
Inborn error of metabolism	Inborn error of metabolism
Glycogen storage disease	Fructose intolerance
Insulinoma	Galactosaemia
Non-pancreatic tumour	Reactive (post prandial)
particularly Mesenchymal	especially after gastric surgery
Hepatoma	
Adrenocortical	
Carcinoma	
Carcinoid	

Investigations

It is first necessary to establish that the subject's symptoms are due to hypoglycaemia, and subsequently to establish its cause.

If an insulinoma is suspected, the serum insulin level must be measured at time of hypoglycaemia, when it is inappropriately high for the low level of blood glucose.

Differential diagnosis

There may be particular difficulty in detecting hypoglycaemia caused by self-administration of insulin or a sulphonylurea (factitious hypoglycaemia).

Treatment

Treatment of individual episodes is with sugar by mouth or, if the patient is unable to swallow, with i.v. glucose or parenteral glucagon. Otherwise, treatment is of the underlying condition, if possible. The drug diazoxide reduces insulin secretion and is sometimes used in the medical management of hypoglycaemia.

CALCIUM AND BONE

The main bone forming cells are the osteoblasts and those that resorb bone are the osteoclasts. The activity of the latter is stimulated by parathyroid hormone (PTH) and inhibited by calcitonin. Vitamin D, either taken in the diet or derived by the action of sunlight on the precursor 7-dehydrocholesterol in skin, is hydroxylated first in the liver and then the kidney to form the active compound 1,25-dihydroxycholecalciferol. Vitamin D promotes calcium absorption in the gut and normal mineralisation of bone. Approximately 50% of circulating calcium is bound to plasma proteins, in particular albumen, the level of which must be considered when assessing the total serum calcium.

HYPERCALCAEMIA

There are many causes of hypercalcaemia (Table 5.15) of which the most common in adults are primary hyperparathyroidism (see p. 201) and a tumour, usually malignant. Tumour-induced hypercalcaemia occurs with bone metastases, from local secretion of osteolytic substances such as prostaglandins, or with primary tumours from the effect of a humoral substance which, with some, has been identified as a PTH-related peptide.

Symptoms and signs

Mild hypercalcaemia (< 3.0 mmol/l) is often asymptomatic, but higher levels, especially of rapid onset, cause nausea, vomiting, polyuria, polydipsia, constipation, confusion and, eventually, coma and death.

Investigations

Once the presence of hypercalcaemia has been established, the most useful investigations in determining its cause are tests for an underlying malignancy, such as chest X-ray and serum immunoglobulins (myeloma), and measure-

Table 5.15. Causes of hypercalcaemia

Main	Rare
Hyperparathyroidism (primary or tertiary)	Acromegaly
	Addison's disease
Malignant tumours particularly carcinoma of breast, bronchus (squamous cell), renal tract or multiple myeloma	Familial hypocalciuric hypercalcaemia
	Immobilisation
	Milk-alkali syndrome
Sarcoidosis	Paget's disease of bone (on immobilisation)
Vitamin D overdose	Thiazide diuretics (? only in patients with primary hyperparathyroidism)
	Thyrotoxicosis

ment of serum PTH levels. Familial hypocalciuric hypercalcaemia is detected by measuring the calcium/creatinine clearance ratio and checking the serum calcium levels of first degree relatives.

Differential diagnosis
In most patients with tumour-associated hypercalcaemia, the tumour has already been diagnosed or is readily detected.

Treatment
Treatment is of the underlying condition, if possible. Acute treatment of symptomatic hypercalcaemia is with i.v. saline, often in large amounts, which may lower the calcium level sufficiently. The most effective drug treatment is with a biphosphonate, given either i.v. or orally. Glucocorticoids are specifically indicated for hypercalcaemia caused by multiple myeloma, vitamin D overdose and sarcoidosis.

HYPOCALCAEMIA

Hypocalcaemia is relatively uncommon. It occurs with hypoparathyroidism, causes of which include autoimmune destruction of the parathyroid glands and thyroid surgery. Other causes include vitamin D deficiency, magnesium deficiency, which reduces the secretion and effect of PTH, and acute pancreatitis.

Symptoms and signs (See Table 5.16)

Investigations
Measurement of serum magnesium and PTH levels may be indicated.

Differential diagnosis
The cause of hypocalcaemia may be evident clinically, for instance shortly after thyroid surgery. Hypocalcaemia in patients presenting with fits is rare but should be considered.

Table 5.16. Symptoms and signs of hypocalcaemia

Symptoms	Signs
Muscle cramps, paraesthesia of extremities and lips	Overt
	Carpopedal spasm
Fits, psychiatric abnormality	Papilloedema*, cataracts*
In children:	Latent
Choking attacks from spasm of muscles of glottis (laryngismus stridulus)	Positive Trousseau's sign
	Positive Chvostek's sign

*After prolonged hypocalcaemia

Treatment

Hypoparathyroidism is treated with either 1-hydroxy or 1,25-dihydroxychole-calciferol. Other causes of hypocalcaemia are treated as appropriate. Acute hypocalcaemia, e.g. after thyroid surgery, requires immediate treatment with i.v. calcium until vitamin D has become effective.

OSTEOPOROSIS

Osteoporosis is thinning of bone from loss of mineral content, the bone itself being of normal architecture. Peak bone mineral content is established between the ages of 20 and 30 and thereafter is reduced in both men and women. Once bones have reached a critical degree of thinness, fractures occur, either spontaneously or with minor trauma, when the diagnosis of osteoporosis is made. The most important factor causing an accelerated decline is oestrogen deficiency at the menopause, or earlier if there is premature cessation of ovarian oestrogen production. Other risk factors include dietary deficiency of calcium, hypercalcuria, thyrotoxicosis, glucocorticoid treatment, smoking, alcohol and thinness.

Osteoporosis predisposes to vertebral fractures and fractures of long bones, particularly the neck of the femur and the wrist.

Symptoms and signs

Vertebral collapse causes back pain and ultimately kyphosis and loss of height.

Investigations

The diagnosis is radiological. Serum biochemistry is typically normal, other than a raised serum alkaline phosphatase for a few weeks following a fracture.

Differential diagnosis. The main differential diagnosis is from diffuse infiltration of the skeleton with a malignancy, particularly multiple myeloma.

Treatment

Every effort should be made to avoid the condition by attention to risk factors. Women with premature cessation of oestrogen secretion, for whatever reason, should receive oestrogen therapy, and women with a normal menopause should be considered for hormone replacement therapy (HRT) according to risk factors for osteoporosis. Bone density can be measured to help in the evaluation of women for HRT. Established osteoporosis is treated either by HRT or by cyclical biphosphonate, the latter for periods of 2 weeks every 3 months, with calcium supplements in between.

PRIMARY HYPERPARATHYROIDISM

Primary hyperparathyroidism is usually from a single parathyroid adenoma, but sometimes from two or more adenomas, hyperplasia or, occasionally, carcinoma. It occurs particularly in middle aged or elderly women and may cause renal calculi or, in the more severe form, bone disease (osteitis fibrosa cystica) and symptoms of hypercalcaemia. Nowadays the condition is commonly detected on routine screening of serum calcium.

Symptoms and signs
Patients with mild hypercalcaemia are usually asymptomatic but may have renal calculi. With more severe disease, patients may experience bone pain and deformities and symptoms of hypercalcaemia (see p. 198).

Investigations
In addition to serum calcium, serum electrolytes, urea and/or creatinine levels should be determined and X-ray of the abdomen for urinary tract calculi undertaken. The pathognomic radiological bone abnormality, seen only with severe hyperparathyroidism, is subperiosteal erosions of the phalanges.

Differential diagnosis
Other causes of hypercalcaemia (Table 5.15) need to be considered, but diagnosis depends upon the absence of clinical or laboratory evidence of a malignant tumour and a serum parathyroid hormone level that is inappropriately high for the level of serum calcium.

Treatment
Treatment is by surgical excision of the underlying parathyroid tumour(s). However, particularly in elderly women, the condition is often benign and managed conservatively. Severe hypercalcaemia, bone disease, renal calculi and possibly osteoporosis are indications for surgery.

OSTEOMALACIA/RICKETS

Vitamin D deficiency causes osteomalacia in adults and rickets in children. Histologically there are widened osteoid seams and the bone is liable to deformity and fracture. Vitamin D deficiency may be dietary in origin and is rare nowadays in the UK except in the Asian population. It can also be caused by a malabsorption syndrome or by impaired production of 1,25-dihydroxycholecalciferol in renal disease.

Symptoms and signs
In children, vitamin D deficiency results in failure to thrive, bone pains and deformities. In adults, the condition is often subtle in its presentation with

non-specific aches and pains, sometimes together with symptoms of a proximal myopathy.

Investigations

The serum calcium level is typically subnormal or in the lower half of the normal range, and the bone isoenzyme of serum alkaline phosphatase is elevated. Radiological changes include pseudofractures (Looser's zones), subperiosteal erosions from secondary hyperparathyroidism and bone deformities, but these all develop late.

Treatment

Dietary vitamin D deficiency responds to relatively small doses of vitamin D (ergocalciferol), e.g. 50 µg (2000 units) daily, without any risk of hypercalcaemia. With malabsorption syndromes, once monthly injections of vitamin D are given. In vitamin D resistant syndromes, it is best to use either 1-hydroxy or 1,25-dihydroxycholecalciferol as they act more rapidly than ergocalciferol and their duration of action is shorter, so any hypercalcaemia is less prolonged.

PAGET'S DISEASE

Paget's disease is a localized bone disorder of unknown aetiology with disturbed bone architecture caused by initial excessive osteoclastic and subsequent osteoblastic activity. The bone is thickened and spongy; both it and the overlying skin have a greatly increased blood supply. The condition is very common in certain parts of the world, including the UK where it affects approximately 3.5% of those over the age of 40.

Symptoms and signs

In most subjects it is asymptomatic. It can, however, cause bone pain and deformity (Fig. 5.6). The skull, femur and tibia are commonly affected causing characteristic enlargement of the skull and bowing of the thigh and leg. The main complications are fractures, otosclerosis and neurological compression syndromes of the cranial nerves (especially the 8th) and the spinal cord. High output cardiac failure, hypercalcaemia on immobilisation and osteogenic sarcoma are rare complications.

Investigations

The serum calcium level is almost always normal but levels of the bone isoenzyme of serum alkaline phosphatase are raised, often grossly. The characteristic radiological changes, which are often detected by chance during other investigations, include coarsening of the trabecular pattern with expansion and cortical thickening.

Differential diagnosis

It is often difficult to distinguish the pain of Paget's disease from other causes of pain affecting an elderly population, such as osteoarthritis.

Treatment

The usual indication for treatment is for bone pain. Courses of up to 6 months of one of the biphosphonates are given by mouth or, less commonly, calcitonin

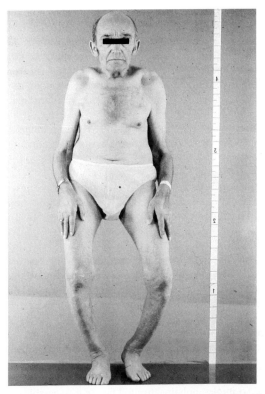

Fig. 5.6 A patient with Paget's disease with marked bone deformities.

given by subcutaneous injection 2–3 times weekly. If pain is not relieved within 4–6 weeks, its cause should be reviewed.

HYPERLIPOPROTEINAEMIA

The major clinical significance of hypercholesterolaemia and, to a lesser extent, of hypertriglyceridaemia, is as risk factors for the development of atheroma affecting, in particular, the coronary arteries and causing ischaemic heart disease (IHD). In addition, they can cause skin, tendon and eye lesions, and severe hypertriglyceridaemia may induce acute pancreatitis.

HYPERCHOLESTEROLAEMIA (WHO classification: Type IIa)

The predominant cholesterol-carrying lipoproteins are the low-density lipoproteins (LDL) and the concentration of both total cholesterol and LDL have been shown to be directly related to the risk of developing IHD. Familial hypercholesterolaemia (FH) is a single gene defect, inherited as an autosomal dominant, resulting in deficiency or abnormality of the LDL receptor and consequent hypercholesterolaemia. Those with homozygous FH have very high total serum cholesterol levels (>10 mmol/l) and develop IHD as children or young adults; the heterozygous form has an incidence of approximately 1 in 500 in the UK. However, in most people with elevated serum cholesterol levels the hypercholesterolaemia is partly environmental (chiefly dietary) and partly genetic (via a polygenic mode of inheritance) in origin.

High-density lipoproteins (HDL) take up cholesterol from the periphery, returning it to the liver, and have a protective effect upon the development of IHD, the level of serum HDL having an inverse relationship with risk of developing IHD.

In a number of diseases, such as hypothyroidism, biliary cirrhosis and the nephrotic system, hypercholesterolaemia exists as a secondary condition.

Symptoms and signs
Most often hypercholesterolaemia is only detected because of the development of arterial disease, usually IHD; however, in some subjects, particularly those with FH, it is associated with skin and/or eye lesions (Table 5.17).

Investigations
Serum cholesterol can be measured on a random (i.e. not necessarily fasting) blood sample. The possibility of secondary hypercholesterolaemia should be considered. Serum HDL cholesterol should also be measured in asymptomatic subjects being considered for hypocholesterolaemic drug treatment.

Treatment
The mainstay of treatment of hypercholesterolaemia is dietary, the essential feature of which is a reduction in total fat intake from the current level in the UK of approximately 42% of total calories to 35% or less. Within this reduction of total fat intake, polyunsaturated fats (e.g. vegetable oils) and monoun-

Table 5.17. Skin and eye lesions associated with hyperlipoproteinaemia

Lesion	Description	Type of hyperlipoproteinaemia
Tendon xanthomata	Nodules of tendons, usually extensors of hands and Achilles	FH
Corneal arcus	Opacity round rim of iris*	Hypercholesterolaemia
Xanthelasmata	Yellow deposits on eyelids or beneath eyes†	Hypercholesterolaemia
Eruptive xanthomata	Yellow–red nodules, particularly on elbows, knees, buttocks	Hypertriglyceridaemia Hyperchylomicronaemia
Palmar xanthomata	Yellow lines on skin creases of palms, fingers	Intermediate density
Lipaemia retinalis	White retinal blood vessels	Hyperchylomicronaemia

* Common in the elderly, unrelated to hyperlipoproteinaemia

† Hyperlipoproteinaemia found only in approximately 50%

Table 5.18. Drugs used in the treatment of hyperlipoproteinaemia

Drug	Comments
Hypercholesterolaemia	
Anion exchange resin	Not absorbed
Cholestyramine	Bind cholesterol/bile salts in gut
Colestipol	Commonly cause GI symptoms
Statin	
Pravastatin	Inhibit HMG-Co A reductase
Simvastatin	May cause rise in hepatic transaminase and (rarely) myositis
Fibric acid derivative	
Bezafibrate	Complicated mechanism(s) of action
Fenofibrate	Potentiate oral anticoagulants
Gemfibrozil	(Rarely) cause myositis
	Avoid in gallbladder disease
Nicotinic acid	Decrease release of non-esterified fatty acids (NEFA) from adipose tissue
	Side-effects common, especially flushing of face
Probucol	Reduces serum HDL
	Nevertheless can cause shrinkage of xanthomata
Hypertriglyceridaemia	
Fibric acid derivative	As above
Nicotinic acid	As above

saturated fats (e.g. olive oil) should be substituted for saturated (animal) fats. Other important dietary changes are reduction of calories in those who are overweight and increase in fibre intake. A variety of hypocholesterolaemic drugs are available for those whose serum cholesterol levels remain too high despite dietary modifications (Table 5.18).

Every attempt should be made to reduce the total serum cholesterol level to < 6.0 mmol/l in subjects with established IHD (secondary prevention) and ideally to 5.2 mmol/l or less. However, it is impractical to try to achieve this degree of cholesterol reduction in everyone with IHD, e.g. the elderly. Asymptomatic subjects with hypercholesterolaemia (primary prevention) should be given dietary advice. If their cholesterol levels remain > 6.5 mmol/l, serum HDL/LDL levels should be determined and drugs considered for those whose total serum cholesterol levels are > 7.8 mmol. Other factors to be considered prior to drug therapy are age, sex and other IHD risk factors, e.g. hypertension, smoking, diabetes. Independent treatment with drugs that adversely affect the serum lipid profile, such as thiazide diuretics and beta-blockers should be avoided.

HYPERTRIGLYCERIDAEMIA (WHO classification: Type IV)

Hypertiglyceridaemia is caused by the elevation of VLDL and is commonly secondary to some other condition, particularly obesity and/or alcoholism.

Symptoms and signs

There may be clinical features of IHD. In addition, hypertriglyceridaemia is associated with skin and eye lesions (see Table 5.17), and those with markedly elevated serum triglyceride levels (>10 mmol/l) are at risk of developing acute pancreatitis.

Investigations

Serum triglyceride levels should be measured on a *fasting* blood sample.

Treatment

Hypertriglyceridaemia commonly responds to treatment of underlying factor(s), such as reduction of weight and/or alcohol intake, and drug treatment (see Table 5.18) is needed far less often than with hypercholesterolaemia.

MIXED HYPERCHOLESTEROLAEMIA AND HYPERTRIGLYCERIDAEMIA (WHO classification: Type IIb)

Mixed hypercholesterolaemia and hypertriglyceridaemia occurs commonly and is associated with an increased incidence of IHD. The clinical features, investigation and management are similar to those of hypercholesterolaemia and hypertriglyceridaemia considered above.

HYPERCHYLOMICRONAEMIA (WHO classification: Type I)

A rare condition of inherited deficiency of lipoprotein lipase. It does not predispose to arterial disease but is associated with skin lesions and a risk of acute pancreatitis. Treatment is with a low-fat diet.

INTERMEDIATE DENSITY HYPERLIPOPROTEINAEMIA (WHO classification: Type III)

This is a congenital abnormality resulting in raised levels of intermediate density lipoprotein (IDL) and is associated with a markedly increased risk of IHD. The condition responds to treatment with dietary modifications and a fibric acid derivative.

MIXED HYPERTRIGLYCERIDAEMIA AND HYPERCHYLOMICRONAEMIA (WHO classification: Type V)

This is a relatively rare condition which may be an extreme form of hypertriglyceridaemia. As with hypertriglyceridaemia, it is commonly associated with overweight and/or alcoholism and may respond to treatment of these; in addition, treatment with a fibric acid derivative is often necessary.

6

DIABETES

Roger Corrall

Diabetes mellitus is a condition characterised by chronic elevation of blood glucose levels. There are two types of primary diabetes. Insulin-dependent diabetes mellitus (IDDM), formerly known as juvenile onset diabetes, is dependent on insulin treatment, has a tendency to ketosis and usually a relatively young age of onset. Non-insulin-dependent diabetes (NIDDM), formerly referred to as maturity onset diabetes, does not require treatment with insulin, is ketosis resistant and the majority of cases are diagnosed beyond 40 years of age. It should be emphasised that these two varieties of diabetes are entirely separate disorders.

Diabetes may be secondary to other conditions which include pancreatic disease and endocrine disease, the latter generally involving hypersecretion of insulin antagonists. It may also be drug induced, most commonly related to thiazide diuretics.

NON-INSULIN-DEPENDENT DIABETES

In NIDDM, insulin secretion from the pancreatic islets in response to food is reduced in amount compared with non-diabetic individuals of comparable obesity and the early rapid phase of secretion is impaired. Secondly, NIDDM is associated with a state of insulin resistance, i.e. a reduced biological effect of circulating insulin on peripheral cells.

The causative mechanisms underlying NIDDM are incompletely understood, although much evidence suggests a strong genetic component. The condition runs in families and identical twin studies show an almost 100% concordance rate. Obesity, which is associated with NIDDM, may cause it to be manifested overtly via an increase in peripheral insulin resistance in those who are genetically predisposed to this condition.

Symptoms

Many patients are asymptomatic and glycosuria is noted on routine medical examination. Patients may complain of thirst, polydipsia, polyuria and nocturia related to a glucose induced osmotic diuresis. Tiredness and weight loss are common. Pruritus vulvae and balanitis are related to candidal infections of the genitalia. Visual disturbance is caused by a temporary lens malfunction. Pain and parasthaesiae in the limbs may be present, caused by a painful neuropathy. The clinical history is typically insidious over months or years.

Signs

Patients are frequently obese. Physical signs related to chronic diabetic complications such as neuropathy or retinopathy are sometimes seen at diagnosis in NIDDM.

Investigations

Although glycosuria arouses suspicion, the diagnosis of NIDDM must be confirmed by demonstrating raised blood glucose levels; accepted limits of normality must be exceeded (Table 6.1). In a glucose tolerance test, circulating glucose levels are determined in the fasting state and 2 hours after the ingestion of 75 g of glucose. In clinical practice, an abnormally raised fasting level or a blood glucose value taken more than 2 hours after a meal in excess of 10 mmol/l (plasma 11.1 mmol/1) is sufficient to confirm the diagnosis.

The condition of impaired glucose tolerance (see Table 6.1), where blood glucose levels fall outside strictly normal limits, is not associated with the specific microvascular complication of diabetes. It is, however, linked with a propensity to premature atheroma and may worsen to frank NIDDM.

Differential diagnosis

This includes other causes of polyuria, weight loss and general tiredness.

Treatment

The aim is to achieve as normal a state of metabolic control as possible without inducing any side-effects or toxicity. Newly diagnosed diabetic patients can generally be categorised on simple clinical criteria as NIDDM or IDDM. Those thought to fall into the former category are treated initially with dietary

Table 6.1. Diagnostic criteria for diabetes

	Venous glucose (mmol/l)	
	Blood	Plasma
Impaired glucose tolerance		
Fasting value	<6.7	<7.8
2 h value of glucose tolerance test	6.7–10	7.8–11.1
Diabetes mellitus		
Fasting value	>6.7	>7.8
2 h value of glucose tolerance test	>10.0	>11.1

modification and taught how to monitor their own state of control. If control is inadequate, they may need oral hypoglycaemic drugs. These may prove successful, although failure may be seen at the beginning (primary failure) or after a period of satisfactory control (secondary failure). In these cases, insulin will be required.

Diet

Diet is the basis of all diabetic treatment. Appropriate diets, which are tailored to individual requirements, are variants of the standard or prudent diabetic diet based on the following principles:
1. Foods containing significant amounts of refined carbohydrates (monosaccharides and disaccharides, foods generally tasting sweet) are forbidden but those containing unrefined carbohydrates (starchy, non-sweet foodstuffs) are allowed.
2. High fibre foods are encouraged.
3. Animal fats (saturated) are reduced and replaced by vegetable oils (polyunsaturates and monounsaturates).

This simple diet alone is sufficient to achieve satisfactory control in many non-obese patients with NIDDM. Obese patients will need to reduce their overall calorie intake by limiting starchy and fatty foods.

Oral hypoglycaemic agents

Sulphonylureas. Act primarily by increasing secretion from the pancreatic beta cells. Pertinent details of individual drugs are given in Table 6.2. It is normal practice to start with a low dose, increasing it until either satisfactory blood glucose control or a maximum tolerable dose is achieved.

Hypoglycaemia is the commonest side-effect and often necessitates a reduction in dosage. Flushing after ingestion of alcohol is specific to chlorpropamide. Other side-effects, including skin rashes and marrow depression, are uncommon. Chlorpropamide should be avoided in the elderly and in those with impaired renal function.

Biguanides. In contrast to sulphonylureas, biguanides act primarily on peripheral cells to enhance insulin sensitivity. They are often the preferred

Table 6.2. Sulphonylurea drugs

Drug	Duration of action (h)	Site of elimination	Initial dose	Maximum dose
Tolbutamide	8	Liver	500 mg	3 g
Chlorpropamide	36	Kidney	100 mg	500 mg
Glibenclamide	12	Liver	2.5 mg	20 mg
Gliclazide	18	Liver	40 mg	320 mg
Glipizide	10	Kidney	2.5 mg	20 mg

option in obese patients. Metformin, the only biguanide used in the UK, is given after food in two or three daily doses. The commonest side-effects are gastrointestinal—predominantly diarrhoea, nausea and vomiting. These effects are lessened by increasing the dose gradually (at not less than weekly intervals) and by taking the medication after meals. The rare potentially fatal complication of lactic acidosis is only encountered if the drug is given to patients with renal or hepatic failure, alcoholism and conditions associated with peripheral cell hypoxia.

Monitoring control

Diabetic control should be monitored both by the patient in the community and at visits to the outpatient clinic. In many centres, urine testing for glucose is still the preferred home method in NIDDM. It is best performed using quantitative reagent sticks such as Diastix. The normal renal threshold is 10 mmol/l and therefore possitivity indicates that blood glucose levels are above the physiological range. In NIDDM, urine specimens tested in the fasting state and at least 2 hours after the main evening meal will suffice in monitoring control. With a normal renal threshold, such tests would generally be negative in a well-controlled diabetic.

There is an increasing tendency to assess control in NIDDM by blood glucose testing, the standard monitoring method for IDDM. In NIDDM, good control is associated with fasting levels lower than 7 mmol/l.

At clinic visits, a retrospective estimate of overall glycaemic control may be made using indices of blood protein glycosylation. Both haemoglobin in red cells and plasma proteins combine chemically with glucose (glycosylation) in both normal and diabetic individuals. The level of glycosylation is increased in diabetes and its magnitude reflects prior metabolic control.

INSULIN-DEPENDENT DIABETES MELLITUS

IDDM is characterised by a virtually total destruction of the pancreatic beta cell mass with very low or zero plasma insulin levels despite hyperglycaemia. The onset usually occurs before 30 years of age. Beta cell destruction is confirmed histologically in the early stages with round cell infiltration characteristic of an autoimmune destructive process. Hyperketonaemia and ketonuria are often present at diagnosis, reflecting the absence of sufficient circulating insulin to suppress lipolysis and hepatic ketogenesis.

IDDM is a familial condition. There is an association of IDDM with the HLA haplotypes DR3 and DR4. When both are present, the relative risk of IDDM is increased 14 times. Identical twins have shown approximately 50% concordance for IDDM, indicating a strong genetic component but raising the possibility of environmental influences. Circulating islet cell antibodies are commonly present at diagnosis. They may be present for several years before the development of clinical diabetes, which manifests overtly when more than 90% of islet cells have been destroyed. It is possible that a viral infection may trigger the autoimmune destructive process in those genetically predisposed. Coxsackie B4, mumps and rubella are possible contenders.

Symptoms and signs

These are similar to those of NIDDM but the history is more acute, often no more than a few weeks. Rarely, patients may present in diabetic ketoacidosis. They often show evidence of weightloss, and obesity is uncommon. Evidence of chronic diabetic complications is extremely rare at diagnosis in IDDM.

Investigations

The condition must be confirmed by blood glucose assay using the same criteria as in NIDDM. Ketonuria is commonly noted.

Treatment

Diet

This is based on the standard diabetic formula described above but quantitatively the starchy, carbohydrate component is more rigorously apportioned to particular meals in order to minimise variation in oral carbohydrate intake. It is customary to allot this carbohydrate as 10 g exchanges, taken at meals and snacks.

Insulin therapy

Insulin preparations. Insulin of bovine, porcine and human origin is prescribable for the treatment of IDDM. Human insulin is generally made by genetic recombinant techniques and is very similar to porcine insulin. When injected subcutaneously, beef insulin is absorbed more slowly into the circulation than human or porcine varieties.

Each variety of insulin has a characteristic time of onset, peak effect and total duration of action and on this basis can be divided into three groups (Table 6.3). Neutral soluble insulin is unmodified insulin in solution at a neutral pH and appears clear. All other insulins have a cloudy appearance.

Table 6.3. Time actions of insulin preparations

Insulin	Time action (h)			Proprietary examples
	Onset	Peak	Total duration	
Short-acting				
Neutral Soluble	0.25–1	2–4	5–8	Velosulin
Intermediate-acting				
Semilente	0.5–1	4–6	8–12	Semitard
Isophane	2–4	6–10	12–24	Protaphane
Long-acting				
Ultralente	3–4	14–20	24–36	Ultratard
Protamine Zinc	3–4	14–20	24–36	

Premixed preparations are also available, such as lente insulin (30% Semilente, 70% Ultralente), Mixtard insulin (30% Velosulin, 70% Protaphane) and Initard insulin (50% Velosulin, 50% Protaphane). The time actions of all insulins after injection are very variable. In practice, most clinical problems can be resolved using a combination of neutral soluble and isophane insulins.

Choice of insulin regimens. In the elderly, a single injection of isophane or a premixed formulation will often achieve acceptable control. In this age group, relatively high blood glucose levels may be acceptable in the absence of symptoms of poor diabetic control.

In younger patients, a greater flexibility and a desire for better diabetic control necessitate the use of multiple injection regimens. Two systems that have proved satisfactory are shown diagrammatically in Figure 6.1. Both regimens are associated with four peak times of insulin action before the four main

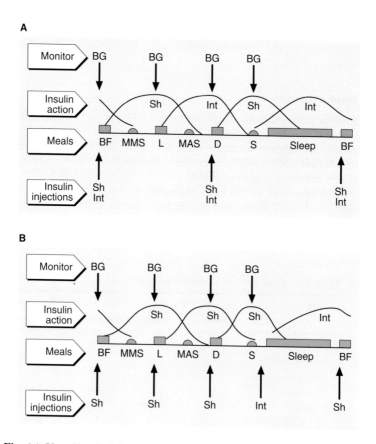

Fig. 6.1 Use of insulin injections in a twice daily **(A)** and four times daily regimen **(B)** BF = breakfast; MMS = midmorning snack; L = lunch; MAS = midafternoon snack; D = dinner; S = supper; BG = blood glucose; Sh = short-acting insulin; Int = intermediate-acting insulin.

meals. In regimen B, the short acting insulin may be given from a cartridge loaded pen device that may be carried in the pocket to facilitate injection.

Monitoring and adjustment of insulin dose. In some elderly patients with IDDM, urinary glucose monitoring with reagent sticks may suffice as an indirect estimate of blood glucose levels. However, in the great majority of patients, direct home monitoring of blood glucose levels after digital puncture is the preferred method of monitoring metabolic control. Perfect control in a young insulin-dependent diabetic would be associated with preprandial blood glucose levels between 4 and 7 mmol/l with an absence of hypoglycaemic reactions. Lesser degrees of metabolic perfection are accepted in many patients, including the elderly, those with low IQ and those prone to or unaware of hypoglycaemia.

Insulin dosage is adjusted to correspond to its peak time of action according to trends in blood glucose levels. In the absence of unprovoked hypoglycaemia or intercurrent illness, only infrequent and small changes are usually required. Clinic monitoring using glycosylated haemoglobin or fructosamine will give additional objective assessment of metabolic control.

Hypoglycaemia

Hypoglycaemia in IDDM is caused by a failure to match correctly food intake, exercise and insulin dosage. Subtle intellectual and psychomotor impairment—mild neuroglycopenia—is experienced as blood glucose levels fall below 3 mmol/l. At levels below 1 mmol/l, severe neuroglycopenia is experienced with confusion, disturbed behaviour, fits and ultimately coma. A generalised autonomic activation is triggered at blood glucose levels below 2 mmol/l which causes acute symptoms, including palpitations, sweating and tremor. Awareness of hypoglycaemia may be chronically reduced or lost in IDDM patients after many years of insulin treatment. In addition, acute intensive insulin therapy may sometimes induce a reversible blunting of hypoglycaemic awareness.

To prevent hypoglycaemia, patients must learn to avoid missed or late meals, cover significant exertion with extra carbohydrate and avoid blood glucose profiles that are bordering on hypoglycaemia. Blood glucose guidelines may have to be relaxed in those with chronic hypoglycaemic unawareness. In conscious patients, hypoglycaemia is usually reversed by 20 g oral glucose. Unconscious patients may respond to glucose gel squirted into the mouth. Glucagon 1mg s.c. or i.m. may be given by doctors or trained relatives or intravenous glucose (30 ml of 20% solution) may be required.

Intercurrent illness

This decreases insulin sensitivity in IDDM and thus tends to cause impairment of diabetic control. Urine should be tested for ketone concentration. Injections of insulin should never be omitted and insulin doses may need to be progressively increased depending on changes in blood glucose levels. If appetite is affected, carbohydrate exchanges should be maintained as liquid equivalents. Vomiting may require the administration of anti-emetics.

DIABETIC KETOACIDOSIS

Diabetic ketoacidosis (DKA) is a life-threatening complication of diabetes with an average mortality of 7%. The commonest recognised causes are acute infection and management errors; it is also seen in newly diagnosed cases of diabetes. DKA is the result of an absolute or relative insulin deficiency associated with an increase in catabolic hormones, particularly glucagon, cortisol and catecholamines. Unrestrained gluconeogensis gives rise to hyperglycaemia with secondary water and electrolyte depletion. Increased hepatic ketogenesis causes raised levels of ketone bodies which are responsible for the acidosis and hyperventilation. Average adult deficits of fluid and electrolytes are listed in Table 6.4.

Symptoms and signs

Symptoms of DKA include increasing polyuria with polydipsia, weight loss, weakness and drowsiness leading to coma. Abdominal pain may be present in the absence of pathology.

There may be evidence of salt and water depletion with tachycardia, hypotension, reduced skin turgor and low intraocular pressure. Hyperventilation may be marked with deep sighing breaths (Kussmaul's respiration). The odour of acetone on the breath is characteristic though not obvious to all.

Investigations

1. Urine will show heavy glycosuria and ketonuria.
2. A blood glucose reagent stick will typically confirm significant hyperglycaemia (usually >22 mmol/l) and centrifuged plasma will read ++ or +++ on Ketostix.
3. Plasma urea and electrolytes should be obtained, a depressed bicarbonate (<5 mmol/l in severe cases) confirms the metabolic acidosis and arterial blood gases may show acidaemia with a depressed arterial pH value.
4. A full blood count commonly shows a neutrophil leukocytosis which in this context may not necessarily indicate acute infection.

Table 6.4. Average fluid and electrolyte deficits in diabetic ketoacidosis (DKA)

Water	5–8 litres
Sodium	400–600 mmol
Potassium	300–1000 mmol
Calcium	50–100 mmol
Magnesium	25–50 mmol
Phosphate	50–100 mmol

Table 6.5. Treatment plan for diabetic ketoacidosis

Fluid and electrolytes

Volume:	Initially 3 litres in first 3 h then according to needs (total in first 24 h: 6–10 litres)
Fluids:	1. Isotonic saline (150 mmol/l) as basic replacement fluid
	2. Hypotonic saline (75 mmol/l) if plasma sodium >150 mmol/l
	3. 5% Dextrose when blood glucose < 14 mmol/l
	4. Sodium bicarbonate (1.4%) if arterial pH < 7.0, 100 mmol over 45 min (with 20 mmol KCL) repeated if necessary
Insulin	By continuous i.v. infusion 5–10 u/h initially 2–4 u/h when blood glucose falls below 14 mmol/l
Potassium	Monitor serum levels regularly, initially 2-hourly. Add following amounts to each 1 litre of fluid:

if plasma K^+ < 3.5 mmol/l, add 40 mmol KCL

3.5–5.5 mmol/l, add 20 mmol KCL

> 5.5 mmol/l, add no KCL

5. Infection should always be actively sought with at least blood and urine culture and a chest X-ray.

Treatment

The essentials of treatment are listed in Table 6.5.

Infection should be treated energetically with appropriate antibiotics. Gastric aspiration is indicated in those with impaired consciousness. Cerebral oedema may rarely occur during treatment and is associated with deepening coma. Thrombo-embolic complications may develop.

Diabetic non-ketotic hyperosmolar coma

Non-ketotic hyperosmolar coma is characterised by the insidious development of marked hyperglycaemia (generally > 50 mmol/l) with marked salt and water depletion but without acidosis. A minor elevation of plasma ketone bodies may be present up to 3 mmol/l (normal 0.05–0.5; DKA 5.0–50.0). The condition has a high mortality rate in excess of 30%. Precipitating factors are often evident, including infections, the administration of diuretics, steroids and phenytoin and an over-enthusiastic ingestion of glucose-rich drinks.

Symptoms of polyuria, intense thirst and progressive clouding of consciousness are characteristic. Coma and severe dehydration are common. Patients are frequently moribund on admission to hospital but Kussmaul's respiration is not seen. Treatment involves rehydration, insulin therapy and electrolyte replacement in a manner similar to that used for DKA.

LONG-TERM COMPLICATIONS OF DIABETES

Diabetics, after many years, are prone to pathological changes in their blood vessels.

1. Premature and widespread atheroma in large and medium sized arteries, which is not specific to diabetes, may be responsible for complications such as myocardial infarction or diabetic foot.
2. Microvascular changes, which are specific for diabetes and do not occur in the absence of long-standing hyperglycaemia, are a major pathogenetic factor in the development of three classical complications: retinopathy, neuropathy and nephropathy. The duration of diabetes and the quality of diabetic control are important determinants of these and constitute the basis for advocating good metabolic control from an early stage in young patients with IDDM.

Diabetic eye disease

Diabetic retinopathy remains the commonest cause of new blind registrations in those under 65. Background retinopathy, the earliest stage of ophthalmoscopy, is characterised by normal visual acuity and minor retinal changes sited maximally at the posterior pole of the eye. This may remain static for many years or develop into either maculopathy (commonest in NIDDM) or proliferative retinopathy (commonest in IDDM). In maculopathy, more advanced changes develop at the posterior pole with oedema and impaired visual acuity. Early treatment with retinal laser may achieve some preservation of visual function and prevent blindness. Proliferative changes may be heralded by new retinal abnormalities characteristic of the pre-proliferative phase. In proliferative retinopathy (PR), abnormal new vessels grow into the vitreous originating from areas of local retinal ischaemia. Early treatment by laser may prevent its progression. If PR is not controlled, the new vessels will bleed into the vitreous; subsequent deposition of fibrous tissue will result in blindness. Vitreo-retinal surgery may improve visual acuity in those with advanced diabetic proliferative complications.

Senile cataract occurs on average 10 years earlier than in non-diabetics.

Diabetic neuropathy

Diabetic neuropathy is thought to result from axonal damage secondary to microvascular ischaemia to peripheral nerves. Abnormal nerve metabolism may also contribute. A classification of neuropathy in diabetes is given below.

1. A *chronic distal symmetric polyneuropathy* is most commonly found and is usually asymptomatic though evidence of impaired sensation of a glove and stocking distribution may be demonstrable on examination. Lower limb deep tendon reflexes may be reduced or absent. There is no proven specific treatment.
2. *Acute painful neuropathy* is typically experienced in the lower limbs and may be very severe. Antidepressants can give symptomatic relief.

3. *Proximal motor neuropathy* leads to weakness and wasting of thigh muscles. It is often asymmetric and knee jerks are reduced or absent. The condition normally reverses within 2 years.
4. *Diabetic mononeuropathy* affects individual nerves. In some instances, this relates to local pressure, e.g. carpal tunnel syndrome; in others, it results from a localised nerve infarction. More than one nerve may be affected (mononeuritis multiplex).
5. *Autonomic neuropathy* typically presents with diarrhoea, postural hypotension, impaired gastric emptying, bladder dysfunction and impotence.

Diabetic nephropathy

1. Proteinuria develops in 40% of IDDM patients of whom two-thirds will develop renal failure.
2. Glomerular capillary basement membrane thickening can be detected within 2 years of diagnosis of IDDM and increases in time but does not cause clinical nephropathy per se. Its development in some patients is characterised by increasing proteinuria (sometimes with a frank nephrotic syndrome) decreasing GFR and hypertension and correlates with a progressive reduction of the filtration surface through expansion of the glomerular mesangium content. When plasma creatine levels rise above normal, end stage renal failure supervenes after an average of 5 years.
3. Microalbuminuria is a subclinical (Albustix negative) increase in urinary albumin excretion in the range 30–300 mg per 24 hours associated with a 20-fold increase in the risk of developing clinical nephropathy.

Treatment
In patients with microalbuminuria, great attention should be paid to meticulous control of diabetes and hypertension if present. In those with frank proteinuria, perfect blood pressure control with diastolic levels below 85 mmHg may greatly delay the advent of uraemia. ACE inhibitors may have a particular role in treatment. Renal supportive therapy-transplantation, haemodialysis or continuous ambulatory peritoneal dialysis should be available for those that develop end stage renal failure.

The diabetic foot

Neuropathy and ischaemia frequently act in combination, often with infection, to predispose to ulceration of the diabetic foot. The typical neuropathic foot is numb and warm with peripheral pulses. Complications include neuropathic skin ulceration and Charcot arthropathy. The ischaemic foot in contrast is cold and pulseless and prone to rest pain, ulceration and gangrene.

Management involves the correction of the relative contributions of neuropathy, ischaemia and infection in a collaborative teamwork exercise.

SURGERY

In diabetic patients undergoing surgery it is important to avoid extremes of hyper- or hypoglycaemia and to maintain normal hydration and electrolyte balance. In IDDM patients a glucose/insulin infusion with blood glucose monitoring is often used during the operation and for a variable time post-operatively until oral intake of food and water can be resumed.

PREGNANCY

Poorly controlled diabetes is associated with macrosomia, pre-eclampsia and hydramnios. The death of foetus or neonate occurred in one third of diabetic pregnancies 30 years ago. Current management with meticulous control of blood glucose levels has achieved results comparable to those with non-diabetic pregnancies.

Diabetes that develops during the course of pregnancy is termed gestational diabetes. Treatment is with diet in the first instance but some patients may require insulin during the pregnancy. NIDDM may develop later in life.

7

NEPHROLOGY

Anthony E. G. Raine

INTRODUCTION

Although diseases specifically affecting the kidneys are relatively rare, proper understanding of many problems encountered in everyday clinical practice requires a working knowledge of renal function and dysfunction. These problems include correct assessment of fluid balance, renal impairment related to surgical procedures, infection, heart and liver failure, and induced by drug therapy. Many common multisystem diseases such as diabetes mellitus also affect the kidney.

The four main functions of the kidneys are excretion of metabolic waste products (e.g. urea and creatinine), maintenance of normal fluid volumes and electrolyte concentrations in the intracellular, extracellular and intravascular compartments, maintenance of acid–base balance, and secretion of renin and erythropoietin and activation of vitamin D. Figure 7.1 represents the normal glomerulus.

The consequences of renal impairment are readily predicted from knowledge of these functions. Impairment of fluid and electrolyte control leads to oedema or, in a minority of cases, to a salt-losing state and hypovolaemia. Loss of renal buffering mechanisms results in systemic acidosis. Impaired ability to excrete waste products results in uraemia. Disturbance of renal endocrine function has several consequences. Inappropriate renin secretion may cause hypertension; loss of activation of vitamin D causes renal bone disease, and inadequate erythropoietin secretion results in the anaemia of renal failure.

Symptoms of renal disease are broadly divisible into those referable to the urinary tract and systemic symptoms which are a consequence of renal failure.

URINARY TRACT

Haematuria may be gross and obvious, or demonstrable only by microscopy or Stix testing. It may come from glomerular bleeding, from the renal tubules, from trauma (e.g. stones) or from a tumour in the ureters or bladder. It is a sign of disease and always requires further investigation.

Proteinuria is the result of either glomerular leakage or tubular protein loss. Heavy proteinuria almost always indicates significant glomerular disease.

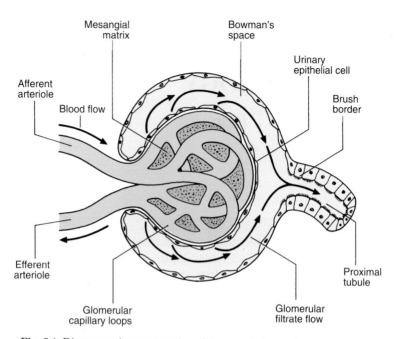

Fig. 7.1 Diagrammatic representation of the normal glomerulus.

Pyuria, white cells in the urine, is usually caused by infection, and some-times inflammation.

Dysuria is painful micturition, again usually caused by infection.

Polyuria and nocturia indicate the passing of excessive volumes of urine, as a result of failure of urinary concentrating mechanisms in renal failure.

SYSTEMIC SYMPTOMS

Oedema is caused by fluid retention and may be worsened by hypoalbu-minaemia, occurring because of urinary protein losses.

Pruritus is common in renal failure and is believed to be from accumulation in the skin of phosphate, calcium and other substances.

Dyspnoea may have several causes, including fluid retention in the lungs, hyperventilation induced by acidosis, and poor cardiac function and hyperten-sion, both of which are common in renal failure.

Bone pain and arthralgia are common and partly due to low vitamin D levels, low serum calcium and, consequently, increased parathyroid hormone secretion.

Nausea is common in severe uraemia, as is disturbance of bowel habit.

Fatigue is very common and has several causes, including accumulation of toxins and anaemia.

Investigations

Urine testing and microscopy for the presence of red cells, protein and casts.

Blood biochemistry (urea, creatinine and electrolytes), as renal failure of any significance results in elevated urea and creatinine levels.

A blood count will confirm whether anaemia is present.

24-hour urine collection enables quantification of protein excretion and determination of creatinine clearance from the formula:

Creatinine clearance (ml/min)

$$= \frac{\text{(urinary creatinine concentration, mM)} \times \text{24-h urine volume, ml/min} \times 0.694}{\text{Plasma creatinine concentration (mM)}}$$

Normal value = 115–125 ml/min/1.73 m^2

This gives a reasonable approximation of the glomerular filtration rate, which may be more accurately assessed by radioisotopic methods (e.g. ^{51}Cr-EDTA clearance). Urinary electrolyte excretion (sodium, potassium, chloride) may also be quantified by a 24-hour urine collection.

Many renal diseases have an immune aetiology, and there are several tests to assess activation of the complement system (serum C_3, C_4, immunoglobulins), and for specific antibodies, e.g. anti-DNA, anti-GBM (glomerular basement membrane); these are discussed under the specific diseases.

Radiology is essential in the diagnosis of renal disease. The key questions are, kidney size; collecting system anatomy; presence of obstruction; renal scarring; presence of calculi (stones). Plain abdominal X-ray and renal ultrasound give immediate information on kidney size, obstruction and presence of calculi. More detailed anatomy is revealed by intravenous urography (IVU). Specialised retrograde and antegrade urography may be performed under anaesthesia. CT scanning gives definitive information on renal cystic lesions and masses, and retroperitoneal disease involving the ureters.

Renal biopsy is performed in specialised centres and enables precise histological diagnosis of renal disease. It is reserved mainly for patients with unexplained renal failure who have normal sized kidneys and for patients with evidence of active nephrotic syndrome or glomerulonephritis. Clotting time and platelet count must be normal and two kidneys confirmed to be present. The biopsy is taken from the lower pole, using a percutaneous biopsy needle under ultrasound guidance.

HYPERTENSION AND THE KIDNEY

There are several important inter-relationships between the kidney and hypertension. There is much evidence that the kidney plays a role in the pathogenesis of essential hypertension. In addition, specific links occur between the kidney and blood pressure in malignant hypertension, renovascular hypertension and hypertension in chronic renal failure.

MALIGNANT (ACCELERATED) HYPERTENSION

This almost always causes renal impairment, which may be severe and irreversible. The pathology within the kidney is of intimal proliferation of the afferent arteriole ('onion skin' appearance) and sometimes fibrinoid necrosis of afferent arterioles and glomerular capillaries.

Symptoms and signs

Headache, malaise and breathlessness on exertion are caused by extreme hypertension. Oedema, pruritus and nausea are seen if renal dysfunction is severe.

Grade III hypertensive retinopathy (flame haemorrhages, soft exudates) or grade IV retinopathy (papilloedema) will be present. Haematuria and proteinuria indicate renal involvement.

Investigations

Renal biopsy will show whether the malignant hypertension is primary or secondary to underlying renal disease, such as glomerulonephritis or renal ischaemia.

Treatment and prognosis

Untreated, the prognosis of malignant hypertension is poor, with a 1-year mortality of 90%. Effective blood pressure reduction greatly reduces this mortality rate and often restores renal function.

Severe cases require ITU management, with i.v. infusion of nitroprusside or labetalol and dialysis, if necessary. Less severe cases receive oral antihypertensive therapy, e.g. beta-blockers or calcium channel blockers. In all cases, smooth and gradual blood pressure reduction is essential to avoid cerebrovascular complications.

RENOVASCULAR HYPERTENSION

Narrowing of one or both renal arteries causes secondary hypertension. In young adults, especially women, this may be the result of fibromuscular hyperplasia of the arterial wall. In the elderly, atherosclerotic disease is the cause. Activation of the renin–angiotension–aldosterone system in the affected kidney results in increased blood pressure (see Ch. 1).

Symptoms and signs

Often, there are no symptoms but there may be angina, claudication or other symptoms indicating vascular disease elsewhere.

If both kidneys are affected, renal failure may develop, causing uraemic symptoms.

The signs are those of hypertension. An abdominal bruit may be heard in a minority of cases.

Investigations

The IVU shows a delayed and dense nephrogram on the stenosed side. Doppler ultrasound may detect the stenosis. Isotope renography shows delayed uptake and excretion on the affected side and renal angiography is the definitive technique for demonstrating the arterial narrowing.

Treatment

This is either surgical or medical. Transluminal angioplasty of the stenosis may be very effective but is less so in the elderly with severe atheroma. In reconstructive vascular surgery there are various approaches, including renal autotransplantation and splenorenal anastomosis.

Medical therapy may be used for hypertension caused by unilateral stenosis or if the patient is unsuitable for surgery. Converting enzyme inhibitors are particularly effective but may cause the glomerular filtration rate (GFR) to fall dramatically, if bilateral stenosis is present.

HYPERTENSION IN CHRONIC RENAL FAILURE

Virtually all patients with renal impairment become hypertensive as renal function declines. The main causes are hypervolaemia from inadequate sodium and water excretion and excessive secretion of renin. It is established that hypertension itself hastens the progression of renal damage and dysfunction, and hence careful blood pressure control is essential.

Treatment

Loop diuretics control the hypervolaemia. Thiazides are relatively ineffective as the GFR falls, and potassium-sparing diuretics (amiloride, triamterene, spironolactone) may cause dangerous hyperkalaemia.

Beta-blockers, calcium channel blockers, vasodilators and converting enzyme inhibitors are used as needed to maintain a normal blood pressure.

GLOMERULONEPHRITIS

The primary lesion in glomerulonephritis (GN) is inflammation of the glomeruli. This results from immunological damage, which may occur in three main ways:

1. deposition of immune complexes within the capillary wall as ultrafiltration of plasma occurs
2. formation of immune complexes within the kidney if circulating free antigen is trapped within the glomerulus and antibodies then bind to it.
3. more rarely, antibodies directed specifically against GBM may arise and cause injury, as in Goodpasture's syndrome.

Although these mechanisms account for patterns of injury seen in GN, confusion often arises from the fact that the clinical syndromes associated with GN —acute nephritis, the nephrotic syndrome, progressive renal failure—bear very little relationship to the underlying glomerular inflammation. In other words, one histological form of GN, such as mesangiocapillary disease, may result in any of these syndromes.

Pathology

Deposition of immune complexes within glomerular capillary wall gives rise to an inflammatory response, i.e. the activation of complement (reduction in circulating C_3, and leukocyte infiltration, leading to damage to the glomerular filtration barrier, and resulting in proteinuria and haematuria.

In some forms of glomerular disease, e.g. those associated with systemic vasculitis or diabetes, there is no evidence of immune complex deposition, and the predisposing factors are thought to be metabolic or vascular.

The main forms of histopathologically identified GN are summarised in Table 7.1. As already stressed, there is no close correlation between these specific pathological definitions and the clinical syndromes associated with them.

Table 7.1. Categories of glomerulonephritis (GN)

	Pathology	Immuno-fluoresence	Common clinical presentation
Proliferative GN	Endothelial and mesangial cell proliferation	C3, IgG deposits	Acute nephritis, SLE
Minimal change GN	Normal	Absent	Nephrotic syndrome
Membranous GN	Thickening of GBM	IgG, C_3 deposits	SLE, nephrotic syndrome, chronic renal failure (33%)
Membrano-proliferative (mesangiocapillary) GN	Thickening of GBM, Mesangial cell proliferation	C_3	Nephrotic syndrome, renal failure (50%)
Focal glomerulos-clerosis	Segmented scarring of glomeruli	? C_3, IgM	Nephrotic syndrome, renal failure (50%)
IgA nephropathy	Mesangial cell proliferation	Mesangial IgA	Recurrent haematuria, renal failure (20%)
Rapidly progressive GN	Crescents	Linear deposits IgG, C_3	Haematuria, proteinuria, renal failure (80–100%)

SLE = systemic lupus erythematosus.

ACUTE GLOMERULONEPHRITIS

This usually follows 10–20 days after an upper respiratory infection with a beta haemolytic Lancefield group A *Streptococcus*. The bacterial antigen becomes fixed in the glomerulus and leads to an acute diffuse proliferative GN. It is seen mainly in children and is fairly rare.

The oedema and hypertension in acute GN are caused primarily by hypervolaemia as a result of enhanced renal sodium retention and impaired renal function.

Symptoms and signs

The symptoms are malaise and fever, oliguria, haematuria from glomerular inflammation, and severe headache, coma and seizures if hypertensive encephalopathy develops.

Oedema is the most obvious sign and characteristically affects the face, eyes and legs. Hypertension may be severe. Proteinuria and haematuria are often very heavy.

Investigations

Urine testing and microscopy show haematuria, proteinuria and red cell casts.

Serum urea and creatinine levels are elevated and creatinine clearance reduced. The anti-Streptolysin O titre may be raised and confirms recent streptococcal infection while a reduced serum C_3 level indicates complement system activation.

Renal ultrasound shows that the kidneys are normal size or large. Renal biopsy is not usually necessary but if performed shows a diffuse and severe proliferative GN.

Treatment and prognosis

This is largely supportive, the major aims being control of fluid retention and hypertension. Principal measures include salt restriction, i.v. loop diuretics (frusemide or bumetanide) and vasodilators, if necessary, for hypertension. Fluid balance is carefully monitored by daily weight charts and fluid balance charts. Serum urea, creatinine and potassium levels are measured daily to monitor renal function. Dialysis is not usually necessary.

If signs of impending hypertensive encephalopathy develop (severe headache, mental slowing, coma) intensive care monitoring is necessary and blood pressure control with i.v. infusion of nitroprusside or labetalol.

The outlook is good, with complete recovery in most cases, although a small minority go on to develop progressive renal failure.

NEPHROTIC SYNDROME

In contrast to acute GN, in which gross haematuria and mild proteinuria are usual, the nephrotic syndrome is defined by the occurrence together of heavy proteinuria (> 3–5 g per 24 hours), oedema and hypoalbuminaemia (< 30 g/l). A number of different forms of GN may result in this syndrome (Table 7.1). It also commonly occurs in conditions such as renal amyloidosis and diabetic nephropathy. The clinical presentation is similar in all patients with nephrotic syndrome, whatever the glomerular pathology, but the outcome will depend very much on the underlying cause of renal damage.

The primary reason for development of the nephrotic syndrome is damage to the glomerular capillary filtration barrier. Plasma proteins leak into the tubular fluid because of the loss of electrostatic and physical barriers to their passage. Intense renal sodium retention is the other main feature of the nephrotic syndrome. The reason for this is unclear; it was previously thought to be caused by intravascular hypovolaemia, resulting in activation of the renin–angiotensin system. It is now considered more likely that there may be a primary intrarenal defect in sodium excretion.

Symptoms and signs

Mild malaise, awareness of swelling, especially in the ankles, genitals and abdomen and symptoms of chronic renal failure (p. 238), if the nephrotic syndrome is associated with serious renal impairment, are the common symptoms.

Pitting oedema of the ankles, worsening with upright posture during the day, and of the thighs and genitals, if the nephrotic syndrome is severe, and ascites, and arm and facial oedema, if very severe, are the major signs.

Investigations

The diagnosis of nephrotic syndrome can only be sustained if a 24-hour urine specimen confirms heavy proteinuria (> 3–5 g per 24 hours and sometimes 20–30 g per 24 hours) and plasma albumin is reduced (< 30 g/l).

Associated abnormalities are usually hypercholesterolaemia and increased low density lipoprotein (LDL) cholesterol and increased plasma α and β globulin levels. Both these are due in part to a compensatory increase in hepatic synthesis.

Urine is examined for red blood cells and casts, indicating active GN.

Serology, including serum C_3, C_4, CH_{50}, ASO titre and antinuclear factor, may give evidence of immunologically-mediated glomerulonephritis or of a cause such as systemic lupus erythematosus (SLE). Serum electrophoresis may show a monoclonal band, indicating myelomatosis or amyloidosis.

Renal biopsy is usually performed in adults, especially if the urinary sediment is active (cells and casts) or renal function is impaired biochemically. It enables determination of the cause, the renal prognosis, and of any appropriate specific therapy.

Differential diagnosis

This is important. It is crucial to differentiate the nephrotic syndrome from other oedematous states such as congestive heart failure and liver disease. In heart failure, the jugular venous pressure is elevated, while in the nephrotic syndrome it is normal or low. In cirrhotic ascites, signs of liver disease are usually obvious.

Treatment

This has several aims, including symptomatic control of oedema and reduction of glomerular protein leak.

Oedema can be dramatic in the nephrotic syndrome, with up to 30 or more litres of fluid retention. Treatment is with bedrest, dietary salt restriction and diuretic therapy. High doses of i.v. loop diuretics are often needed to initiate a diuresis, together with amiloride or metolazone in refractory cases. Oral diuretics are substituted once a diuresis is established. The goal is to lose about 1 litre (1 kg weight) of fluid daily. High protein diets have traditionally been given but there is little evidence that they help.

Immunosuppressive therapy. In minimal change disease, which accounts for almost all childhood cases and is common in adults, proteinuria is virtually always steroid-responsive. Prednisolone 40–60 g per 24 hours is given initially, tapering down over several weeks. Repeated relapses and remissions occur over the years. Cyclophosphamide and cyclosporine have both been used successfully recently in steroid-resistant minimal change disease.

The role of immunosuppressive therapy to reduce proteinuria is less clear in other causes of nephrotic syndrome. Membranous GN responds at times to combination treatment with prednisolone and azathioprine or chlorambucil.

No specific therapy appears helpful in membranoproliferative GN or focal glomerulosclerosis.

Converting enzyme inhibitors (captopril, enalapril) are capable of reducing proteinuria through renal haemodynamic effects in diabetic nephropathy and in most other glomerular diseases. Heparin is given prophylactically if prolonged bedrest is needed, because patients with the nephrotic syndrome, particularly membranous GN, are at increased risk of venous thrombosis.

Prognosis

This depends on the underlying disease. For patients with minimal change disease, the prognosis for renal function is very good. For most other forms of GN, there is a 50% or more chance of progression to end stage renal failure.

OTHER GLOMERULAR DISEASES

IgA nephropathy

This is a form of glomerulonephritis (Table 7.1) which occurs especially in young adult males. Bouts of recurrent gross haematuria develop, often precipitated by upper respiratory infection. Microscopic haematuria persists between these bouts and proteinuria is not marked. There is no effective treatment. Previously considered a benign disease, IgA nephropathy is increasingly recognised as a common cause of progressive renal failure.

Henoch-Schönlein purpura

Mesangial IgA deposition also occurs in this condition which mainly affects children, and is characterised by recurrent episodes of arthralgia, abdominal pain and purpuric rash on the legs and buttocks. Renal failure develops in a minority of cases.

Rapidly progressive glomerulonephritis

This is distinguished histologically by the presence of epithelial cell crescents in Bowman space, which progressively obliterate the normal glomerular tuft. As the name implies, this form of glomerulonephritis leads rapidly to end stage renal failure, within weeks to several months, especially if more than half the glomeruli display crescent formation.

Crescentic change may be seen in many forms of GN but is especially associated with systemic vasculitis (microscopic polyarteritis, Wegener's granulomatosis) and Goodpasture's syndrome, and it may occur in SLE (lupus nephritis). These are all conditions characterised by development of antibodies causing damage within the kidney and elsewhere and are discussed in Chapter 13. They have certain similarities; all may have widespread multiorgan involvement, depending in which tissues antibody-mediated damage arises and may progress rapidly to end stage renal failure, or failure of other organs, if untreated. However, there is often a very good response to intensive immunosuppression with prednisolone and other agents, especially cyclophosphamide. Repeated plasma exchange (plasmapheresis) may help in particularly resistant cases.

Diabetic nephropathy

This is a major and feared complication of both insulin-dependent and non-insulin-dependent diabetes. It arises in 30% of patients and leads inexorably to end stage renal failure. The mortality rate is very high owing to cardiovascular complications. The nephropathy is caused by diabetic microvascular disease, and most patients also have severe diabetic retinopathy.

The pathology is of glomerulosclerosis, with basement membrane thickening and increased mesangial matrix. Although the progression to a nephrotic syndrome and then to endstage renal failure is usually invariable, recent trials have shown that strict control of hypertension may slow this process. Converting enzyme inhibitors appear particularly effective.

RENAL INVOLVEMENT IN SYSTEMIC DISEASE

In addition to SLE and systemic vasculitis, other systemic diseases may also affect the kidney.

Systemic sclerosis

Marked thickening of the arterial intima occurs and results in ischaemic glomerular damage and histological appearances indistinguishable from malignant hypertension. Adequate control of hypertension is very important in minimising renal damage.

Sickle cell anaemia

The kidney may be affected in several ways. Sickling of erythrocytes in the renal medulla, where oxygen tension is low, causes haematuria which is often heavy. Renal failure in sickle cell disease is caused by renal cortical necrosis from vasculopathy or by a specific glomerulopathy.

Haemolytic–uraemic syndrome (HUS) in children and thrombotic thrombocytopenic purpura (TTP) in adults

These are related disorders in which there is intravascular haemolysis, sometimes triggered by a viral infection, with fragmentation of red cells, fibrin deposition in small blood vessels and thrombocytopenia. In the kidney this process, called microangiopathic haemolytic anaemia, causes oliguria, haematuria and uraemia. Short-term support by dialysis may be required. Recovery from HUS is usual but the outlook is worse in adults, who often also develop neurological complications and failure of other organs.

Myeloma

Renal failure is common in this condition and has several possible causes, including hypercalcaemia, secondary hypovolaemia and tubular accumulation of myeloma paraprotein. Renal amyloidosis may complicate myeloma.

Amyloidosis

This may also be primary (cause unknown) or arise in patients with longstanding chronic inflammation or infection (e.g. rheumatoid arthritis or empyema). In amyloidosis, abnormal sheets of amyloid fibrils are deposited, with development of heavy proteinuria and a severe refractory nephrotic syndrome leading to progressive renal failure.

Hepatorenal syndrome

This may complicate chronic ascites and liver failure. There is oliguria, hyponatraemia, intense sodium reabsorption and a reduction in GFR.

URINARY TRACT INFECTION

Urinary tract infection (UTI) is much more common in women than in men, probably because of the short length of the female urethra and proximity to the anal region, allowing ascending infection by bowel organisms. The commonest infecting organism in UTI is *Escherichia coli*. Bladder infection (cystitis) is facilitated by poor bladder emptying, previous damage to the bladder epithelium and low urinary flow rates. Ascent of infection up the ureters is aided by vesico-ureteric reflux which occurs when normal valvular action at the uretero–vesical junction during bladder contraction is defective. Ascending infection results in renal parenchymal infection (pyelonephritis).

Symptoms

The symptoms of lower urinary tract infection are dysuria, together with cloudy and offensive-smelling urine and urgency of micturition. Suprapubic pain or tenderness, urinary frequency and nocturia are also present.

In pyelonephritis there may also be marked pyrexia and rigors, loin pain on the affected side, nausea and vomiting.

Investigations and treatment

Urine microscopy will show pyuria, and organisms may be seen on gram staining.

IVU is performed in women only for repeated infection but in all men with UTI, as an underlying structural abnormality or stone is likely

A urine specimen for culture should be obtained before starting treatment. More than 10^5 organisms/ml are significant, lower counts or mixed growths are not. Suprapubic bladder aspiration may be necessary when in doubt. A 5-day course of amoxycillin, trimethoprim or nitrofurantoin is given, and a high fluid intake is maintained. In women with relapsing infection, prophylactic antibiotics may be required for 12 months for eradication of infection. Relapsing infection in men may be caused by prostatitis. Pyelonephritis is a serious infection which usually requires parenteral antibiotics, such as an aminoglycoside (e.g. gentamicin) or a cephalosporin.

The presence of malaise, fever and sterile pyuria may indicate renal tuberculosis, diagnosed by positive culture of an early morning urine specimen. Treatment is with combination anti-tuberculous therapy.

TUBULO-INTERSTITIAL NEPHRITIS

After chronic GN, chronic inflammation of the renal tubules and interstitium, with relative glomerular sparing, is the second commonest finding in patients with chronic renal failure. It was once assumed that virtually all of these cases were caused by repeated urinary infection with reflux—'chronic pyelonephritis'. However, repeated infection with reflux in adult women does not cause renal impairment, although it may do so in infancy. In half of all adult patients who have histologically proven chronic tubulo-interstitial nephritis, no cause is established. Of the remaining 50%, a proportion are caused by infection and reflux in childhood.

Papillary necrosis accounts for another group of patients with tubulo-interstitial nephritis. In this condition there is ischaemic injury to the papillae, which may slough and pass into the ureter, causing obstruction. Diagnostic changes of calyceal clubbing are seen on IVU. The best-known cause of papillary necrosis is analgesic nephropathy—ingestion over years, of large quantities of analgesics including salicylate, paracetamol and especially its metabolite phenacetin. Causes of papillary necrosis are analgesic nephropathy, diabetes mellitus, sickle cell disease and toxin exposure, e.g. to lead or cadmium.

Acute increases in serum uric acid level (hyperuricaemia) occur when chemotherapy of lymphomas and other tumours leads to massive cell lysis and generation of urate. This may precipitate in the renal tubules, causing obstruction and uraemia. There is no strong evidence that chronic hyperuricaemia, the cause of gout, leads to renal failure. However, increased uric acid secretion may cause development of uric acid stones.

RENAL STONE DISEASE

Up to 5% of the population develop calculi at some stage. These may occur in the collecting system of the kidney (nephrolithiasis) or within the ureters and bladder (urolithiasis). Much more rarely, the renal parenchyma becomes calcified (nephrocalcinosis) as a result of hypercalcaemia, or as a consequence of medullary sponge kidney or renal tubular acidosis. Most calculi contain calcium and oxalate. Their formation is a physical process, depending on concentration of their constituents in the urine and conditions such as urine pH. Most renal stone formers have 'idiopathic hypercalciuria', with increased urinary calcium excretion and normal serum calcium concentration. Increased urinary calcium excretion occurs also when serum calcium is increased (hyperthyroidism, sarcoidosis, vitamin D ingestion). Calcium oxalate stones are radio-opaque, in contrast to uric acid stones which are radiolucent.

'Staghorn' calculi which enlarge slowly, outlining the renal pelvis, may develop in association with chronic UTI, especially with *Proteus mirabilis*. They also develop in cystinuria, an inborn tendency to excrete excessive urinary cystine.

Symptoms
Passage of a stone into the ureter causes renal colic with sharp severe flank pain radiating to the groin, and accompanying nausea, vomiting and sweating. There is no postural relief and it is worsened by increased urine flow rate.

Investigations
The diagnosis can be rapidly established by urine testing, microscopy and culture for haematuria, pyuria and coexistent UTI, abdominal X-ray and tomography for radio-opaque calculi, IVU to localise ureteric calculi. 24-hour urine is performed for excretion of calcium, oxalate and uric acid, and serum electrolytes to exclude hypercalcaemic disorders.

Differential diagnosis
This is wide and includes any cause of acute and severe abdominal pain, such as cholecystitis, pancreatitis or bowel pathology. In practice, the history of renal colic is usually typical and the diagnosis confirmed by abdominal X-ray demonstrating a stone, and coexistence of microscopic haematuria.

Treatment
Acute management of renal colic is conservative with adequate pain relief (opiates). Stones not passed spontaneously require urological removal. When possible this is endoscopic, involving percutaneous nephrolithotomy (kidney puncture), or urethroscopic removal of lower ureteric stones.

Extracorporeal shock wave lithotripsy (ESWL) is increasingly performed; in this technique high-frequency shock waves are focused to shatter the calculus, enabling passage of fragments.

Prevention of recurrent stone formation involves ensuring a high daily fluid intake (3–4 litres per 24 hours) to reduce urinary mineral concentration. Dietary calcium intake is reduced, and if necessary thiazide diuretics, which reduce tubular calcium excretion, are given. Uric acid stone formers are given the xanthine oxidase inhibitor allopurinol.

URINARY TRACT OBSTRUCTION

Obstruction of urinary outflow may cause either acute or chronic renal failure. Acute obstruction may result in severe uraemia but full recovery is usually possible, provided the obstruction is rapidly relieved. In contrast, chronic obstruction, as in prostatic hypertrophy, may lead to unsuspected chronic renal failure with limited scope for recovery. Obstruction may occur at any point in the urinary tract, and potential sites are shown in Table 7.2. The blockage may be intraluminal (e.g. clot, calculus), or from abnormal urinary tract narrowing (stricture) or external compression (e.g. tumour). Obstruction above the level of the bladder must be bilateral to cause anuria or uraemia.

Table 7.2. Sites of urinary tract obstruction

Tubules	Precipitation, e.g. urate or sulphonamide crystals
Collecting system	Sloughed papilla Staghorn calculus Tumour Pelvic–ureteric junction obstruction Blood clot
Ureters	Stricture (previous calculus, tuberculosis) Calculus Blood clot Compression (retroperitoneal fibrosis, tumour)
Bladder	Tumour Blood clot Ureterovesical stricture Neuropathic bladder
Urethra	Prostatic hypertrophy (males) Stricture

Acute obstruction causes dilatation above the blockage and back pressure which ultimately nullifies glomerular filtration pressure. If it persists, tubular and interstitial atrophy occur with eventual glomerular sclerosis. The tubular damage also interferes with urinary concentrating mechanisms, and many patients with prolonged obstruction have polyuria and nocturia.

Symptoms and signs
Loin pain and anuria occur in complete acute obstruction. Chronic partial obstruction causes polyuria, urinary retention and incomplete bladder emptying. Dysuria and frequency occur if there is accompanying infection.

The kidneys are palpable if they are enlarged by acute obstruction. Prostatic enlargement is present in prostatic hypertrophy. The bladder is enlarged and palpable in bladder outflow obstruction.

Investigations
In contrast to GN, urine microscopy shows no cellular casts. Renal ultrasonography will rapidly show whether a dilated collecting system is present, confirming obstruction.

The IVU will show a delayed nephrogram and excretory phase on the affected side. Isotope renography will show a similar delay. Cystoscopy with retrograde ureteric catheterisation will define precisely the site of a ureteric lesion. Alternatively, antegrade pyelography will visualise the upper ureter.

Abdominal CT scanning will demonstrate extrinsic compression from tumour or retroperitoneal fibrosis, a condition in which the ureters become encased in fibrous tissue, there is low back pain and the erythrocyte sedimentation rate (ESR) is raised.

Differential diagnosis
This is with the other causes of uraemia (p. 235).

Treatment

The principles are relief of the obstruction and decompression of the collecting system.

Prostatic obstruction is relieved by passage of a urinary catheter, until definitive transurethral prostate resection. Ureteric obstruction is bypassed with 'double J' stents at retrograde urography. If this is not possible, a percutaneous nephrostomy is inserted at antegrade pyelography, under local anaesthesia, with insertion of a drainage catheter into the renal pelvis. This will maintain urine flow and renal function pending a definitive procedure.

In retroperitoneal fibrosis the ureters are freed surgically (ureterolysis) and steroid therapy may help prevent relapses.

Prognosis

There is complete recovery of renal function if acute obstruction is rapidly relieved. Unsuspected chronic obstruction may lead to irreversible renal failure, requiring long-term dialysis.

CYSTIC RENAL DISEASES

There are several forms of inherited or congenital cystic disease of the kidney. In all of them, cysts develop within the renal parenchyma but the outcomes differ greatly. Small renal cysts also arise with ageing, and in long-term dialysis patients.

ADULT POLYCYSTIC KIDNEY DISEASE (APKD)

APKD is an autosomal dominant condition and is by far the commonest inherited cause of renal failure. Minute cysts, present from birth, progressively enlarge, causing loss of function as the cysts obliterate normal nephrons. The cysts are apparent on ultrasound examination by late adolescence. Significant renal impairment usually develops by the fourth or fifth decade, although it may not arise until late in life.

Symptoms and signs

Bleeding or infection within the cysts causes fever, loin pain or tenderness. There is dull flank pain when the kidneys are large and ureteric colic from blood clots.

Grossly enlarged and irregular kidneys are usually easily palpable on abdominal examination. Hypertension is especially common in APKD. Associated hepatic cysts lead to liver enlargement.

Investigations

The diagnosis is readily made by ultrasound scanning, or alternatively by IVU or abdominal CT scan. Renal function is accurately assessed (serum urea and electrolytes, and creatinine clearance). Urine culture is performed to exclude coexistent infection.

Treatment

The major principles of management in APKD are effective treatment of both urinary infection and hypertension, to maximise maintenance of renal function. Cyst infection may lead to severe septicaemia and requires parenteral antibiotics and cyst aspiration and drainage. Cyst debris or blood clots may cause acute ureteric obstruction.

A complication of APKD is an association with berry aneurysms of the cerebral circulation, a potentially fatal cause of subarachnoid haemorrhage. Development of severe headache and focal neurological signs in a patient with APKD should always arouse suspicion of this complication, with cerebral angiography and neurosurgical intervention if appropriate.

Prognosis

Patients with APKD and significant renal impairment will progress slowly but steadily to end stage renal failure over a period of years.

Although antenatal diagnosis of APKD is now possible by genetic linkage analysis, the case for therapeutic abortion in this condition, in which the quality and duration of life may be near-normal, remains highly controversial.

MEDULLARY CYSTIC DISEASE

In medullary cystic disease, inheritance may be recessive or dominant and end stage renal failure develops in late adolescence. Development of small medullary cysts results in tubulo-interstitial scarring and secondary glomerular sclerosis.

In contrast, medullary sponge kidney is not inherited but is a sporadic and benign disorder in which medullary cysts develop and often calcify. Patients are prone to ureteric colic and urinary infection but renal function is preserved.

ACUTE RENAL FAILURE

Acute renal failure is characterised by rapid loss of renal function and the development of uraemia within hours or days. Usually, though not always, it is reversible. In contrast, chronic renal failure is the final outcome of many glomerular and tubulo-interstitial diseases and is slowly progressive, but irreversible loss of renal function occurs. The functional consequences of renal failure are similar whether acute or chronic and include uraemia, with loss of renal excretory function, loss of fluid and electrolyte balance, loss of acid–base balance, and abnormal endocrine function. However, the distinction between acute and chronic renal failure can usually be made using the guidelines summarised in Table 7.3.

In practice, the two most useful pointers to longstanding chronic renal failure are demonstration of small kidneys on ultrasound scan and evidence of secondary hyperparathyroidism (phalangeal erosions, hypocalcaemia, raised serum alkaline phosphotase levels) as neither occur in acute renal failure.

Traditionally, the aetiology of acute renal failure is divided into pre-renal, renal and post-renal causes (Table 7.4). Although inexact, it is a useful cate-

Table 7.3. Differentiation of acute and chronic renal failure

	Acute renal failure	Chronic renal failure
Duration of uraemic symptoms	Short (days)	Weeks or months Nocturia and cramps precede more severe symptoms
Signs Hypertension Anaemia	Infrequent Variable	Usual Present (except polycystic disease)
Investigations Renal size	Normal	Small (except in amyloidosis, myeloma or polycystic kidney disease)
Secondary hyperparathyroidism	Absent	Present

Table 7.4. Causes of acute renal failure

Pre-renal	
Impaired renal perfusion	Hypotension, septic shock, volume depletion (haemorrhage, burns, gastrointestinal fluid loss)
Renal artery occlusion	Atherosclerotic thrombo-embolism, aortic dissection
Hepatorenal syndrome	
Renal	
Glomerular disease	Acute proliferative GN (post-streptococcal), rapidly progressive GN, vasculitis, anti-GBM disease, haemolytic–uraemic syndrome
Acute interstitial nephritis	Penicillins, thiazides, non-steroidal anti-inflammatory drugs
Rhabdomyolysis + myoglobinuria	Trauma
Systemic infections	Viral infection, leptospirosis, legionella, HIV
Post-renal	
Urinary tract obstruction	Intrarenal, renal pelvis, ureters, bladder, urethra

gorisation, as it helps determine management. Pre- and post-renal failure (obstruction) in particular may respond rapidly to therapy if recognised and treated sufficiently early. The common factor in pre-renal failure is impaired renal perfusion, which causes a compensatory fall in the GFR and very avid sodium and water reabsorption. If renal perfusion remains impaired, acute tubular necrosis (ATN) supervenes. This is a progressive decline in both glomerular and tubular function, whose pathogenesis remains poorly under- stood. On renal biopsy there is patchy tubular necrosis and the glomeruli appear normal. Once ATN is established, there is an obligatory period of olig- uria and renal failure, usually lasting 2–4 weeks, and followed by a diuretic phase as renal function recovers.

Symptoms and signs

These depend on the cause of acute renal failure, e.g. loin or back pain in uri- nary tract obstruction, haematuria and oedema in acute GN. Uraemic symp- toms (anorexia, nausea, malaise, clouding of consciousness) may be marked in severe acute renal failure.

The signs also depend on the cause; hypotension and tachycardia are seen with haemorrhage or septicaemia, and hypertension and oedema in acute GN or rapidly progressive GN.

Investigations

Assessment of volume status is crucial in patients with acute renal failure, to determine whether the intravascular volume is decreased (hypovolaemia) or increased (hypervolaemia). The guidelines for this are outlined in Table 7.5. The most sensitive parameter is the blood pressure (BP) and heart rate response to standing.

Urine microscopy shows urine virtually free of protein, cells or casts in pre- renal uraemia or obstructive uropathy. With ATN proteinuria, pyuria and tubular cell casts appear. Red cell casts indicate GN.

In pre-renal uraemia, the urine has a high osmolality and urea concentration and low sodium concentration (<20 mmol/l) because of marked renal sodium and water retention. Once ATN is established, urine osmolality falls and sodium concentration rises.

Urgent ultrasound scanning is essential to determine kidney size and to exclude obstruction. An abdominal X-ray may show urinary tract calculi.

Renal biopsy is not indicated in obstruction and not necessary in ATN, unless the diagnosis is uncertain. It should be performed when vasculitis,

Table 7.5. Assessment of volume status

	Hypovolaemia	Hypervolaemia
Supine blood pressure	Normal or low	High
Postural BP fall	> 20 mmHg	< 20 mmHg
Postural tachycardia	> 20/min	< 20/min
Tissue turgor	Reduced	Normal
Jugular venous pressure	Low	High
Pulmonary oedema	Absent	Present
Peripheral oedema	Absent	Present

accelerated hypertension or drug-induced acute interstitial nephritis is suspected.

Treatment

The need for urgency in evaluation of the cause of acute renal failure has already been stressed. This enables correct management.

Pre-renal uraemia

To minimise the likelihood of progression to ATN, hypovolaemia is corrected by volume expansion with saline, albumin or blood, as appropriate. Central venous pressure is monitored, and maintained in the range 5–10 cmH$_2$O. Frusemide 40–120 mg i.v. may be given once hypovolaemia is corrected, together with low-dose dopamine infusion to encourage urine output. Failure of response to these measures, and higher dose frusemide (250–500 mg i.v.) indicate that ATN is established.

Renal and post-renal acute renal failure

Outflow obstruction is relieved as soon as possible. If acute GN or vasculitis is diagnosed serologically or on renal biopsy, intensive immunosuppression is given.

Acute interstitital nephritis is a drug-induced hypersensitivity reaction, in which renal tubulo-interstitial inflammation may be accompanied by an erythematous skin rash, arthralgia and fever. The drug implicated is withdrawn and a short course of steroids is given. Complete recovery is usual.

Established acute renal failure

Meticulous management is essential, paying attention to several aspects:

Fluid and electrolyte balance. Stability is maintained by monitoring daily weight (1 litre of fluid lost/gained is 1 kg change in bodyweight), BP and pulse, central venous pressure and fluid balance. Plasma urea and electrolyte levels are measured daily. The fluid intake allowed is 500 ml added to the previous 24-hour output. Daily sodium and potassium intake is restricted. In the polyuric phase of recovery from ATN, large volumes of i.v. fluids are needed to replace urinary losses.

Nutrition. Protein intake is reduced to minimise protein catabolism and urea load and 2000 kcal daily given as carbohydrate and fat.

Sepsis is avoided. Bladder catheterisation is unnecessary and should not be used.

Dialysis. If plasma urea and creatinine levels continue to increase despite the above measures, renal support is commenced. Other indications for dialysis are pulmonary oedema, pericarditis, hyperkalaemia (serum potassium > 6.5 mmol/l) and severe acidosis (pH < 7.2). Three main modes of renal support are used:

1. acute peritoneal dialysis
2. intermittent haemodialysis
3. continuous arteriovenous or venovenous haemofiltration (CAVH or CVVH), which may be combined with dialysis (CAVHD, CVVHD). The patient's blood is circulated continually through a porous filter; up to 20 litres per 24 hours of plasma ultrafiltrate is removed and replaced by electrolyte solution. Filtration is driven by the patient's own blood pressure (CAVH) or by an external pump (CVVH).

Prognosis

With adequate dialysis support during the oliguric–uraemic phase, full recovery often occurs in acute renal failure. However, many patients with ATN have other serious problems, including septicaemia, postoperative complications or shock, and so the overall mortality of acute renal failure remains 50% or more.

CHRONIC RENAL FAILURE

Chronic renal failure is the end result of many of the different forms of renal injury already described. It refers to a progressive and usually irreversible loss of renal function. Once this is insufficient to sustain life (usually when GFR is 5% or less of normal), end stage or terminal renal failure has occurred. The rate of decline depends on the underlying disease. It may be several weeks in rapidly progressive GN and many years in polycystic kidney disease and chronic pyelonephritis.

Although there are many possible causes of chronic renal failure, most fall into a few categories and the commonest, in order, are chronic GN, chronic pyelonephritis/tubulo-interstitial nephritis, diabetic nephropathy, APKD, and renovascular hypertension.

End stage renal failure is fairly rare. In the UK, 50–80 patients per million population commence renal replacement therapy each year. Not all patients receive treatment; some are very elderly and infirm. At present, approximately 19 000 patients receive replacement therapy in the UK, half of whom have a functioning kidney transplant and the remainder are divided equally between haemodialysis and continuous ambulatory peritoneal dialysis (CAPD).

Prognosis

The reasons for renal injury, once initiated, leading to progressive nephron loss and renal scarring remain uncertain, although they are the subject of intensive research. Current interest focuses on the mechanisms of hypertrophic and inflammatory responses in the glomeruli and tubulo-interstitium. The rate of loss of renal function usually follows a predictable course in each patient. The GFR declines linearly, but the corresponding increase in the serum creatinine level is hyperbolic (Fig. 7.2). A reciprocal plot of serum creatinine level against time gives an approximately straight line with negative slope (Fig. 7.3) from which the likely onset of end stage renal failure can be predicted.

The onset of chronic renal failure is usually insidious and over half the renal function may be lost before any symptoms develop. Severe uraemia may cause

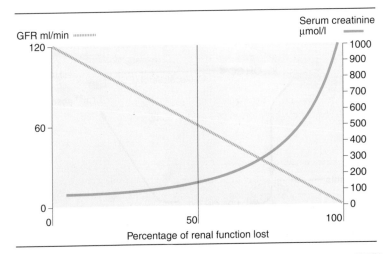

Fig. 7.2 Relationship between the linear decline in glomerular filtration rate (GFR) and exponential rise in serum creatinine levels as renal function is lost.

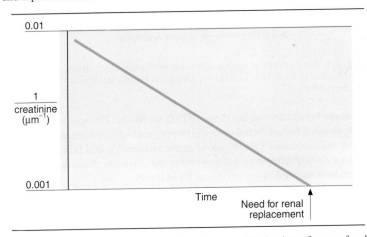

Fig. 7.3 Use of the reciprocal creatinine plot to predict the time of onset of end stage renal failure.

symptoms referable to virtually every organ system, as shown in Table 7.6 but some deserve special mention.

Anaemia is largely caused by the failure of production of erythropoietin and accounts for much of the fatigue, lethargy and dyspnoea. It also worsens symptoms of dyspnoea and ischaemic heart disease.

Hypertension and hyperlipidaemia predispose renal failure patients to atherosclerosis; they also have a very high risk of stroke, myocardial infarction and heart failure.

Secondary hyperparathyroidism (Fig 7.4) is due to lack of renal activation of vitamin D, which causes hypocalcaemia; both lead to a compensatory

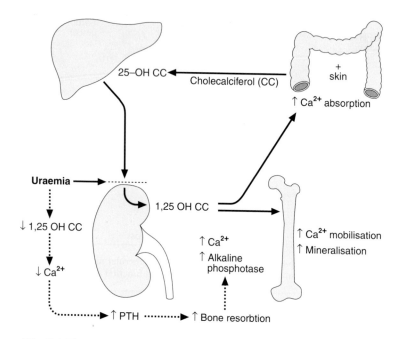

Fig. 7.4 The pathway of normal activation of vitamin D (cholecalciferol) and its interruption in renal failure. PTH = parathyroid hormone; OHCC = hydroxy-cholecalciferol.

increase in parathyroid hormone (PTH) secretion. The spectrum of bone disease in renal failure (renal osteodystrophy) includes osteomalacia (inadequate bone mineralisation) from lack of active vitamin D, and bone resorption and bone pain with subperiosteal erosions in the clavicles, phalanges (Fig. 7.5) and elsewhere, caused by excess serum PTH levels.

Symptoms and signs

The symptoms are many and relate to the organ systems involved (Table 7.6). The early symptoms of chronic renal failure (nocturia, polyuria, leg cramps and pruritis) may give a guide to its duration. Nausea, fatigue, oedema and other 'characteristic' uraemic symptoms arise relatively late.

Signs may be few or absent in early chronic renal failure. In severe disease they are widespread and include oedema and hypertension from hypervolaemia, anaemia, peripheral neuropathy and uraemic fetor. In severe life-threatening uraemia there may also be pericardial rub, confusion and metabolic flap.

Investigations

Ultrasound examination will show kidney size and parenchymal loss. If the kidneys are less than 9 cm in length, irreversible scarring has almost certainly occurred and renal biopsy is not indicated. If they are over 9 cm, renal biopsy is usually performed to enable a diagnosis to be made.

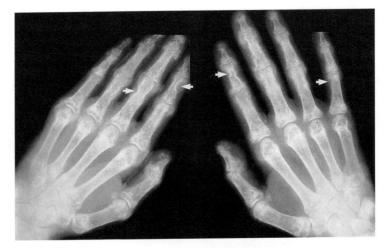

Fig. 7.5 Hand X-rays of a male long-term haemodialysis patient showing changes of severe renal osteodystrophy. Arrows indicate marked subperiosteal erosions.

Table 7.6. Clinical features of chronic renal failure

System	Symptoms	
Cardiovascular	Hypertension, Heart failure	Uraemic pericarditis, Oedema, Ischaemic heart disease
Central nervous	Confusion, coma (severe uraemia), Autonomic neuropathy	Peripheral neuropathy
Endocrine & Metabolic	Glucose intolerance, infertility, Hyperlipidaemia	Amenorrhoea, Hyperparathyroidism
Skin	Pruritus	Pigmentation
Musculo Skeletal	Muscle cramps Bone pain (renal osteodystrophy)	Myopathy
Blood	Anaemia	Platelet dysfunction

Renal function is monitored initially by serial measurement of creatinine clearance or isotopic GFR and later by serum creatinine measurement.

The anaemia of renal failure is normochromic and normocytic. Serum ferritin, vitamin B_{12} and folate levels are measured in case deficiency of these is worsening the anaemia.

A low serum calcium level, high alkaline phosphatase, increased serum PTH, and X-ray of the hands for subperiosteal erosions confirm secondary hyperparathyroidism.

Treatment

The principles of conservative management are similar to those for acute renal failure. To minimise the rate of progression and to lessen uraemic symptoms, dietary protein restriction is introduced, at around 0.6–0.8 g/kg per 24 hours. This reduces the catabolic load imposed on the kidney.

Effective control of hypertension is essential. This also reduces the rate of loss of renal function and lessens the risk of cardiovascular complications.

To maintain fluid balance, high doses of loop diuretics may also be needed.

The anaemia of renal failure could until recently be treated only by repeated blood transfusion, with attendant risks of iron overload and sensitisation, prejudicing future transplantation. Recombinant human erythropoietin is now widely used and is very effective in reversing renal anaemia.

Hyperphosphataemia causes pruritis and promotes vascular calcification in uraemia. Phosphate binders are given with meals to reduce gut phosphate absorption. Aluminum hydroxide preparations are now avoided if possible because of the risk of long-term aluminium overload. Calcium carbonate preparations are an alternative.

Secondary hyperparathyroidism is treated with active vitamin D analogues (calcitriol or alfacalcidol). If tertiary (autonomous) hyperparathyroidism develops, parathyroidectomy is usually necessary.

END STAGE RENAL FAILURE

When GFR is below 10 ml/min, patients develop increasingly severe uraemic symptoms. Renal replacement therapy should begin before this state is reached. This corresponds in general to a serum urea level of 30 mmol/l, a creatinine level of 800–1000 μmol/l, or severe hyperkalaemia or acidosis. The options for treatment are haemodialysis, CAPD and renal transplantation. Careful planning and an integrated approach are required for all of these.

Haemodialysis

This in essence involves circulation of the patient's blood and of dialysis fluid on opposite sides of a semipermeable dialysis membrane. The principle is shown in Figure 7.6. The membrane allows the passage of water, electrolytes and small molecules, but not large molecules (over 20 kD), proteins or cells. Urea, creatinine, other waste products and potassium diffuse down their concentration gradients. Water removal is achieved by applying negative pressure to the dialysis fluid circuit.

Access to the circulation is usually achieved by formation of an arteriovenous fistula between the radial artery and cephalic vein, which provides an accessible site for insertion of needles. Most patients undergo haemodialysis for 4 or 5 hours three times weekly, either in their own homes with an installed control unit which pumps and monitors blood flow, or in hospital. Many patients have now been maintained in relatively good health for 20–25 years by haemodialysis, although long-term complications have arisen such as aluminium overload and amyloidosis from deposition of β-2 microglobulin, which is not cleared from plasma by conventional dialysis.

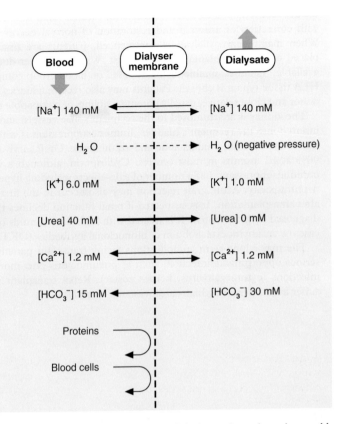

Fig. 7.6 The principle of haemodialysis. The dialysis membrane is semipermeable, allowing passage of water, ions and small molecules.

Continuous ambulatory peritoneal dialysis

CAPD has been available as an alternative to haemodialysis for over a decade. A soft silastic (Tenckhoff) catheter, implanted through the abdominal wall, is used to enable instillation of a 1.5–2.0 litre bag of sterile dialysis fluid into the peritoneal cavity. After dwelling for 4 hours, the fluid is drained out and a new bag drained in. These 'exchanges' are usually performed four times daily. Electrolytes and waste products equilibrate across the peritoneal membrane, between the fluid and adjacent blood vessels. Water removal occurs through osmosis, as CAPD fluid is available in varying strengths of hypertonicity.

CAPD is simple and effective, rapidly learnt, and allows greater patient independence than haemodialysis. The major drawback is the risk of peritonitis, although this is reducing with introduction of newer 'no-touch' sterile connection systems. Treatment is by intraperitoneal antibiotics.

Renal transplantation

Successful renal transplantation is the optimal mode of treatment for most patients with end stage renal failure. It removes the need for dialysis and dietary restrictions and if fully successful, returns renal function to normal with correction of anaemia and restoration of normal energy and fertility. When maintenance dialysis is commenced, patients are tissue-typed and placed on the transplantation waiting list. When a cadaver donor kidney is available, the most suitable recipient based on blood group compatibility and HLA tissue typing is chosen. Patients may also receive a kidney from a living donor and close relative, usually parent or sibling, of compatible tissue type.

The kidney is anastomosed to the recipient's iliac vessels, and the ureter is inserted into the recipient's bladder. Immunosuppression is with a combination of cyclosporin, prednisolone and azathioprine. Graft survival is now over 90% at 12 months in most centres. Cyclosporin, although a very effective immunosuppressant, has a number of side-effects including hypertension and nephrotoxicity. Acute graft rejection may also occur in the first 2–3 months after transplantation. It is suspected if renal function declines rapidly and is diagnosed by graft biopsy. It is treated with high-dose steroids or in resistant cases by antithymocyte globulin or monoclonal antibodies (OKT3).

The major long-term complications facing transplant patients are risk of serious opportunistic infection, such as pneumocystis pneumonia, and viral infections (cytomegalovirus, herpes zoster). Renal transplant patients also suffer from a persisting high cardiovascular mortality.

8

WATER, ELECTROLYTE AND ACID–BASE BALANCE

David Stansbie

Water accounts for over 60% of the bodyweight; the major part (70%) lies within the cells and constitutes the intracellular volume (ICV). The remainder is the extracellular volume (ECV) and can be divided into an interstitial component (22%) and the plasma (8%). Water intake is mainly from food and drink but a small amount is produced by the oxidation of foodstuffs. Water is lost in urine, faeces, sweat and expired air. The distribution of body water in a 70-kg man is illustrated in Figure 8.1.

The concentrations of the main intra- and extracellular ions are shown in Table 8.1. Sodium is the predominant extracellular cation. Intake is largely from food and losses are in urine, sweat and faeces. Total body sodium in a 70-kg man is approximately 3000 mmol.

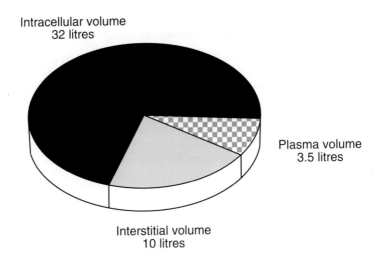

Intracellular volume
32 litres

Plasma volume
3.5 litres

Interstitial volume
10 litres

Fig 8.1 Distribution of body water.

Table 8.1. Intracellular and extracellular ion concentrations

Intracellular concentration (mmol/l)		Extracellular concentration (mmol/l)	
Na^+	10	Na^+	145
K^+	140	K^+	5
H^+	8×10^{-5}	H^+	4×10^{-5}
Ca^{2+}	1.5	Ca^{2+}	2.5
HCO_3^-	8	HCO_3^-	25
Cl^-	2	Cl^-	100
SO_4^{2-}	10	PO_4^{2-}	1
Organic PO_4^{2-}	50		

Potassium is the main intracellular cation; a 70-kg man has approximately 4500 mmol. Energy-dependent pumps maintain the gradient of sodium and potassium across the cell membrane.

WATER AND SODIUM BALANCE

Under normal circumstances the ECV is determined by the total body sodium and its distribution between the intra- and extracellular compartments. The maintenance of blood volume and the regulation of sodium and water home-ostasis is controlled by aldosterone, atrial natriuretic peptide (ANP), anti-diuretic hormone (ADH; also known as arginine vasopressin) and thirst.

Aldosterone and the renin–angiotensin system

A decreased ECV results in a decreased renal blood flow; this stimulates the release of renin from the juxtaglomerular apparatus of the kidney. Renin is an enzyme which acts on an alpha-2-globulin produced by the liver to produce the decapeptide angiotensin I.

Angiotensin converting enzyme (ACE) cleaves angiotensin I to the octapep-tide angiotensin II, which stimulates the release of aldosterone, a steroid pro-duced by the adrenal cortex; this promotes the uptake of sodium in exchange for potassium or hydrogen ions in the distal tubule of the kidney (Fig. 8.2).

Antidiuretic hormone and thirst

ADH is normally secreted in response to changes in extracellular osmolality. An increase in plasma sodium concentration, the main determinant of plasma osmolality, results in the recognition by the osmoreceptors of an increase in the ratio of extracellular to intracellular osmolality and stimulates ADH secretion. The major effect of ADH is to increase the permeability to water of the distal tubules and collecting ducts of the kidney. The hypertonicity of the medulla of

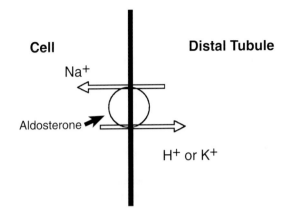

Fig 8.2 Aldosterone mediated sodium transport mechanism.

the kidney which surrounds the collecting ducts ensures that in the presence of ADH water is reabsorbed.

Thirst receptors, located near the osmoreceptors in the hypothalamus, stimulate drinking in response to an increased osmotic gradient across their cell membranes. Depletion of vascular volume may also stimulate thirst and ADH secretion independently of changes in osmolality.

Atrial natriuretic peptide

ANP is produced by the atria of the heart in response to an increased blood volume and results in a natriuresis; its place in sodium and water balance remains to be defined.

Overall the net effect of a reduction in renal blood flow is to promote sodium retention which tends to increase ECV osmolality. This is turn stimulates ADH release which promotes water reabsorption and increases the circulating blood volume thus restoring renal blood flow.

DISORDERS OF WATER AND ELECTROLYTE BALANCE

Accurate measurement and recording of fluid intake and output is the key to understanding and resolving most fluid balance problems. Insensible loss of water in sweat and expired air is about 900 ml per 24 hours; 500 ml per 24 hours is produced by metabolic processes and, therefore, the net insensible loss is 400 ml per 24 hours. The daily requirement of water for an average adult is 2.5 litres, of which just over 2 litres is derived from food and drink.

Pyrexial patients or patients being ventilated have greater insensible losses.

Assessment of water and electrolyte balance requires the history, clinical and laboratory findings to be taken into account. Laboratory tests that are useful for assessing hydration are total plasma protein concentration or the haematocrit. The finding of elevated levels implies a loss of water but depends upon the assumption that protein concentration and haematocrit were normal before the water loss. The estimation of sodium and potassium concentrations in plasma and urine are the basis for assessing water and electrolyte balance.

Hypernatraemia

The clinical effects of hypernatraemia depend more upon its rate of development than the absolute value of the plasma sodium concentration. They are caused by the cerebral cellular dehydration that results when the brain is bathed in a hyperosmolar fluid.

Clinical features of hypernatraemia are thirst, confusion, coma and ultimately death.

Water deficit is the commonest cause of hypernatraemia; a deficit of 2.5 litres will result in an increase in plasma sodium concentration of about 10 mmol/l. Some of the causes of hypernatraemia are given in Table 8.2.

Inadequate water intake

Failure of adequate water intake leads to the development of hypernatraemia, a hyperosmolal state and, normally, thirst. Hypernatraemia from water depletion leads to a shift in water from the cells to the extracellular space and consequently the plasma volume does not shrink unduly; blood pressure and renal blood flow are initially maintained. As the water deficit increases, renal blood flow falls and uraemia develops.

Excess water loss

In diabetes insipidus (DI) a lack of ADH results in excessive secretion of dilute urine and a failure to conserve water. It may be caused by a failure of secretion of ADH (cranial DI) or end organ failure to respond to ADH (nephrogenic DI). The net effect is that the kidneys lose their ability to produce a concentrated urine.

The disorder is characterised by the production of a dilute urine in the presence of hyperosmolal plasma due to hypernatraemia. Patients complain of

Table 8.2. Causes of hypernatraemia from water deficit

Inadequate water intake	Excess water loss
Lack of availability of water	Patients on a ventilator and/or with a fever and unable to replenish loss
Physical or mental illness which prevents drinking e.g. stroke or coma	Diabetes insipidus
Neglect at the extremes of age	Vomiting or diarrhoea
	Osmotic renal loss
Loss of appreciation of thirst	

thirst and polyuria and hypernatraemia is usually only present when the patient is deprived of water. Since this is both unreasonable and may be dangerous, water deprivation tests to establish the diagnosis of DI should only be performed under strictly controlled conditions.

Loss of hypotonic fluids by vomiting, diarrhoea or loss through fistulae will lead to water loss and hypernatraemia. Loss of excess water in the urine because of a high solute load may also lead to hypernatraemia.

Sodium excess

This is usually iatrogenic from the administration of excessive amounts of sodium in the form of hypertonic intravenous infusions, or the use of oral sodium chloride solutions as emetics.

Investigation of hypernatraemia

The distinction between hypernatraemia from water depletion and that from sodium excess is most easily made from the clinical history. A raised haematocrit or total plasma protein concentration suggests water depletion. A failure to produce a concentrated urine (> 700 mosmol/l) in the presence of water deprivation, and the subsequent response to the synthetic ADH analogue desmopressin, will identify DI and allow a distinction to be made between its cranial and nephrogenic forms. Beware of artefactual causes of an elevated plasma sodium concentration as a result of blood being collected into a syringe containing sodium heparin or elevations caused by sampling from or near the cannula used to administer hypertonic sodium bicarbonate during resuscitation procedures.

Hyponatraemia

The clinical consequences are the result of the reduction in plasma osmolality that is normally a feature of hyponatraemia. This causes the osmotic uptake of water by cells, including those of the brain. Cerebral cellular oedema and a rise in intracranial pressure may occur if the hyponatraemia develops rapidly. As with hypernatraemia, the rate of development of hyponatraemia, rather than the absolute value of the plasma sodium concentration is the main determinant of the clinical features. These may be present where the plasma sodium has fallen to 125 mmol/l over the course of a few hours, yet remain absent at 115 mmol/l if this level has been reached gradually over several days.

Clinical features of acute hyponatraemia are confusion and lethargy, nausea and vomiting, and seizures leading to coma and death.

Water excess (dilutional hyponatraemia)

Dilutional hyponatraemia occurs when the kidney is unable to dispose of a water load by producing a dilute urine. The increased ECV inhibits renin–aldosterone secretion and stimulates ANP. This condition is often included under the blanket diagnosis of the syndrome of inappropriate antidiuretic hormone secretion (SIADH) although serum ADH levels are not invariably increased.

Common causes of chronic dilutional hyponatraemia are ADH production by tumours, inflammatory lung disease, CNS disorders, trauma and surgery, and drugs, e.g. carbamazepine, chlorpropamide, cytotoxics, thiazides and tricyclic antidepressants.

The criteria for diagnosis are hypoosmolal hyponatraemia with an inappropriately concentrated urine (urine osmolality > plasma osmolality) containing sodium at a concentration of >10 mmol/l (implying no sodium deficit) in the presence of normal renal and adrenal function. The plasma urea and total protein concentrations and the haematocrit are usually low. Acute dilutional hyponatraemia is often iatrogenic and most commonly occurs postoperatively following inappropriate fluid regimens. Compulsive water drinking is another cause and here the excessive fluid intake is associated with an impaired ability to excrete water.

Management of chronic hyponatraemia from water excess depends upon the clinical state. Water restriction to 500 ml per 24 hours is always effective if adhered to but changes take place slowly and sodium supplements may be required. Demeclocycline, which impairs the effects of ADH on the kidney, is useful in patients with inappropriate ADH secretion by tumours since this allows some relaxation in the water restriction schedule.

Patients who have the severe neurological manifestations of acute water intoxication often show a marked improvement in response to hypertonic saline but this treatment should be used with extreme caution since it may precipitate acute pontine myelosis and, in susceptible patients, heart failure.

Sodium depletion

Hyponatraemia is seen in Addison's disease partly as a result of a lack of aldosterone. In addition, these patients lack cortisol, which is necessary in order to excrete a water load. The hyponatraemia of Addison's disease is therefore due in part to relative water excess.

Pseudohyponatraemia

Plasma with a high lipid or protein content may lead to an underestimate of the sodium concentration in the plasma water.

Spurious hyponatraemia

The commonest cause of spurious hyponatraemia is a blood sample collected from an arm into which a dextrose drip is flowing.

Hyperkalaemia

Hyperkalaemia is a potentially life-threatening metabolic abnormality. Plasma levels above 6.5 mmol/l are associated with an increased risk of cardiac arrest; levels above 7.0 mmol/l must be reduced as a matter of urgency. This may be achieved by slow i.v. infusion of 5–10 ml of 10% calcium gluconate followed by 100 ml of 50% glucose with 20 units of short-acting insulin. Clinical features are non-specific and development of a cardiac arrhythmia may be the first manifestation.

Pseudohyperkalaemia caused by release of potassium from cells in vitro is more common than true hyperkalaemia. Haemolysis of red cells, a high white cell or platelet count, storage of blood at 4°C or collection of blood from a 'drip arm' may all result in pseudohyperkalaemia. If there is any doubt, another sample should be collected before instituting potassium lowering measures.

Causes of hyperkalaemia are factitious (pseudohyperkalaemia), excess potassium administration, renal failure, acidosis, drugs (e.g. spironolactone, amiloride), ACE inhibitors, hypoaldosteronism and tissue necrosis.

Several mechanisms lead to hyperkalaemia in vivo: cell destruction and release of intracellular potassium by trauma, burns or tumour chemotherapy; displacement of potassium from the intracellular compartment by acidosis; impaired excretion by the kidney because of acute or chronic renal failure; failure of exchange of sodium for potassium ions in the distal tubule caused by impairment of the aldosterone-mediated transport mechanism.

Hypokalaemia

Total body potassium depletion is the usual cause of hypokalaemia. The clinical effects are muscle weakness, hypotonia, paralytic ileus and cardiac arrhythmias.

The concentration of potassium in intestinal secretions may be 10 times that of plasma and their loss by prolonged vomiting, watery or secretory diarrhoea or from fistulae leads to hypokalaemia. Villous adenomas of the rectum and laxative abuse are other causes of loss by this route. Diuretics increase renal losses of potassium by increasing the delivery of sodium to the distal tubule where potassium is lost secondarily to preferential sodium reabsorption. Hyperaldosteronism from Conn's syndrome and the mineralocorticoid effects of steroids administered or produced endogenously as a result of Cushing's syndrome also result in hypokalaemia secondary to increased sodium reabsorption in the distal tubule.

Mild hypokalaemia is treated by oral potassium supplements and potassium-rich food (bananas). Severe hypokalaemia (≤ 2.5 mmol) may require intravenous KCl therapy. It should be given very cautiously at no more than 20 mmol per hour. In all cases, the cause of the potassium loss must be corrected. If diuretics are the cause, then potassium-sparing diuretics should be added to the existing potassium-losing drugs, e.g. amiloride to frusemide.

ACID–BASE BALANCE

The extracellular fluid (ECF) pH is maintained at about 7.4 (40 nmol/l of H^+) despite the production of up to 100 mmol of hydrogen ion (H^+) each day by the average adult. The H^+ is mainly derived from ureagenesis, anaerobic glycolysis and ketogenesis. Homeostasis is maintained by short-term mechanisms in the form of buffers; long-term compensation involves the kidney and depends on normal lung function. Buffering mechanisms in the blood include the bicarbonate and phosphate systems and haemoglobin. They are most effective at maintaining the free H^+ concentration when faced with an acid load. Acids dissociate to produce H^+; alkalis dissociate to form hydroxyl ions (OH^-). The action of the bicarbonate/carbonic acid system is illustrated below.

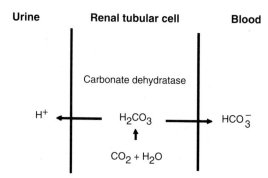

Fig 8.3 Mechanism of renal hydrogen ion production.

Bicarbonate/carbonic acid buffer system

$$H^+ + HCO_3^- \rightarrow H_2CO_3 \rightarrow CO_2 + H_2O$$

An increase in H^+ concentration results in the combination of H^+ with HCO_3^- to form undissociated carbonic acid. The free H^+ concentration decreases as does the bicarbonate ion concentration. The carbonic acid dissociates in turn to produce carbon dioxide and water. Some cells, notably erythrocytes and renal tubular cells, contain an enzyme called carbonate dehydratase which speeds this process (Fig. 8.3).

The kidney is responsible for the elimination of H^+ produced during metabolism. It is able to secrete H^+ against a concentration gradient of about 800 : 1 and consequently the urine pH may fall to 4.5. The kidney's ability to secrete an alkaline urine is very limited and the maximum urine pH is 7.8. The H^+ in the urine is mainly buffered by the $HPO_4^{2-}/H_2PO_4^-$ buffer system.

Although the kidneys are responsible for H^+ elimination, whole body H^+ homeostasis also involves the lungs. The H^+ eliminated by the kidneys is derived from CO_2 which is hydrated to form carbonic acid which in turn dissociates to form H^+ and HCO_3^-. The secretion of H^+ is associated with the return to the circulation of HCO_3^-.

Investigation of acid–base balance

This is essentially an investigation of kidney and lung homeostatic mechanisms and depends upon the measurement of partial pressures of oxygen (PO_2) and carbon dioxide (PCO_2) as well as pH and HCO_3^- concentration in blood. Arterial blood is used for 'gas' measurements but PO_2 is not part of the acid–base assessment and will not be considered further.

The pH of blood determines absolutely whether the patient has an acidosis or an alkalosis. Compensatory mechanisms which act to restore blood pH towards normal always cease before normality is reached and overcompensation does not occur. The direction of the original pH perturbation may therefore be recognised.

The PCO_2 measures the respiratory component of an acid–base disturbance. Part of a normal blood gas analysis is the standard bicarbonate. This is the HCO_3^- concentration which would be present in the blood sample at 37°C and normal barometric pressure if the PCO_2 was normal (40 mmHg or 5.3 kPa). It is a measure of non-respiratory or metabolic components of an acid–base disturbance. A change in PCO_2 or standard bicarbonate may be the primary event in an acid–base disturbance or a secondary compensatory mechanism. It is not possible to determine which from an inspection of the PCO_2 or standard bicarbonate value alone.

In order to use these values to evaluate an acid–base disturbance the following simplified scheme may be helpful. The principal buffer in blood is the bicarbonate/carbonic acid system and PCO_2 is a reflection of the carbonic acid concentration. The lungs determine the PCO_2; the kidneys determine the HCO_3^- concentration. The relationship between them and pH may be expressed in the following way:

$$pH \propto \frac{[HCO_3^-]}{PCO_2}$$

This may be used to define the main acid–base disturbances found in practice.

Respiratory acidosis

Acute respiratory failure, e.g. from an impacted foreign body in the bronchial tree, will result in an increase in PCO_2 and decrease in pH.

$$\blacktriangledown pH \propto \frac{[HCO_3^-]}{\blacktriangle PCO_2}$$

compensation leads to

$$\downarrow pH \propto \frac{\uparrow [HCO_3^-]}{\blacktriangle PCO_2}$$

If the cause of the respiratory failure is a long-term problem, e.g. chronic obstructive airways disease, the kidney compensates for the hypercapnia by excreting H^+ in the urine and at the same time, increasing the HCO_3^- concentration of blood. This increase is over and above that due to the increased PCO_2 and results in an increase in the standard bicarbonate.

Metabolic acidosis

Acute metabolic acidosis caused by lactic acid accumulation, for example, will lead to the production of H^+ which will be buffered by the bicarbonate/carbonic acid system and lead to a fall in HCO_3^- concentration. The H^+ will eventually be excreted by the kidney but in the short term the respiratory rate will increase (air hunger) and the PCO_2 level will fall; the blood pH will tend to return towards normal.

$$\blacktriangledown pH \propto \frac{\blacktriangledown [HCO_3^-]}{PCO_2}$$

compensation leads to

$$\downarrow pH \propto \frac{\downarrow [HCO_3^-]}{\downarrow PCO_2}$$

Respiratory and metabolic acidosis

A patient with respiratory failure and carbon dioxide retention who also develops a metabolic acidosis will have a raised PCO_2 associated with a decreased standard bicarbonate; blood pH will be depressed by both mechanisms.

$$\blacktriangledown pH \propto \frac{\downarrow [HCO_3^-]}{\blacktriangle PCO_2}$$

The inter-relationship between blood pH, standard bicarbonate and PCO_2 are summarised in Table 8.3. It should be emphasised that while the student may find this approach useful it is didactic and simplistic and must only be used as an introduction to the understanding of acid–base disturbances in patients.

Table 8.3. Relationship between pH, standard bicarbonate (std HCO_3^-) and PCO_2

	PH	PCO$_2$	std HCO$_3^-$
Respiratory acidosis (compensated)	↓↓ / ↓	↑↑ / ↑↑	— / ↓
Metabolic acidosis (compensated)	↓↓ / ↓	— / ↓	↓↓ / ↓↓
Respiratory and metabolic acidosis	↓↓↓	↑↑	↓↓

9

GASTROENTEROLOGY

Alan E. Read

Gastroenterology includes the study of the gut and associated glands like the liver and pancreas. It has progressed at a remarkable rate, and most of the gut, biliary and pancreatic ducts can be visualised or opacified using endoscopy and radiology, whilst biopsy, absorptive studies and breath tests using ^{14}C-labelled bile salts or hydrogen production can detect small intestinal bacterial contamination and measure gut transit time. Simple tablet tests can be used to detect chronic pancreatic disease, and scanning, both ultrasonic and CT, have revolutionised the detection of hepatobiliary and pancreatic disease, whilst viral and autoimmune tests have helped to compartmentalise chronic liver-disease.

DISORDERS OF THE OESOPHAGUS

OESOPHAGEAL REFLUX AND REFLUX OESOPHAGITIS

Reflux of gastric and duodenal contents into the oesophagus is common and may cause heartburn and pain. Pathologically, oesophagitis, stricture formation and peptic ulceration can occur. It is encouraged by the following:

1. a defective lower oesophageal sphincter (LOS), as when a hiatus hernia destroys LOS function, or with relaxation of a normal LOS in the obese, in pregnancy, with smoking and stooping,
2. impaired lower oesophageal 'clearing' which allows gastric juice retention in the oesophagus,
3. impaired gastric emptying or increased gastric acid production.

Pathology

There is oesophageal inflammation, ulceration and sometimes stricture formation. Gastric mucosal islands may be found in the lower oesophagus (Barrett's oesophagus) which may be premalignant. Ulcers may bleed, perforate and penetrate, and there may be a hiatus hernia.

Symptoms and signs

1. Heartburn is a burning sensation from the epigastrium up to the neck and jaws. It is worse on lying, bending, straining, in pregnancy and after food, and is accompanied by acid regurgitation.

2. Dysphagia from oesophagitis or a stricture.
3. Gastrointestinal (GI) bleeding may be from oesophagitis or an ulcer.
4. Severe pain may be caused by oesophageal spasm, and aspiration of gastric contents into the lungs can cause pneumonia and wheezing.
   Usually there are no signs.

Investigations

Endoscopy reliably assesses the severity of oesophagitis, allows biopsy and detects complications such as stricture.

Radiology gives similar but less precise information; 24-hour oesophageal pH monitoring can be correlated with the patient's symptoms and is a valuable ambulatory method of recording reflux incidence (low pH values < 4).

Treatment

A lot can be achieved by the manoeuvres listed in Table 9.1. Where symptoms are resistant or where complications such as bleeding occur, surgery may be required. The operation is usually a fundoplication to restore the function of the LOS or the positioning of a soft plastic collar (Angelchik's prosthesis) around the lower oesophagus. Ulcers may require resection and vagotomy to control gastric secretion.

ACHALASIA OF THE CARDIA

This is a diffuse oesophageal disease caused by intramural autonomic nerve plexus degeneration. The disease results in the failure of LOS relaxation with dysphagia, oesophageal dilatation and retention oesophagitis. It occurs at all ages but is more common in young adults.

Symptoms and signs

There is a gradual onset of lower oesophageal dysphagia with regurgitation, initially relieved by drinking fluids with meals. Weight loss is moderate.

Severe attacks of central chest pain, often nocturnal and mimicking ischaemic heart disease, are caused by muscle hyperactivity in the denervated

Table 9.1. Medical therapy of oesophagitis

Altered behaviour	Drugs
Stop smoking (it reduces LOS function)	Simple antacids
Lose weight	H_2-blocking agents, e.g. ranitidine 150 mg at night (to control gastric acid)
Avoid stooping	Cisapride 10 mg 8-hourly (releases
Prop up head of bed at night	acetylcholine and stimulates oesophageal clearing)
Avoid heavy meals (particularly at night)	Omeprazole 20–40 mg per 24 hours (a proton pump inhibitor. Blocks almost
Avoid constipation	completely gastric acid production

gullet. Cough, recurrent chest infections and wheezing from bronchial aspiration are seen. Rarely, clubbing of the fingers and chest signs are observed.

Investigations
A chest X-ray may show a grossly dilated oesophagus, an absent gastric air bubble and possibly pneumonia or lung fibrosis. Barium studies confirm oesophageal dilatation and define the smoothly narrowed distal oesophagus (c.f. the irregularity seen with oesophageal cancer).

Endoscopy with preliminary oesophageal lavage confirms mega-oesophagus, detects oesophagitis and the narrowed distal segment. When supplemented by oesophageal manometry, it confirms a raised LOS pressure and disorganised oesophageal muscular activity.

Differential diagnosis includes lower oesophageal cancer and peptic oesophagitis. Ischaemic heart disease may be mimicked by the pain.

Treatment
The preferred treatment is pneumatic dilatation of the LOS under general anaesthesia and endoscopic control. This usually gives satisfactory relief and can be repeated.

Surgical treatment is by cardiomyotomy (Heller's operation) in which the muscular coat of the lower oesophagus is incised down to the mucosa.

Successful treatments relieve dysphagia, allow the oesophagus to return to normal size and hopefully prevent oesophageal cancer which may complicate achalasia.

HIATUS HERNIA

Two major types of this common abnormality occur where part of the stomach is within the thoracic cavity. A sliding hernia (70%) is accompanied by an altered and thoracic site of the LOS, and may cause major reflux although it is small; a large rolling herniae in which the LOS is not displaced may or may not cause symptoms. The disease is more common in women in whom obesity, multiple pregnancies and ageing are important aetiological factors. Herniae contain gastric mucosa, and peptic ulceration with all its complications may occur within them (Fig. 9.1).

Symptoms and signs
Large herniae may be asymptomatic but there may be attacks of severe chest pain mimicking myocardial ischaemia, whilst complicating ulcers cause dyspepsia and vomiting. Bleeding, causing haematemesis or anaemia, also occurs. Small sliding herniae may cause severe heartburn and dysphagia from peptic oesophagitis.

Signs are usually absent, although there may be obesity.

Investigations
A barium meal demonstrates a pouch of stomach in the chest. With large herniae there may be a retrocardiac shadow on a plain chest film. Complications such as a stricture or ulcer within the gastric pouch are well demonstrated.

Endoscopy is valuable and allows a more precise identification of oesophagitis and its severity, and allows histology and cytology of ulcers.

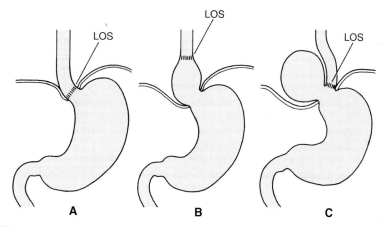

Fig. 9.1 Types of hiatus hernia: **(A)** normal structure; **(B)** sliding hiatus hernia; and **(C)** rolling hiatus hernia.

Treatment

Control of symptoms is outlined in the section on reflux (Table 9.1). Rarely, surgery may be required for persistent symptoms, and ulcer perforation or bleeding. Hernia repair with fundoplication and highly selective vagotomy are the usual approaches; large herniae may require surgery because of the risk of volvulus.

CARCINOMA OF THE OESOPHAGUS (see Table 9.7)

OTHER DISORDERS OF THE OESOPHAGUS (see Table 9.2.

DISORDERS OF THE STOMACH AND DUODENUM

The stomach acts as a hopper delivering premixed and predigested food to the small bowel. Lined with columnar epithelium forming pits or glands, it produces mucus, hydrochloric acid (HCl) and intrinsic factor (in the body of the stomach). The pyloric region produces gastrin from G cells.

The secretion of HCl is under humoral and vagal control. The final common stimulus to acid production is histamine while gastrin is an important intermediate. Released by vagal and food stimulation, it exists in several molecular forms. Gastrin release is inhibited by H^+ ions (HCl) and by hormones like somatostatin. Vagal stimulation excites a gastrin response. The mucosa of the stomach is protected from acid damage by a thin layer of mucus through which bicarbonate is secreted.

PEPTIC ULCER

This includes both gastric and duodenal ulcers, acute or chronic. Though chronic gastric and duodenal ulcers show significant differences, the two conditions are described together. Peptic ulcer is common, about 4500 people die

Table 9.2. Other diseases of the oesophagus

Lesion	Cause	Effect	Treatment
Candida oesophagitis	Candida infection of oesophagus in immunosuppressed or antibiotic treated or diabetic patients	Painful dysphagia Plaques of white material seen on endoscopy	Drug therapy nystatin, miconazole, fluconazole
Mallory-Weiss syndrome	Mucosal tear at the oesophagogastric junction, often following vomiting	Haematemesis Tear seen by endoscopy	Conservative
Barrett's oesophagus	Gastric mucosa lines part of the lower oesophagus	Oesophageal reflux	Treatment of reflux Monitor for cancer
Systemic sclerosis	Involvement of oesophagus is common	Dysphagia Dilated aperistaltic oesophagus with secondary peptic oesophagitis	Conservative
Oesophageal web	Anteriorly placed shelf of epithelial tissue at level of cricoid cartilage Often associated with iron deficiency	Mild dysphagia May be a risk of subsequent carcinoma	Dilate endoscopically Treat iron deficiency
Diffuse oesophageal spasm	Uncertain—middle-aged and elderly patients show diffuse spasm of oesophagus on barium swallow (corkscrew oesophagus)	Chest pain mimicking angina Dysphagia	Nitrates or calcium channel blockers, e.g. nifedipine occasionally dilatation

annually from it in Great Britain and 10% of adult males are sometime sufferers. The death rate is rising, particularly in elderly women, because of non-steroidal analgesic consumption. The incidence of the disease varies from country to country and there are major differences within countries, e.g. in India. In the UK it is more common in men and more commonly duodenal than gastric. The incidence in females has increased and in them the relative proportion of duodenal ulcers has fallen. The 'cause' of peptic ulcer is unknown. The following are major aetiological factors:

1. Gastric acid/pepsin. Whether an injury of the epithelium is required before gastric acid/pepsin can produce ulceration is uncertain. Ulcerogenic drugs like aspirin and other non-steroidals probably act in this way and allow acid/pepsin to potentiate damage. Acid levels are generally high in duodenal ulcer and normal or low in gastric ulcer, but there is considerable overlap with levels in normal subjects.
2. Recently, *Helicobacter pylori* infection of the gastric mucosa in duodenal ulcer, and less often in gastric ulcer and gastritis, has been demonstrated. Eradication of infection seems to be important in preventing ulcer relapse. The level of 'mucosal cytoprotective' prostaglandins is also a further factor protecting the mucosa.
3. Genetic factors which determine ulcer susceptibility include a family history of ulcer, inheritance of blood group O and the existence of non-secretor status in duodenal ulcer sufferers.
4. Acquired factors include smoking which prevents healing of ulcers, but is a less certain cause of ulcer formation. Chronic obstructive airways disease and alcoholism are frequent accompaniments.

Pathology
Chronic ulcers are commonly found on the gastric lesser curve and duodenal anterior wall and rarely occur in the second part of the duodenum. Chronic ulcers cause fibrosis and local deformity and can penetrate through the stomach or duodenal wall. The base of the ulcer often contains large blood vessels where protective arteritis obliterans helps to prevent vessel erosion. Malignant change may be found in gastric ulcers but modern opinion suggests that this type of ulcer is malignant from the start rather than as a change in a benign ulcer.

Symptoms and signs
Endoscopy has shown that ulcers may be present with no or minimal symptoms. Usually there is pain, often epigastric and localised by the patient with a fingertip. It is often burning, may radiate to the back or shoulders if the ulcer penetrates, and it is periodic, i.e. it may be present for 2–3 weeks and then disappears to recur after a pain-free interval. Classically worse before or just after meals, and at night, it is relieved by food, alkalis and vomiting, and patients may induce vomiting for relief.

Vomiting is common and, if persistent and copious, suggests pyloric (outflow) obstruction.

Heartburn, nausea and anorexia are further symptoms, and weightloss results.

Often there are no signs except for epigastric tenderness. Physical signs result from complications.

Investigations

Peptic ulcers in the lower oesophagus in a hiatus hernia or in the stomach or duodenum are readily demonstrated by a barium meal or endoscopy. Endoscopy also allows brush cytology and biopsy for all gastric ulcers to ensure they are benign. Histology, the detection of urease activity (change in pH on incubation), and detection of antibodies can confirm *H. pylori* infection.

Anaemia and iron deficiency, and (positive) faecal occult bloods suggest ulcer bleeding.

Hypoalbuminaemia occurs in debilitated patients with large chronic gastric ulcers, and electrolyte deficiency in those with vomiting.

The *differential diagnosis* is ulcerating gastric cancer which may be diagnosed radiologically and proved by endoscopy and biopsy.

Complications

The following important complications occur with gastric and duodenal ulcer:

1. Penetration into the pancreas, posterior abdominal wall, etc. may cause pack pain.
2. Perforation of an ulcer into the peritoneal cavity causes an abdominal emergency with severe pain, vomiting and shock.
3. Ulcers may penetrate large blood vessels with intestinal bleeding, either haematemesis, melaena or both, or chronic anaemia.
4. Local fibrosis and contraction of scar tissue results in hour-glass deformity from a lesser curve gastric ulcer, or more importantly pyloric obstruction with gastric outflow constriction. A previous history of ulcer dyspepsia then gives way to vomiting as a more important symptom. Characteristically, the vomitus is copious, projectile and contains stale food eaten 48 hours or more before. Abdominal examination shows the outline of a distended stomach, visible peristalsis and a succussion splash.

Hypokalaemic alkalosis and mild uraemia is found in the blood. Gastric washouts, fluid replacement and surgical correction (gastroenterostomy and a highly selective vagotomy) are usually required.

Treatment

The principles for treating chronic peptic ulcers are:

1. Patients should not smoke and should take regular small but tasty meals to ensure maximal food buffering. Biscuits and a glass of milk or alkalis by the bedside relieve night pain.
2. Pain is helped by antacids, e.g. aluminium hydroxide 1–2 tablets chewed 3–4 times daily, and on retiring. Ulcerogenic drugs, e.g. aspirin and other non-steroidals, are avoided, and in patients with gastric ulcer, malignancy must be excluded by complete ulcer healing at endoscopic follow-up. Ulcers heal by the use of the drugs shown in Table 9.3.

Once healing has been achieved, maintenance therapy, usually with a nightly H_2-blocker, such as ranitidine 150 mg, or cimetidine 400 mg, is required. Unless maintenance treatment is continued, 80% of ulcers will

Table 9.3. Drug treatment of peptic ulcer

Drug	Mode of action	Side-effects	Dose
Sucralfate (an aluminium hydroxide compound)	? Coats and protects ulcer from acid and pepsin	Minimal	Tablets of 1 g 2 g 12-hourly
De Nol (tripotassium dicitratobismuthate)	? Coats ulcer Eradicates *H. pylori*	Pungent odour (liquid) Black stools Theoretical risk of bismuth absorption (encephalopathy)	Liquid 5 ml 6-hourly (diluted with water) for 28 days Tablets 1 tab 6-hourly
H₂-blockers (cimetidine, ranitidine famotidine, etc.)	Reduction of gastric acidity by blocking histamine in stomach	*Cimetidine* Gynaecomastia Reversible liver and blood dyscrasia Confusion Inhibits drug metabolism *Ranitidine* No important side-effects *Famotidine* No important side-effects	400 mg 12-hourly or 800 mg at night 150 mg 12-hourly or 300 mg at night 40 mg at night
Proton pump inhibitors (omeprazole)	Inhibits gastric acid by blocking H⁺–K⁺ ATPase of parietal cells	No important side-effects ?Long-term danger of gastric tumours	20–40 mg 12-hourly (not for long-term use)
Prostaglandin analogues (Misoprostol)	Inhibits gastric acid production and may be cytoprotective	Diarrhoea Abnormal menstrual bleeding	200 μg 2–4 times per 24 hours

relapse. *H. pylori* infection in patients with recurrent peptic ulcer dyspepsia should also be treated following ulcer healing, with antibiotics such as ampicillin and metronidazole.

Ulcers that fail to heal are dealt with by using higher doses of ulcer-healing drugs, perhaps in combination and by making sure that factors such as smoking, alcohol intake, work stress, drug compliance and dietary indiscretions are controlled. The possibility of a Zollinger-Ellison syndrome (see Table 9.8) should also be remembered. Relapse is most important in the elderly and in those with serious chronic diseases. Surgery is now required for only a few troublesome ulcers. The operations of choice are local ulcer resection and a highly selective vagotomy for gastric ulcers and a highly selective vagotomy and pyloroplasty for duodenal ulcers. Partial gastrectomy is now very rarely required.

GASTRITIS

Inflammation of the gastric mucosa may be acute or chronic.

Acute gastritis

Acute gastritis is caused by alcohol, aspirin and other non-steroidal drug injury, intracranial disease and subarachnoid haemorrhage. It is also common after major trauma, burns and shock. It can lead to serious bleeding from multiple acute gastric ulcers and will require blood transfusion and treatment with H_2-blocking drugs.

Chronic gastritis

Two forms are recognised.

Gastric atrophy in the antrum and body is an autoimmune lesion. Vitamin B_{12} malabsorption results from intrinsic factor deficiency causing pernicious anaemia. Gastric atrophy is also associated with an increased incidence of gastric carcinoma and carcinoid tumours, and due to the achlorhydria, to an increased incidence of bacterial infections of the gut.

Chronic superficial gastritis is virtually universal with ageing. It is common in the antrum and can complicate gastric surgery when it is due to reflux of bile into the stomach. It is not a primary autoimmune disorder, although patients may have parietal cell antibodies in the blood. The precise cause or causes are uncertain, but they include bile reflux, alcohol, smoking, hot spicy food, aspirin, other non-steroidals and *H. pylori* infection.

Symptoms vary from none to severe ulcer-type pain with nausea, vomiting and flatulence. Treatment is by avoiding risk factors, and with alkalis, or in severe cases H_2-blockers with antibiotics for *H. pylori* infection.

Ménétrièr's disease is a rare condition with rugal hyperplasia. The cause is unknown and there is a risk of malignant change.

THE SMALL BOWEL—MALABSORPTION

The small bowel digests and absorbs nutrients and is a major endocrine organ producing secretions that act locally or stimulate neural transmission.

Malabsorption can also affect haematinics such as iron, folic acid and vitamin B_{12} and electrolytes such as sodium, potassium and calcium.

Causes of malabsorption

Malabsorption can results from:

1. liver or pancreatic disease, e.g. cirrhosis, obstructive jaundice, chronic pancreatitis
2. intestinal or gastric resection, post-gastrectomy, short bowel syndrome, etc.
3. abnormalities of luminal secretions, e.g. bacterial overgrowth, disaccharidase deficiency, abnormal small bowel pH (as in Zollinger-Ellison syndrome)
4. disease of the small bowel mucosa, e.g. coeliac disease, tropical sprue, Whipple's disease
5. disease of the small bowel wall, e.g. destruction of intramural nerve plexuses (aganglionosis), infiltration with lymphoma
6. systemic disease, e.g. amyloidosis, thyrotoxicosis, etc.

More than one cause may operate, as in extensive Crohn's disease where there may be mucosal disease and bacterial overgrowth from stricturing.

Symptoms and signs

Diarrhoea is the major symptom with pale, bulky, frothy, fatty offensive stools (with excessive rectal wind), flushing with difficulty. Weightloss results from anorexia and malabsorption (though in some patients the appetite is preserved or even excessive, e.g. chronic pancreatitis).

Abdominal distension is related to excessive gas formation from fermentation of unabsorbed starches. There is fluid retention and usually ankle oedema from hypoproteinaemia.

Anaemia with dyspnoea and lassitude are caused by deficiency of iron, folic acid and vitamin B_{12}. Iron and folate are absorbed in the upper small bowel, while vitamin B_{12} deficiency is a feature of ileal disease, resection, or small intestinal bacterial contamination. Weakness and lassitude are also often related to electrolyte disorders like hypokalaemia and hypomagnesaemia.

Tetany (painful cramps and paraesthesiae in the hands) is from hypocalcaemia and hypomagnesaemia. Metabolic bone disease, usually osteomalacia, is related to impaired absorption of vitamin D; sometimes there is osteoporosis.

There are also other factors related to specific types of malabsorption, e.g. abdominal pain, a feature of Crohn's disease; lymphadenopathy in Whipple's disease, etc.

Investigations

The following are helpful in the diagnosis of malabsorption:

1. Estimation of 24-hour faecal fat excretion on a known and preferably high intake of fat (fat balance). After an equilibration period, faeces are collected for 3–5 days (normal excretion < 23 mmol fatty acid per 24 hours).
2. Radiology will show the general changes of malabsorption, such as dilated small bowel. Specific features may suggest Crohn's disease, intestinal fistulae, a blind loop or coeliac disease.
3. Anaemia, either hypochromic (iron deficiency) or macrocytic (folate or vitamin B_{12} deficiency). Vitamin B_{12} and folate absorption tests may then be helpful.
4. Serum protein levels may be low and the serum albumin 30 g/l or less in oedematous subjects.
5. Plasma electrolyte levels may be reduced (particularly sodium and potassium) and a raised alkaline phosphatase and a low calcium level may signify the presence of osteomalacia, verified by bone biopsy.
6. Biopsy of the small bowel mucosa, either via a Crosby capsule or at upper gastrointestinal endoscopy, can diagnose coeliac disease, tropical sprue and Whipple's disease, etc.
7. A blind loop syndrome may be suggested by ^{14}C-labelled bile salt or hydrogen breath tests.

SPECIAL TYPES OF MALABSORPTION

Coeliac disease

This genetic disorder in which small bowel mucosal damage (partial or subtotal villous atrophy) results from exposure to dietary gluten, a protein found in wheat, rye, oats and barley, is found in about 1 in 2000 of the population in Western Europe. It is more common in women and sufferers are four times more likely than normals to have the histocompatibility antigens HLA B8/DW3. Mucosal damage is probably immunologically determined.

Biopsies of the small bowel show virtually diagnostic partial or total villous atrophy (Fig. 9.2). However, in the UK similar changes are found in cow's milk hypersensitivity, tropical sprue and some cases of intestinal lymphoma.

Seen classically in infancy with first exposure to dietary gluten, the disease may be delayed in onset until adult life. Weightloss, diarrhoea, anaemia, oedema and anorexia usually accompany a low serum folate level. Anaemia, often chronic iron deficiency, worse with each pregnancy, is sometimes the only feature. Aphthous ulcers (small, painful superficial ulcers) of the mouth can occur and the symptoms may be precipitated by gastric surgery or intestinal resection. Other autoimmune diseases may also occur in the coeliac patient.

Complications

Dermatitis herpetiformis, a vesicular skin rash, causes severe itching. Lymphoma is the most serious complication and presents with abdominal pain, weightloss and perhaps intestinal perforation. Chronic ulceration of the small bowel may cause abdominal pain and intestinal obstruction due to structuring.

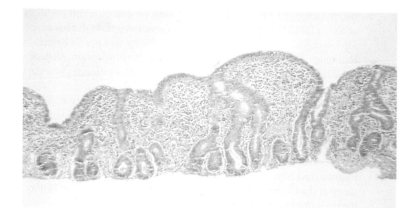

Fig. 9.2 The small bowel mucosa in coeliac disease. This jejunal biopsy shows blunting of villi, increased cellularity of the submucosa and crypt hyperplasia. Higher power changes include important epithelial disorganisation and lymphocytic infiltration. These changes are all corrected by a gluten-free diet.

Central nervous system disorders, including cerebellar and pyramidal tract damage, are of uncertain cause.

Atrophy of the spleen causes changes in the peripheral blood count, like the presence of Howell-Jolly bodies (nuclear remnants).

Treatment
Coeliac disease is treated with lifelong gluten restriction and excludes wheat flour in bread, cakes, biscuits and in a large variety of prepared foods where it is present in sauces, soups, ice cream, etc. Gluten-free products, including flour and bread mix, are available on an NHS prescription and gluten-free foods are marked for easy recognition. Some resistant patients may need corticosteroids and a lactose-free diet additionally, although poor compliance is the usual cause of failure to respond.

Biopsy appearances return to normal with complete gluten exclusion. The risk of lymphoma is the reason for persisting with a strict gluten-free diet throughout adult life.

Other causes of malabsorption
See Table 9.4

GASTROINTESTINAL BLEEDING

Rapid bleeding from the GI tract may cause haematemesis (vomiting of blood, either fresh or like coffee grounds) or melaena (passage of black, tarry stools) or both. Bleeding from the distal colon and anal region causes the passage of fresh blood, i.e. rectal bleeding. Insidious bleeding may cause anaemia, and

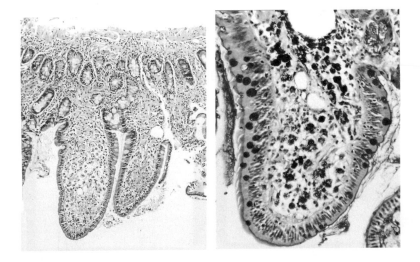

Fig. 9.3 Whipple's disease. **(A)** Ballooning of the villi which, in the PAS stained photograph **(B)**, show many bacteria which have been identified.

although the stools appear normal they contain occult blood on stool testing. The causes of GI bleeding are given in Table 9.5.

UPPER GI BLEEDING

Symptoms and signs

The symptoms are haematemesis and melaena. If bleeding is severe, shock, faintness, nausea and sweating also occur. In elderly patients, loss of blood volume may cause blindness (retinal artery thrombosis) or stroke or myocardial pain.

The important signs are pallor, sweating, tachycardia and hypotension. If patients have underlying chronic liver disease, signs of liver cell failure (see p. 297) will appear.

Abdominal signs are usually absent unless there is liver disease (hepatosplenomegaly, etc. Severe abdominal pain should suggest perforation as an accompaniment to bleeding. When taking the history, the following *must* be included:

1. Does the patient suffer from chronic dyspepsia? This may suggest peptic ulcer/hiatus hernia, etc.
2. Does the patient have a history to suggest chronic liver disease—previous jaundice, known alcoholism, etc?
3. Does the patient take drugs such as aspirin, NSAIDs, anticoagulants, etc?
4. Does the patient drink alcohol—was he drinking immediately prior to the bleed?
5. Has the patient bled before? If so:
   a. When?

Table 9.4. Other Disorders causing malabsorption

Lesion	Cause	Symptoms and signs	Treatment
Tropical sprue	Acquired bacterial infection of small bowel causing villous atrophy Occurs after or during residence in tropical areas	Malabsorption with diarrhoea and anaemia? Vitamin B_{12} deficient neuropathy	Antibiotics Vitamin B_{12} (curable)
Whipple's disease (Fig 9.3)	Acquired bacterial infection of the gut and other tissues Causes villous atrophy with PAS+ve bacterial remnants in mucosa	Malabsorption Arthritis Lymphadenopathy Pigmentation	Antibiotics (curable but can relapse)
Intestinal lymphangiectasis	Genetic disorder with dilated lymphatics in gut and in other situations	Malabsorption Protein-losing Pitting oedema, e.g. of limbs Thickened yellow nails Pleural effusions	Low fat diet Medium chain triglyceride supplements (MCTs) Can be controlled
Radiation enteritis	Radiotherapy to gut, e.g. from irradiated cervix or abdominal lymph nodes Causes telangiectasia, bleeding, stricturing and obliterative vasculitis	Abdominal pain, diarrhoea, bleeding and malabsorption depending on situation	Resection if localised Otherwise symptomatic treatment
Stagnant loop syndrome	Bacterial colonisation of stagnant small bowel Follows surgery or complicates conditions like scleroderma or jejunal diverticulosis	Malabsorption Vitamin B_{12} deficiency	Antibiotics Vitamin B_{12} ? Corrective surgery

Table 9.5. Causes of upper and lower gastrointestinal bleeding

Upper

Common	Chronic peptic ulcer	60%
	Acute peptic ulcer ⎫ Acute erosive gastritis ⎭	20%
	Hiatus hernia ⎫ Oesophagitis ⎬ Oesophageal varices ⎭	10%

Rare	Mallory-Weiss syndrome (see Table 9.2)
	Osler's disease (haemorrhagic telangiectasia)(hereditary—dominant inheritance with bleeding from GI tract and nose; facial, lip, tongue and hand telangiectasia)
	Pseudoxanthoma elasticum (hereditary—dominant inheritance; deficient elastic tissue in skin and in blood vessels; gastrointestinal bleeding, 'chicken breast' skin (pseudoxanthoma) and impaired vision (angioid streaks)
	Gastric tumours

Lower

Common	Haemorrhoids
	Rectal and colonic polyps
	Rectal and colonic tumours
	Diverticular disease

Rare	Angiodysplasia (dilated submucosal vessels—found in the elderly, sometimes associated with aortic stenosis, commonest in the colon)
	Meckel's diverticulum—due to ulcer in contained gastric mucosa; treated surgically

  b. Was he in hospital and where?
  c. Did he need a blood transfusion and how many units?
  d. Was surgery performed?
  e. What was he told concerning the cause?
6. Does he have any other serious disease, e.g. chronic bronchitis, coronary artery disease, etc?

Investigations

Providing the patient's condition is stable, an attempt should be made to determine the site of bleeding, but where bleeding has been severe (tachycardia > 100, blood pressure < 100 systolic) emergency supportive treatment is first required (see below).

The haemoglobin and packed cell volume (PCV) should be measured and blood sent for grouping and crossmatching. The patient's haemoglobin level may be falsely high in the first 24 hours because of the lack of haemodilution. Estimation of the blood urea and electrolyte levels may help in the assessment of severity (pre-renal azotenia). The blood urea level may also be high when there is proximal GI bleeding with subsequent small bowel metabolism and absorption of protein.

Liver function tests (LFTs) and coagulation studies are important in suspected liver disease.

The definitive tests to find out the source of bleeding are:

1. Endoscopy: upper GI endoscopy should be performed once the patient's condition is stable and certainly within 24 hours for maximal diagnostic yield. All varieties of oesophageal, gastric and duodenal pathology can be found and where chronic ulcers occur, fresh clot or a prominent vessel in an ulcer suggests further bleeding is likely. Gastric ulcers should be brushed and biopsied if this is feasible.
2. Barium studies: these are valuable, particularly if endoscopy is not available, and with double-contrast technique the diagnostic yield is 90% or more. Ulcers, both acute and chronic, erosions and small polyps are readily demonstrated.
3. Angiography: if after endoscopy and barium studies the source of bleeding is still uncertain, coeliac, superior mesenteric and inferior mesenteric angiography should be performed looking for a source of bleeding or ectatic vessels.
4. Scintigraphy: using the patient's labelled red blood cells given intravenously, this is indicated where there is chronic blood loss of uncertain cause.

Treatment

Resuscitation is vital. In severe cases, the foot of the bed is raised, i.v. plasma expanders such as Haemaccel are given prior to liberal transfusion of cross-matched blood. In the elderly and those with serious bleeds a central venous line helps to monitor venous pressure and avoids overtransfusion. The aim of transfusion is to return the blood pressure, pulse rate and urine volume to normal. Sedation may be required for the anxious but not in those with liver disease . Monitoring of the pulse rate, blood pressure and the patient's general condition is mandatory. About 80% of patients will respond to this treatment and will not rebleed.

Bleeding is more likely to recur if the patient is elderly, suffering from chronic ulcers, particularly gastric, or bleeding from oesophageal varices.

Serious underlying disease, such as chronic bronchitis, heart failure, liver cell failure, also increase the likelihood, and the endoscopic features described above in these situations. In some centres, adrenaline is injected around the ulcers via the endoscope or the bleeding points are treated with lasers. Usually, early consultation with a surgical colleague experienced in dealing with gastrointestinal bleeding is required.

Acute erosive gastritis is treated with blood transfusion and H_2-blockers or omeprazole; gastric surgery may rarely be required.

If chronic ulcers fail to respond to conservative therapy, blood transfusion and a course of H_2-blockers (or omeprazole) (see Table 9.3) and surgery are required (the latter if the patient's condition allows). Local resection of the ulcer is performed or even ligation and oversewing of the ulcer, i.e. the simplest possible surgery that is likely to be effective.

Prognosis

The mortality remains at about 8% despite advances in investigation, post-operative care and in endoscopic techniques because of the larger number of elderly patients who have serious underlying disease, and who are unable to withstand bleeding or subsequent surgery. In some centres the mortality has been reduced by more early surgery.

DISORDERS OF THE GALLBLADDER AND BILE DUCTS

The gallbladder stores and concentrates hepatic bile via the biliary cannuliculae and biliary duct system. Passage of bile down the biliary tree depends on osmotic forces from bile salts (bile salt dependent fraction) and partly on a sodium-dependent transport mechanism (bile salt independent fraction). Secretin, acting on bile ducts, contributes water and bicarbonate with a total flow of 500–600 ml per 24 hours. Gallbladder contraction is caused by food-released cholecystokinin.

GALLSTONES

These form in the gallbladder or the bile duct. They are composed of cholesterol alone (pure cholesterol stones), or are mixed with calcium salts (mixed cholesterol stones), or consist of bile pigments (pigment stones). The circumstances under which they are found are shown in Table 9.6. In the Western World, the cholesterol stones and mixed cholesterol stones are the most important. Cholesterol stones develop because bile becomes supersaturated with cholesterol, the bile salts being unable to keep it in solution. They are more common in females and increase with age, so at the age of 60 years 15–20% of normal women will have them. Pigment stones occur where there is excessive haemolysis and in cirrhosis. Important differences are seen in stone composition and site of formation in the Far East, where mixed duct stones rather than gallbladder cholesterol stones result from duct infection and infestation.

Symptoms and signs
Patients may be asymptomatic, or pain may occur when stones occlude the cystic duct, migrate into the common bile duct or cause pancreatitis. Pain is then severe, constant, in the right upper abdomen and epigastrium, radiating to the back and angle of the right scapula, with vomiting.

Table 9.6. Gallstones—risk factors

Cholesterol-containing stones
    Obesity ⎫
    Diabetes ⎭ Increased hepatic cholesterol synthesis
    Female sex/multiple pregnancies
    Drugs—oral contraceptives (c.f. pregnancy), clofibrate
    Ileal disease—reduction of bile salt level

Pigment stones
    Haemolysis—increased pigment load
    Liver disease—increased pigment load (minor haemolysis)

Obstructive jaundice may occur with migration into the common bile duct. Flatulence and dyspepsia are common in this group of patients but equally so in subjects without gallstones.

Important signs are right upper abdominal tenderness and guarding. A positive Murphy's sign when the patient experiences inspiratory right upper abdominal pain on palpation may be found. Rarely, a mucocele or empyema makes the gallbladder palpable. Fever, rigors, jaundice and collapse with hypotension may occur from complicating cholangitis and septicaemia.

Investigations

Plain films of the abdomen may show mixed but not pure cholesterol or pigment stones. Ultrasound is the best way of demonstrating gallbladder stones.

Routine LFTs are often normal, though mild elevations of alkaline phosphatase and gamma glutamyl transferase may occur. With cholangitis, more florid changes occur, e.g. raised bilirubin, alkaline phosphatase, etc. The blood count may show a polymorph leukocytosis. A serum amylase is required to rule out accompanying pancreatitis.

Complications

See Figure 9.4.

Treatment

Symptomless gallstones, despite possible complications, are generally not treated. Attacks of gallstone cholecystitis are treated conservatively with analgesics, including non-steroidals and sometimes with antibiotics. Once the attack has settled, a decision is made on procedure. Cholecystectomy is a safe

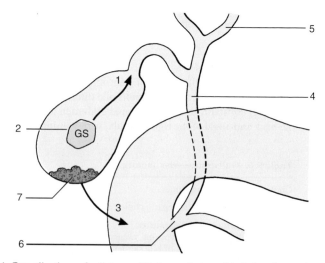

Fig. 9.4 Complications of gallstones. (1) Acute cholecystitis (migration to the cystic duct); (2) empyema or mucocele; (3) rupture into the duodenum—gallstone ileus, or peritoneal cavity—biliary peritonitis; (4) common bile duct migration (obstructive jaundice); (5) ascending sepsis (hepatic abscess, cholangitis, septicaemia); (6) pancreatitis; (7) carcinoma of the gallbladder.

operation which relieves acute symptoms with a low mortality (< 5%), even in the elderly. It can now be carried out at laparoscopy, thus reducing hospital stay, and has become the most usual method of gallbladder removal for uncomplicated cases.

Non-surgical treatment of gallbladder stones

1. Bile salts (chenodeoxycholic) or (chenodeoxyocholic plus ursodeoxycholic acid) continuously by mouth will dissolve cholesterol gallstones 15 mm or less in diameter after 18 months. Symptoms should be minimal. Relapse after treatment is common.
2. Methylene terbutyl ether (MTB) is infused directly into the gallbladder located and punctured under ultrasound control. After the contents have been aspirated, infusion is repeated. Again, cholesterol stones only can be treated. Further, follow-up therapy with oral bile salts may be required.
3. Stones may be fragmented by shock waves produced by an external lithotripter, or under laparoscopic control the gallbladder may be punctured, the entry point dilated and endoscopic examination of the gallbladder carried out. Stones may be removed, broken up with forceps or by a lithotripter introduced into the gallbladder.

Gallstones in the common bile duct or common hepatic ducts may cause biliary obstruction with jaundice and pain. Complications include hepatic abscess formation, cholangitis and septicaemia. Detection of common duct stones may not be conclusive with ultrasound and visualisation of the duct system by endoscopic retrograde choledochopancreatography (ERCP) or fine-needle cholangiography may be required. Surgical removal and T-tube drainage with choledochoduodenostomy or sphincterotomy under endoscopic control are ways of removing or facilitating the removal of duct stones.

CHOLANGITIS

This is an infection of the biliary tree with pyogenic organisms. It occurs where there is a nidus of infection in the obstructed biliary tract, most usually with common duct stones. Patients are usually ill with a high swinging fever and obstructive jaundice. There is tender hepatomegaly. Investigations show a polymorph leukocytosis and liver function tests, an obstructive pattern. Hypotension, tachycardia and septic shock indicate septicaemia. Treatment is with i.v. antibiotics such as gentamicin and/or a cephalosporin like cephradine, fluid replacement and where required, relief of biliary obstruction either surgically or by endoscopic stenting.

ACUTE CHOLECYSTITIS

This is an acute inflammation of the stone-containing gallbladder, often with a stone impacted in the cystic duct. Rarely, pus may form to produce an empyema, or a stone may ulcerate through the gallbladder into the duodenum later to obstruct the ileum (gallstone ileus). Patients are likely to have the risk factors for gallstones (see Table 9.6), but no group is immune.

Symptoms include abdominal pain, sometimes radiating to the shoulder or angle of the right scapula, with vomiting. Signs are of right upper abdominal tenderness with a positive Murphy's sign. Ultrasound allows the detection of gallbladder thickening and detects the presence of stones. Treatment consists of analgesia, non-steroidals for the anti-inflammatory action, and antibiotics. Generally, patients who are not too ill are treated conservatively and subsequent treatment of gallstones is usually by cholecystectomy (see p. 273). When patients are very ill, urgent surgery may be required and when complications such as perforation of the gallbladder or empyema are suspected this is the required approach.

OTHER DISORDERS OF THE GALLBLADDER

Sclerosing cholangitis
This is an immunological disorder with thickening, stenosis and dilatation of the biliary tract. It causes obstructive jaundice with or without cholangitis. Diagnosis is by ERCP. It is associated with inflammatory bowel disease and can be associated with AIDS.

Choledochal cyst
A congenital dilatation of the common bile duct, a choledochal cyst causes obstructive jaundice, fever and abdominal mass. The risk of cancer is increased. Treatment is surgical.

Carcinoma of bile ducts
Slowly growing adenocarcinoma is associated with ulcerative colitis, choledocal cyst and in the Far East, with liver fluke infestation. It causes progressive obstructive jaundice. Surgical removal (rare), stenting and internal radiotherapy are possible treatments.

Carcinoma of the gallbladder
This is usually a complication of chronic cholecystitis with gallstones. It causes progressive obstructive jaundice and is usually inoperable but partial hepatectomy is a possibility.

THE PANCREAS

Secretion follows the presence of food in the upper small bowel which leads to the release of secretin and pancreozymin (cholecystokinin, CCK). Secretin is released in response to acid in the duodenum with the production of pancreatic fluid rich in bicarbonate. Cholecystokinin is particularly stimulated by fat in the small bowel lumen and results in the production of fluid rich in pancreatic enzymes.

ACUTE PANCREATITIS

This is an acute inflammation of the pancreas with a high mortality. The inflammation and necrosis are caused by activation of destructive pancreatic enzymes. In the UK, there are two common causes of acute pancreatitis: alcoholism and the presence of gallstones. Rarer causes are trauma (particularly postoperative trauma), drugs (e.g. corticosteroids, oral contraceptives, thiazide diuretics), hyperparathyroidism, hyperlipidaemia (types IV, V or I) and infections such as mumps.

Symptoms and signs

Severe abdominal pain, usually epigastric, radiating to the back, shoulders or generally throughout the abdomen, is persistent and sometimes relieved by sitting forward. Vomiting is almost universal and there may be haematemesis.

Signs are of abdominal tenderness and rigidity. Abdominal swelling may occur, usually caused by small bowel distension (paralytic ileus), or more rarely by the presence of fluid in the lesser sac or abdominal cavity (pancreatic ascites).

Jaundice may be present, particularly in alcoholics or from complicating gallstones.

The pulse may be rapid and the patient hypotensive.

Rare physical signs include a pleural effusion on the left side. Grey-Turner's sign (a violaceous discoloration in the flanks) and Cullen's sign (a similar appearance around the umbilicus), both due to the extravasation of inflammatory pancreatic fluid can occur.

Patients may be short of breath because of pulmonary adult respiratory distress syndrome (ARDS) with low arterial PO_2 levels. Cardiac dysrhythmias, hypotension and ECG changes may also occur.

Investigations

1. The serum amylase is elevated, usually >1000 Somogyi units/l. Levels twice this are pathognmonic of the disease but other intestinal disorders cause moderately elevated levels.
2. LFTs may be abnormal, particularly in alcoholics.
3. A sample of abdominal or pleural fluid taken by fine-needle aspiration may show very high amylase levels.
4. The serum calcium level may be low from loss into the inflammatory exudate and the glucose level may be raised due to transient insulin deficiency.
5. Blood urea and electrolyte levels may be abnormal because of fluid losses and hypotension.
6. Serial estimations of arterial gases detect and monitor complicating ARDS.
7. Ultrasound shows the enlarged pancreas, the extravasation of fluid and may reveal associated abnormalities in the liver, e.g. cirrhosis, gallbladder stones.

Complications

The complications of acute pancreatitis are shown in Figure 9.5.

Treatment

There is no specific treatment. Pain is treated with pethidine, and shock is vigorously treated by fluid replacement with blood if there has been intestinal bleeding. Monitoring of the pulse, blood pressure and urine volume (catheter) is important, and a central venous line helps. Abnormal levels of blood calcium and glucose need treatment. Nasogastric suction allows gastrointestinal rest and helps to control any ileus. Oxygen is administered and a decision may be

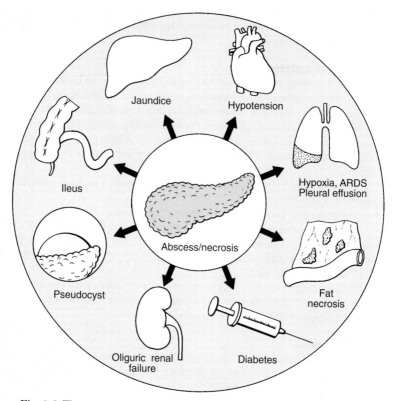

Fig. 9.5 The complications of acute pancreatitis.

required about ventilatory help (PEEP ventilation). There is no evidence that any other form of therapy helps, but where the course is prolonged, intravenous feeding will be required. Surgery and manipulative endoscopy may be needed when there are common duct stones or pancreatic necrosis. On the assumption that some of the damage is generated by leukocyte release of destructive free radicals, treatment with vitamin E is under trial.

Prognosis

The disease has a 20% mortality. Bad signs include hypocalcaemia, hypotension, a raised blood urea level and tissue anoxia. Recurrent attacks are a possibility unless a cause is found and eradicated.

CHRONIC PANCREATITIS

This is not usually the result of recurrent attacks of acute pancreatitis and seems to develop de novo. The gland becomes fibrosed and possibly calcified. The parenchyma, islets and the duct system are involved, and pseudocystic changes may occur. The major causes are alcoholism and, world wide, the effects of malnutrition when calcification is prominent. Rare causes include pancreas divisum. There is also a hereditary form. Some patients with chronic pancreatitis develop pancreatic cancer.

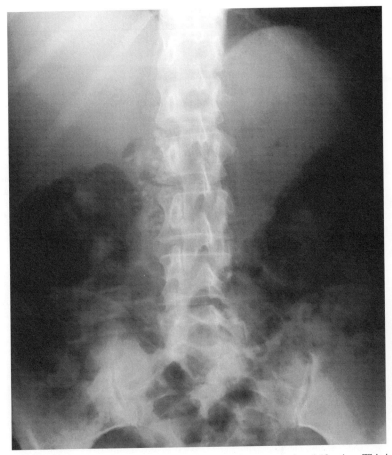

Fig. 9.6 Plain X-ray of the abdomen showing massive pancreatic calcification. This is best seen to the left of the midline at L2.

Symptoms and signs

Attacks of abdominal pain, usually epigastric and episodic, with vomiting, are sometimes exacerbated by food and alcohol. Diarrhoea is often seen with severe steatorrhoea.

Weightloss is not usually a marked feature but it may be caused by food-induced pain, malabsorption and diabetes.

Attacks of obstructive jaundice may occur from constriction of the lower end of the bile duct in the thickened pancreas, or in alcoholics from intrahepatic cholestasis or parenchymal disease.

There are few signs; rarely, a pseudocyst may be palpable, otherwise there is merely abdominal tenderness. Sometimes there is hepatomegaly.

Investigations

1. Reduced pancreatic exocrine function can be shown by tubeless screening tests, backed up by a Lundh or pancreozymin test. Glycosuria and a raised random blood glucose level indicate diabetes.

Table 9.7. Malignant tumours of the GI tract

	Type	Atiological factors
Oesophagus	Squamous cell carcinoma also secondary invasion of lower third by gastric adenocarcinorna	Iron deficiency, Smoking, Alcohol, Coeliac disease ?Barrett's oesophagus, Common in China and Transkei in South Africa
Stomach	Adenocarcinoma Ulcerating, polypoid or superficial (confined to mucosa) Rarely linitis plastica (Fig. 9.9) (leather bottle stomach) or infiltrating	High nitrate content of food (smoked) and water Chronic gastritis Pernicious anaemia Commonest in Japan
Colon and rectum	Adenocarcinoma From pre-existing adenomatous polypoid (60% in rectum and sigmoid)	Familial polyposis coli Relatives with large bowel cancer. Large adenomatous polyps Chronic IBD ?Cholecystectomy
Pancreas	Adenocarcinoma of pancreas also from ampulla of Vater or duct	Chronic pancreatitis ?Smoking, diabetes, coffee

ERCP = endoscopic rectangle cholangiopancreatography; IBD = inflammatory bowel disease
FOBs = faecal occult bloods.

2. Characteristic calcification may be seen on a plain abdominal X-ray (Fig. 9.6), and fibrosis and pseudocyst formation on CT scanning.
3. A definitive diagnosis can also be made at ERCP when stricturing, dilatation and ectasia of the pancreatic ducts are seen.

Treatment

Control of this disease is difficult. Alcohol is forbidden and pain treated without rendering the patient addicted to strong analgesics. Antidepressants may be helpful. Steatorrhoea is treated with a low-fat diet and enteric coated replacement therapy such as Nutrizym GR, Creon or Pancrease are taken with meals. Adequate vitamins, including A, D and K are given. Diabetes is treated by carbohydrate restriction, oral hypoglycaemic agents and sometimes insulin.

Symptoms and signs	Diagnosis	Treatment	Prognosis
Progressive dysphagia Profound weightloss, signs of mediastinal and hepatic secondaries	Endoscopy Cytology Biopsy	Radiotherapy for upper third Resection and calonic transplantation	Poor
Ulcer type dyspepsia, GI bleeding, Wasting, Anaemia, Epigastric mass, Possibly pelvic masses	Endoscopy Cytology Biopsy	Surgical resection	Poor, except superficial cancer
Abdominal pain, Anaemia, Bowel upset, Rectal bleeding or bloody discharge, Abdominal or rectal mass	Sigmoidoscopy Colonoscopy, Biopsy, Barium enema, FoBs, Surgical resection	Surgical resection	?
Head Obstructive jaundice, Weightloss Intestinal bleeding *Body and tail* Weightloss, Abdominal and back pain, Thrombophlebitis migrans	Ultrasound with guided biopsy ERCP	If resectable, Whipple's operation, If not, ?endoscopic stenting or cholecystenterostomy	?

If pain is severe, a coeliac axis block may be tried and repeated if successful.

If symptoms are intractable, surgery should be considered. The gland can be resected (pancreatectomy), when long-term insulin is required, or where there is pancreatic duct obstruction, drainage proximal to a strictured area can follow partial resection and pancreatico-jejunostomy.

MALIGNANT TUMOURS OF THE GASTROINTESTINAL TRACT, LIVER AND PANCREAS

This is not the place for a full description of the malignant tumours of the bowel and intestinal glands, or their therapy. Nevertheless, the student must be knowledgeable about the aetiology, symptomatology and investigations which are appropriate (Table 9.7).

NEUROENDOCRINE TUMOURS

These tumours secrete one or more hormones (Table 9.8). It has been suggested because of their neuroendocrine properties that they are derived from embryonic neural crest cells, and they are also referred to as APUD tumours (*amine precursor uptake decarboxylation*) because of their content and staining properties, although others argue a local (gut) origin. They all have malignant potential.

HEPATOMA

See page 300.

INFLAMMATORY BOWEL DISEASE(IBD)

This section includes Crohn's disease (CD) and ulcerative colitis (non-specific proctocolitis, NSP). Although there are differences (see Table 9.9), sometimes a definite diagnosis may be impossible.

Major epidemiological similarities exist. Both are more common in whites, in urban as opposed to rural dwellers and in Jews. Both show a familial tendency in up to 30% of cases. Both are more common in young adults but occur and may be serious in the elderly. Both demonstrate humoral and cellular immunological abnormalities, of uncertain role in disease initiation and progression. Changes include the presence of anti-colon antibodies and of circulating lymphocytes cytotoxic to cultured colon epithelial cells. IBD has defied a search for an infective cause. In CD, atypical acid-fast bacilli are noted in some cases.

The incidence of the two diseases is different and variable: in North Europe CD has an incidence of $2–5/10^5$ population and a prevalence of about 30. NSP figures are about three times higher. In Third World countries IBD is rare. There are differences in eating and smoking habits. Refined carbohydrate consumption is higher and fibre intake lower in CD, whilst patients with NSP are less likely than normals to smoke. Smoking may actually be more common in Crohn's patients.

Pathology See Table 9.9.

CROHN'S DISEASE

The symptoms of CD are usually colicky-abdominal pain, most often in the right iliac fossa, diarrhoea, sometimes with features of malabsorption (blood is noted by 25% of patients, particularly in colonic disease), and abdominal distension, weightloss, fever and general ill health.

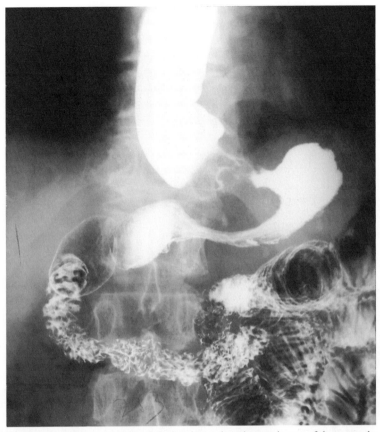

Fig. 9.7 A barium meal radiograph showing an invasive carcinoma of the stomach (linitis plastica). The lumen of the stomach is narrowed due to the thickened rigid infiltrated gastric wall. The oesophagus is dilated because of oesophagogastric involvement.

Signs include anaemia, weightloss, sometimes finger clubbing, fever and a tender right iliac fossa mass. Ankle oedema may occur with hypoproteinaemia. Retarded growth is seen in children.

When dealing with patients who may have CD, the following should always be examined:

1. the mouth for ulceration or hypertrophic gingivitis;
2. the perineum for ulceration, fistulae and skin tags;
3. the joints and spine for arthritis and spondylitis;
4. the skin and eyes for lesions such as pyoderma or erythema nodosum and iritis;
5. the rectum for palpable thickening of the anal and rectal mucosa.

CD can also present as a pyrexia of unknown origin or symptomless weight-loss, or with fistulae into the perineum, bladder or another part of the gut. Patients with colonic disease have a higher incidence of rectal bleeding, more perianal disease and more diffuse abdominal pain.

Table 9.8. Neuroendocrine tumours of the gut

Tumour	Site	Secretion	Effects	Treatment
Carcinoid	Gut, lung May metastasise to liver 'carcinoid syndrome'	5-hydroxytryptophan Histamine and others	Flushing Diarrhoea Right-sided heart lesions Bronchospasm (carcinoid syndrome)	Serotonin antagonists for diarrhoea, e.g. methysergide—consider somatostatin Hepatic artery embolisation
Insulinoma	Pancreas	Insulin	Fits/attacks of stupor due to hypoglycaemia	Resection or streptosotocin and somatostatin
Zollinger-Ellison syndrome	Pancreas	Gastrin	Duodenal and jejunal ulceration Diarrhoea/steatorrhoea	Omeprazole (to inhibit gastric acid production)
Vipoma	Pancreas	Vasoactive intestinal polypeptide	Perfuse watery diarrhoea Hypokalaemia Acidosis	Resection or streptosotocin and somatostatin
Somatostatinoma	Pancreas	Somatostatin	Steatorrhoea Diabetes Gallbladder stones	Resection and/or streptosotocin
Glucagonoma	Pancreas	Glucagon	Steatorrhoea Weightloss++ Diarrhoea Diabetes Characteristic skin rash of perineum, thighs, etc.	Resection

Table 9.9. The pathology of Crohn's disease (CD) and ulcerative colitis

	Crohn's disease	Ulcerative colitis
Site of disease	Ileocaecal commonest Small bowel and upper GI tract sometimes	Total or left-sided, proctocolitis may extend proximally Rectum invariably involved
Inflammatory process	Transmural (all coats of gut) Walls thickened, deep ulcers, lumen narrowed, normal 'skip' areas between involved segments	Superficial and continuous with shallow ulceration
Histology	Transmural inflammation, deep fissures, granulomata, crypt abscesses	Superficial inflammation Crypt abscesses Mucus (goblet cell) depletion
Pathological consequences	Intestinal obstruction, abscess formation fistulae, carcinoma	Carcinoma Pseudo (inflammatory) polyps

Investigations

A blood count shows mild anaemia, a leukocytosis and elevated platelets. The plasma protein levels may be low and with oedema, the serum albumin may be 30 g/l or less.

Barium studies of the small bowel may show thickening and narrowing of the ileum with caecal and ascending colonic deformity. There may be deep ulceration and a cobblestone mucosa. A barium enema detects colonic involvement (Fig. 9.8). Changes similar to those in the small bowel are seen and small multiple ulcers of the mucosa are readily demonstrated.

Endoscopy, either sigmoidoscopy or colonoscopy, will demonstrate inflammation, aphthous ulceration, and thickening and inflammation of the bowel. In CD, comparatively normal areas (skip areas) may be interspersed between areas of Crohn's inflammation. Endoscopy allows biopsies to be taken, crucial in the diagnosis of CD; granuloma formation and deep inflammation are particularly helpful findings.

Activity of the disease is assessed by measuring the erythrocyte sedimentation rate (ESR), plasma viscosity or acute phase proteins such as C-reactive protein. A further technique is the injection of the patient's indium-labelled white cells which 'home' to areas of active inflammation where they can be detected by scanning.

Differential diagnosis

This is wide, particularly where there is an acute onset, and includes:
1. infective dysentery (i.e. *Shigella*, *Salmonella*, enteroinvasive *Escherichia coli*, amoebiasis), *Campylobacter enteritis*, pseudomembranous enteritis, gonococcal enteritis
2. vascular-ischaemic colitis

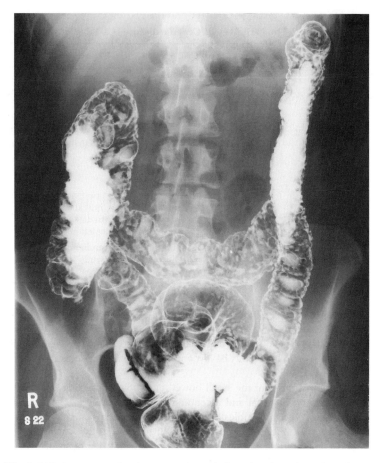

Fig. 9.8 Barium enema showing gross mucosal ulceration throughout the colon and ileum caused by Crohn's disease.

3. post-radiotherapy radiation colitis
4. Others: diverticular disease, carcinoma.

Treatment
Treatment is either medical or surgical by a joint team of specialist physicians and surgeons. The principles are:

1. Immunosuppressant drugs. Corticosteroids, usually given as oral prednisolone, suppress but do not cure this disease. Abdominal pain, fever and diarrhoea may all respond to short courses of corticosteroids, providing abscess formation can be excluded. It may be difficult to withdraw therapy because symptoms return. The side-effects of corticosteroids in this largely young group of patients are serious and the dose can be reduced by using azathioprine as a corticosteroid sparing agent.

2. Other drugs. Azathioprine may be effective in severe cases, particularly for fistulae. Sulphasalazine and other 5-amino-salicyclic acid derivatives are helpful (see p. 287), particularly in Crohn's colitis. Metronidazole sometimes produces healing of troublesome perineal ulceration.

3. Surgery. Resection is only used where there is a failure to control symptoms by medical treatment and must conserve healthy bowel. It is also used where complications like abscess, fistulae or carcinoma have occurred. The standard operation for CD is a right hemicolectomy and ile-ectomy with ileo-transverse colostomy. Conservative surgery such as sphincteroplasty is helpful in those subjects who have had resections.

4. Nutrition is preserved by encouraging the appetite and adding high calorie, high protein liquid feeds; in addition enteral 'space diet' feeding by a small-bore tube and pump and, on occasions, parenteral feeding may be helpful.

5. Symptomatic treatments with anti-diarrhoeals and antispasmodics are used, and anaemia is treated appropriately.

Prognosis
Despite many complications, the long-term prognosis is surprisingly good. Once surgery is required, however, the chances of further symptoms and surgery are about 50%. Many patients have a long and chronic course before their disease eventually burns itself out.

ULCERATIVE COLITIS

Symptoms vary with the amount of colon involved (see Fig. 9.9) but usually include diarrhoea with blood mixed in the stools many times per day, cramping abdominal pain relieved by bowel actions, anorexia, lethargy and weight-loss.

Signs include weightloss, anaemia, fever and occasionally finger clubbing. There is often abdominal tenderness. On inspection of the anus there may be soreness, piles and abscess formation. Sigmoidoscopy shows mucosal reddening, loss of the normal vascular pattern, granularity with touch bleeding and purulent discharge.

In less severe cases, although diarrhoea with blood is still the major symptom, there is less constitutional upset, whilst in the least severe cases (proctitis) bleeding may be accompanied by constipation.

Investigations
A blood count may show anaemia, usually from iron deficiency, leukocytosis and increased platelets. C-reactive protein, the ESR and plasma viscosity are raised because of inflammatory activity. LFTs are often abnormal as a variety of liver disorders may accompany ulcerative colitis (Table 9.10).

The diagnosis rests essentially on the endoscopic appearances of the colonic mucosa supplemented by biopsy and histology. The classical histology is of

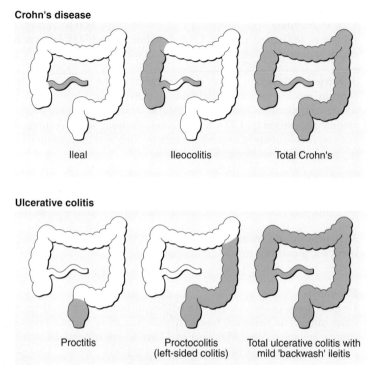

Fig. 9.9 Crohn's disease and ulcerative colitis: the site and pattern of gut involvement.

Table 9.10. Complications of ulcerative colitis and Crohn's disease

Local	Abscess, fistula, haemorrhage, perforation, toxic megacolon, carcinoma
General	
(1) Related to disease activity	
Skin	Erythema nodosum, pyoderma, gangrenosum
Eyes	Scleritis, iritis
Joints	Arthralgia, arthritis of large joints, spondylitis (HLA B27 + ve)
Blood	Hypercoagulability of blood, risk of pulmonary emboli
(2) Not related to disease activity	
Kidney	Renal stones, right hydronephrosis from ileocaecal mass
Liver	Hepatitis, cholestasis, cirrhosis, sclerosing cholangitis, bile duct cancer
Others	Amyloidosis

superficial mucosal inflammation, crypt abscesses and goblet cell (mucus) depletion.

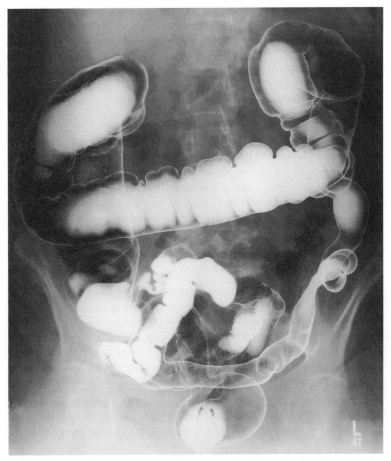

Fig. 9.10 Ulcerative colitis in the rectosigmoid region. The colon here is narrowed and featureless, contrasting with the rest of the normal-looking bowel.

A double-contrast barium enema shows fine mucosal granularity of variable extent. In total chronic cases the bowel may be shortened and featureless due to lack of haustra, with stricturing or the presence of pseudopolyps (Fig. 9.10).

Treatment

Patients with proctitis may respond to treatment of underlying constipation with a high-fibre diet. More diffuse disease is treated with anti-inflammatory drugs: long-term sulphasalazine or mesalazin are useful. Sulphasalazine has many side-effects, including headache, anorexia, skin rashes and in males temporary azospermia, all due to the sulphapyridine portion. The modern approach is to use drugs lacking this portion, such as mesalazin. These drugs suppress colonic inflammation and although relatively ineffective in treating acute disease, they prevent relapses. Corticosteroids can be given locally by enema or as a foam or suppository, and are useful for treating proctitis and left-sided disease. Corticosteroids can also be given systemically and are required in patients who are ill. Short courses are preferred, but there are problems, as in CD, in weaning patients off corticosteroids. Symptomatic treatment of pain, diarrhoea and of anaemia is also important.

In those whose disease is not controlled by medical therapy, surgery must be considered. Surgery is also important for the treatment of some complications (see Table 9.10). The operations that are used are total colectomy with removal of the rectum and ileostomy (as patients with bad symptoms invariably have total colonic involvement) but this is now being replaced by a so-called 'pouch' operation. This procedure forms a reservoir from the distal ileum which allows continence and preserves the normal route of evacuation, thus avoiding the need for a permanent ileostomy. However, it cannot be used in Crohn's colitis.

Ileostomy is well tolerated; adhesive bags are used and emptied regularly several times a day and most patients lead a totally normal life. A patients' society known as the Ileostomy Association and the skilled attention of stoma nurses available in many hospitals are of great help.

Complications of NSP and CD

These are listed in Table 9.10. However, one or two need further explanation:

1. Toxic megacolon is a serious disorder, usually seen in patients with total ulcerative colitis. It is sometimes precipitated by instrumentation of the bowel and the use of antispasmodic drugs. Abdominal distension pain accompanied by vomiting and clinical deterioration occur, although diarrhoea may actually lessen. The pathology is a spreading inflammation into the muscle walls of the colon and destruction of the autonomic plexuses. If suspected, regular abdominal radiographs assess colonic and subsequent small bowel dilatation.

Treatment is as a medical emergency: high-dose steroids, intravenous nutrition, a drip and suck technique, and antibiotic cover may reverse the situation. Otherwise, total colectomy and ileostomy is required as a surgical emergency.

2. Carcinoma. This is a complication of longstanding, and usually total, colitis. It is also seen in the colon and small bowel with longstanding CD. An estimate of the likelihood of cancer can be made by regular colonoscopic monitoring of patients with total colitis by looking for warning histological dysplastic change in the mucosa. Cancer is highly invasive and multicentric; the symptoms are no different from those of ordinary colitis and therefore clinically it is often missed.

3. Sclerosing cholangitis is described on page 274 but the interesting increased incidence of bile duct cancer in patients with NSP and CD can be seen even in patients who have had total removal of their diseased bowel.

OTHER DISORDERS OF THE GASTROINTESTINAL TRACT

THE IRRITABLE BOWEL SYNDROME

This is extremely common. One survey showed that 14% of apparently normal subjects have symptoms but do not seek medical advice. Symptoms are thought to be caused by abnormal intestinal motility and pressure generation. There is no pathological change in the bowel. Some patients have purely colonic symptoms, but in others there is evidence of small bowel, gastric or oesophageal dysfunction.

Patients are more likely than controls to be anxious, depressed or neurotic, and in some there is an increased sensitivity to intestinal pain. Diverticular disease of the colon is thought to represent an end stage of the disease, but this is arguable. Irritable bowel syndrome may also follow an acute attack of gastroenteritis and symptoms may be grafted on to those of another disease such as IBD.

Symptoms and signs
The hallmark of the disorder is abdominal pain and a disturbance of bowel function—either diarrhoea, constipation or both. The diagnosis in many patients is one of exclusion, but the following positive features are often present.

1. Pain is usually lower abdominal, colicky and relieved or rarely worsened by a bowel action. The pain may be upper abdominal and related to the taking of food and be mistaken for dyspepsia.
2. The stools may be small and pellety, or there may be diarrhoea. Often these alternate.
3. The patient may pass mucus from the rectum.
4. There may be abdominal distension and a sensation of incomplete bowel evacuation.
5. Proctalgia fugax (attacks of severe rectal pain) can occur.

Signs, apart from abdominal tenderness, are absent. There may be evidence of neurotic or depressive illness and identical pain may occur with air insufflation on sigmoidoscopy.

Investigations
1. If the patient is young and a normal clinical, rectal and sigmoidoscopic examination is accompanied by a negative faecal occult blood test, no further investigation is necessary.
2. In middle-aged or elderly patients, if symptoms are of short duration and if weightloss is a feature, then additionally radiological examination of the large bowel (barium enema), and possibly of the stomach and small bowel are required. Small bowel radiology is important for the detection of CD, and barium enema for the detection of colonic polyps, carcinoma and IBD.
3. A full blood count, plasma viscosity or ESR, together with LFTs are helpful in excluding organic disease.

Treatment
A positive attitude must be taken by the clinician and some explanation of the way in which symptoms arise and the fact they are not due to organic disease, including cancer, must be conveyed to the patient. Reassurance and explanation are essential and may have to be repeated. Factors which seem to aggravate symptoms are identified and corrected. These include fear of cancer, anxiety, depression, the stresses of work and family life and food allergy. This

latter has led to the use of exclusion diets with subsequent identification and exclusion of offending foods. Some patients, in the hands of unscrupulous practitioners, may become malnourished and totally neurotic. Patients often seek many medical opinions and the temptation for repeated unnecessary investigation must be resisted.

Symptomatic treatment. Diarrhoea is treated by agents such as Imodium and codeine phosphate, and constipation by the use of a high-fibre diet and a stool-bulking agent such as ispaghula (Fybogel, Isogel, etc.). Abdominal pain may be relieved by the use of antispasmodics such as Mebeverine and Pro-Banthine. Hypnosis may be helpful.

Prognosis
Symptoms tend to be recurrent but about 25% will respond completely to simple explanation, dietary and medicinal therapy. Others will have a more troublesome refractory illness.

DIVERTICULAR DISEASE

This common condition found particularly in the middle-aged and elderly causes outpouching of the colonic mucosa through the colonic muscle to occur along the length of the colon, maximally in the sigmoid colon.

Symptoms and signs
Symptoms may be absent or identical to those of the irritable bowel syndrome with attacks of lower abdominal pain accompanied by diarrhoea, constipation, or both. It is the complications of diverticular disease that produce dramatic symptoms:

1. Bleeding from dilated peridiverticular arteries causes anaemia with positive faecal occult bloods, or severe rectal bleeding with shock and collapse. This is treated conservatively, although emergency resection of the diseased bowel may be required.
2. Perforation causes acute abdominal pain and evidence of local or generalised peritonitis. Emergency surgery is required.
3. Abscess formation is by local extension of peridiverticular inflammation with abdominal pain and a tender mass. Drainage and resection of the affected area of colon are required.
4. Portal pyaemia from infection spreading from a diverticular abscess and causing septic embolisation of the portal circulation may result in one or more hepatic abscesses or septic portal vein thrombosis and portal hypertension (see p. 301).

JAUNDICE

Jaundice, the retention of bilirubin in the tissues, can be caused by:

1. haemolysis, when breakdown of red blood cells overwhelms hepatic conjugating capacity
2. obstruction, where the exit of conjugated bilirubin from the biliary tree is prevented

3. liver cell or hepatocellular dysfunction, where there is defective cellular metabolism of bilirubin by the liver cells.

HAEMOLYTIC JAUNDICE

Haemolytic jaundice is mild, with bilirubin levels < 5 mg/100ml (85 mmol/l). The retained pigment is unconjugated and does not appear in the urine, but excessive urobilinogen does. LFTs, apart from the raised serum bilirubin level, are normal but pigment stones may complicate haemolysis and cause a secondary obstructive picture. Causes are those of haemolytic anaemia (see Chapter 11).

OBSTRUCTIVE JAUNDICE

Obstructive jaundice may be mild, moderate or severe. The urine is dark because of the presence of conjugated bilirubin, and the stools are pale from steatorrhoea (bile salt deficiency) and diminished stercobilinogen. Usually there is pruritis, probably owing to bile salt deposition in the skin. Signs include hepatomegaly, an enlarged palpable gallbladder when obstruction is below the cystic duct, and occasionally splenomegaly. LFTs show raised serum bilirubin and alkaline phosphatase (> 30 KA units) levels and moderately elevated serum transaminases.

The obstruction may be:
1. extrahepatic, i.e. of the common bile duct or common hepatic duct, and can be caused by:
   a. duct stones;
   b. malignant tumours of bile ducts, gallbladder, head of pancreas, or ampulla of Vater;
   c. sclerosing cholangitis;
   d. biliary strictures (usually following surgical injury).
2. intrahepatic, i.e. at the level of the biliary cannaliculae, and also has several causes. Acutely it may be caused by viral hepatitis or by certain drugs; it is sometimes seen in the third trimester of pregnancy, or it may be recurrent and of uncertain cause (recurrent idiopathic cholestasis). Chronic causes of intrahepatic cholestasis include primary biliary cirrhosis (see p. 299) and some persistent cholestatic drug reactions (e.g. chlorpromazine).

The site of biliary obstruction cannot be reliably detected clinically although pancreatic tumours can cause intestinal bleeding, and lesions obstructing below the cystic duct may cause gallbladder enlargement. Patients with gallstones may have attacks of biliary pain and fever, and with tumours there is often striking weightloss and back pain.

Investigations
Hepatic ultrasound confirms dilatation of the intrahepatic bile ducts in extrahepatic obstruction. Occasionally patients with extrahepatic obstruction from gallstones may not show this change. Ultrasound may also show a cause for obstruction, such as a pancreatic mass or gallstones.

CT scans can also show bile duct dilatation in extrahepatic obstruction and can demonstrate causes such as hepatic or pancreatic tumours, pancreatitis, etc.

ERCP identifies the site of obstruction, e.g. from bile duct stones, or can place the lesion in the head of the pancreas by identifying pancreatic duct obstruction.

Fine-needle cholangiography will also demonstrate the biliary tree above an obstructive lesion and thus help to define its extent and site.

In patients with intrahepatic obstruction, liver biopsy offers the only possible way of identifying the cause—apart, that is, from the history and viral studies. Even then distinction between drugs and hepatitis may not be clearcut. An ERCP in such cases would confirm a patent but non-dilated biliary tree.

Surgery and biliary obstruction

Patients with extrahepatic obstruction may require surgery. Although ampullary tumours may be resectable, other cancers often are not and a cholecystenterostomy is performed to relieve jaundice. In the elderly and weakened patient, a stent may be placed endoscopically through a stenosing tumour, without recourse to surgery, or it may be performed as a preliminary to surgery to improve the patient's preoperative status. Adequate hydration and vitamin K therapy are important before surgery so that renal failure and bleeding are prevented. Cholangitis and septicaemia are other possible complications which must be vigorously treated.

Intrahepatic biliary obstruction is important because it is not amenable to surgery.

Chronic biliary obstruction

The important cause of this is primary biliary cirrhosis (see p. 299). Patients with chronic biliary obstruction develop:
1. Severe itching, treated by bile salt chelation, e.g. with cholestyramine.
2. Secondary melanin pigmentation of the skin which may require careful cosmetic make-up.
3. Metabolic bone disease, both osteomalacia from vitamin D deficiency (malabsorption and the effects of skin pigmentation) and osteoporosis. Prophylactic supplements of vitamin D (1 µg per 24 hours) and supplementary calcium are given.
4. Bleeding, spontaneous and postoperative from prothrombin deficiency and vitamin K malabsorption, treated with prophylactic intramuscular vitamin K.
5. Hypercholesterolaemia with xanthoma formation and occasional peripheral neuropathy, and bone cholesterol deposits. Treatment is difficult and may require plasmaphoresis.
6. Night blindness and dry skin from malabsorption of vitamin A, treated with vitamin A prophylaxis.
7. Postoperative renal failure (see above).
8. Neuropathy and brain disease from vitamin E deficiency, particularly likely in children.

HEPATOCELLULAR JAUNDICE

Two types of disorder are seen:
1. jaundice without light microscopic liver cell damage, i.e. the congenital hyperbilirubinaemias
2. that due to generalised liver cell disease, e.g. viral hepatitis or cirrhosis.

The congenital hyperbilirubinaemias are caused by defective metabolism of bilirubin. The retained pigment may be unconjugated bilirubin (as in Gilbert's syndrome and Crigler-Najjar syndrome), in which case no pigment is seen in the urine, or conjugated bilirubin (as in Dubin Johnson syndrome and Rotor's syndrome), where pigment is present in the urine. In both types, the serum bilirubin levels are raised.

1. Gilbert's syndrome is a common (5% of population) autosomal dominant condition. LFTs are normal. Bilirubin uptake and conjugation may be defective. Bilirubin rises with fever, trauma and starvation.

2. Crigler-Najjar syndrome is a rare inherited disorder. Severe cases are fatal because of kernicterus; less severe cases are compatible with life.

3. Dubin-Johnson syndrome is a rare inherited disease. The liver contains black (melanin) pigment. Serum alkaline phosphatase levels are raised.

4. Rotor syndrome is a variant of Dubin-Johnson syndrome but the liver does not contain melanin pigment.

Hepatocellular jaundice from liver cell disease

The jaundice is mild, moderate or severe. Stools are pale and the urine dark. Itching, if present, is usually transient. The liver may be enlarged, of normal size or smaller than usual (hence the clinical importance of percussion). Splenic enlargement is common and in chronic cases the cutaneous signs of hepatocellular disease occur (see Table 9.14).

LFTs show raised serum bilirubin, greatly raised transaminase and normal or somewhat raised alkaline phosphatase levels. The prothrombin time is prolonged. The diagnosis of the cause of liver cell jaundice (Table 9.11) rests on a full history, clinical examination, immunological tests for causative viruses, an autoimmune profile, and, if there is no risk from clotting problems, a liver biopsy.

Table 9.11. Some common causes of hepatocellular jaundice

Acute	Hepatitis (viral, drugs and alcohol)
	Fatty infiltration (drugs and alcohol)
	Hepatic necrosis (viruses, drugs)
Chronic	
Chronic hepatitis	Autoimmune, viral, drug induced
Cirrhosis	Alcoholic, post viral, metabolic

Table 9.12. The main causes of viral hepatitis

Virus	Type	Incubation period	Detecting infection
A	Picornavirus (RNA)	2–3 weeks	Virus A IgM antibody
B	DNA	6–9 weeks	HBsAg HBeAg anti-HBc
D	RNA (incomplete virus)	?	anti-Delta + anti-HBc
C	RNA	6–9 weeks	anti-virus C antibody
E	?RNA	—	Nil
EBV	DNA (herpes)	—	Antibody to viral capsid antigen (VCA) EB virus specific IgM
CMV	DNA (herpes)	2–6 weeks	Complement fixation IgG CMV IgM (fluorescent antibody test)

EBV = Epstein-Barr virus; CMV = Cytomegalovirus

VIRAL HEPATITIS

Several viruses cause hepatitis, and viruses A, B, C, D and E are the most important. Viral hepatitis is a world-wide condition and in the case of B and C infection probably accounts for much of the chronic non-alcoholic liver disease and primary hepatic cancer. Despite the number of viruses involved, the clinical picture and some of the complications are common to all. The incubation period is, however, variable (Table 9.12).

Types of viral hepatitis (See also Table 9.12)

Virus A causes infective hepatitis. This is common in childhood within the family unit. Epidemics are common where hygiene is poor. It is spread by oral–faecal contamination. It does not cause chronic liver disease, although fatal acute hepatic necrosis occasionally occurs.

Virus B (HBV) (Table 9.13) is spread by contaminated blood and blood products. Subjects at special risk include homosexuals, those given infected blood or blood products, intravenous drug users, the newborn of infected mothers, patients and staff of mental deficiency and renal dialysis units, and the immunocompromised. The disease is widespread in the Third World and approximately 300 million chronic carriers may exist. Virus B is an important cause of chronic liver disease and hepatic cancer (Fig. 9.11). About 0.1% of subjects in the UK carry the virus, but in Africa and the Far East the rate reaches 15%. The important immunological tests used in the monitoring of

Table 9.13. The immunology of virus B infection

Blood test	Significance
HBs antigen +ve	Indicates infection or carrier state
HBs antibody +ve	Indicates past infection and immunity
HBe antigen +ve	Indicates infectivity and, if persistent, chronicity
HBe antibody +ve	Indicates low infectivity and recovery
HB core antigen +ve	Not detected in serum
HB core antibody +ve	Indicates recent infection (IgM) even if other tests are –ve. If persistent (IgM) chronic liver disease
HBV DNA +ve	The most sensitive test of viral replication and chronicity

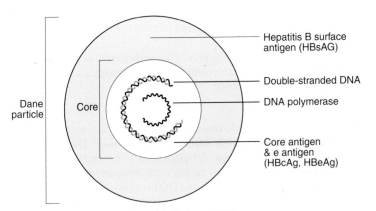

Fig. 9.11 The structure of hepatitis B virus (HBV).

virus B infection are shown in Table 9.13. Mutants of hepatitis B have been described and are of importance in protection therapy with HBV vaccination.

Virus C (HCV). Blood donated for transfusion is HBV tested and thus HCV has become the overwhelming cause of post-transfusion hepatitis. Subjects at risk include patients transfused with blood or blood products, drug addicts, and renal dialysis unit staff and patients. The virus causes an acute hepatitis and, in up to 50%, chronic hepatitis or cirrhosis. Hepatoma is also thought to be an important sequela. An antibody test for infection is available and is positive in up to 3% of Europeans and in 5–10% of the Third World population. Its sensitivity is variable, and better tests are awaited.

Virus D (delta) only exists in association with virus B. It therefore occurs as a combined infection or as a secondary delta infection in a virus B carrier. First described in Italy, it is particularly related to intravenous drug abuse, causes acute hepatitis and renders the virus B carrier more likely to develop hepatic cirrhosis.

Virus E is found in India and the Far East and behaves like virus A. It does not cause chronic liver disease but can cause fulminant hepatitis in pregnancy.

Symptoms and signs

These are of fairly sudden onset. In the pre-icteric phase the symptoms are malaise, fever, upper right abdominal and epigastric pain, and discomfort with nausea and vomiting. After a few days, these symptoms remit and the patient becomes jaundiced. However, jaundice may be absent (anicteric hepatitis).

Apart from the clinical jaundice, the signs are tender, moderate hepatomegaly, splenomegaly, and sometimes enlarged lymph nodes in the neck. The urine contains bile, even before there is jaundice.

Jaundice lasts 7–10 days, improvement is then rapid, appetite returns and LFTs normalise. Many patients, however, suffer from continuing debility, lethargy, abdominal discomfort and fat intolerance: 'post-hepatitis syndrome'.

Investigations

The blood count shows a normal haemoglobin level with leukopenia and a relative lymphocytosis. The ESR and plasma viscosity are raised.

LFTs are abnormal, the serum bilirubin is raised, and serum transaminases elevated, sometimes markedly so—1000–2000 iu/l. The serum albumin level is normal in uncomplicated cases, but total globulin level is raised, with hyper-gammaglobulinaemia.

A liver biopsy, performed only if coagulation is normal, shows hepatic damage to be maximal in the centrilobular areas with a scattered lobular and portal lymphocytic infiltration.

Complications

Resolution without chronic changes in the liver is usual and invariable in virus A or E infection. Chronicity is a feature of virus B, C or D infections.

1. Acute fulminant hepatitis. An acute and severe necrosis of the liver can complicate hepatitis caused by any virus with deepening jaundice, hepatic coma, bleeding and renal failure. The liver becomes smaller and there is an 80% mortality without hepatic transplantation.
2. In virus B infection, immune complex disease may occur either in the pre-icteric phase, with arthralgia and skin rashes, or later as an acute polyarteritis nodosa or glomerulonephritis. Bone marrow involvement with severe aplastic anaemia is also a rare complication of any viral hepatitis. Patients with viral hepatitis can also develop an obstructive picture—cholestatic hepatitis—which may cause diagnostic difficulty.
3. Chronic active hepatitis. Here symptoms continue, there is hepatosplenomegaly and the cutaneous signs of liver disease (see Table 9.14). LFTs do not normalise, liver biopsy shows piecemeal necrosis, bridging necrosis between portal tracts and the centrilobular areas, fibrosis and cellular infiltration.

Treatment

Bedrest and a sensible nutritious diet usually lead to uneventful resolution of the disease. The treatment of acute fulminant liver failure is discussed elsewhere. Patients with chronic hepatitis following viral infection with virus B, C or D may require antiviral therapy. This is currently carried out by injections of alpha-interferon three times weekly over a 6-month period. A preceding course of corticosteroids is sometimes given.

Prophylaxis

Vaccines are available for virus A and, more importantly for virus B. A recombitant yeast-derived virus B vaccine is used. Large-scale vaccination of children in the Third World would be an important way of diminishing hepatic cirrhosis and cancer, were it not for the expense. At present vaccination is with three injections, given at 1 and 5 months intervals, to those at risk, e.g. family and contacts of sufferers, uninfected homosexuals, medical and dental personnel, etc.

Liver cell failure

Impaired hepatocyte function leads to hepatocellular jaundice, fluid retention, bleeding and hepatic encephalopathy. Other important associations include abnormal drug sensitivity, certain endocrine changes and the development of cutaneous signs of liver disease.

Hepatocellular jaundice. This is variable, depending on the severity of liver cell damage. There is no specific treatment.

Fluid retention. This causes ankle oedema, ascites, particularly if portal hypertension exists, and is sometimes generalised. Although hypoalbuminaemia is a factor, the major cause is excessive renal sodium retention.

Treatment is by bedrest, sodium restriction and the use of potassium-sparing diuretics (potassium deficiency is common in liver cell disease). Despite this precaution, electrolyte disturbances are common. Hyponatraemia and a rising blood creatinine level herald the onset of renal failure. Infusions of salt-poor human albumin may reverse this situation. Ultrafiltration and re-infusion of ascitic fluid has its advocates but may not help, and a LeVeen shunt which drains ascitic fluid into the major veins in the neck is sometimes useful in refractory cases.

Acute cases clear easily with improvement in liver function but diuretics may be required.

Bleeding. Spontaneous bleeding may occur into the skin or from mucous membranes. Important causes include failure of hepatic synthesis of coagulant factors, particularly vitamin K-related ones, thrombocytopenia and increased thrombolytic activity.

Bleeding is treated with intramuscular injection of vitamin K and correction of platelet deficiency with platelet infusion. Other clotting defects are treated with fresh frozen plasma.

Hepatic encephalopathy. Confusion, somnolence leading to coma, a flapping tremor of the outstretched hands and a sweetish smell of the breath (fetor hepaticus) are the main features. It is caused by the intoxication by protein-derived breakdown products of the reticular formation and basal ganglia of the brain. The syndrome can occur with rapid onset of coma from acute hepatic necrosis, but in more chronic conditions consciousness is retained, whilst dysarthria, tremor, confusion and constructional apraxia are more obvious.

Alimentary bleeding, infection (anywhere), surgical trauma, paracentesis, a high protein meal, and drugs (analgesics, sedatives and diuretics) may precipitate hepatic encephalopathy.

Protein restriction to < 40 g per 24 hours, preferably of vegetable origin, and the use of non-absorbable antibiotics such as neomycin 1 g 8-hourly reduce bacterial protein breakdown in the gut. Drugs known to aggravate hepatic encephalopathy, such as diuretics which cause hypokalaemia and all sedative drugs, are stopped. Lactulose, a non-absorbable liquid carbohydrate, or lactitol—a tablet form—soften the stools, lower faecal pH and inhibit ammonia-producing organisms (NH_3 is one of the known toxic nitrogenous breakdown products).

Abnormal drug metabolism. Patients with liver cell disease are sensitive to drugs, particularly to sedatives. The reasons for this include slower hepatic metabolism, altered binding to serum albumin, altered distribution volume and diminished first pass metabolism. The sensitivity to sedative drugs is also related to latent hepatic encephalopathy. Drug therapy needs to be carefully monitored in subjects with liver disease and reduced dosing is advised.

Endocrine changes. Both feminisation and impotence occur in males with chronic liver cell failure; changes in females are less obvious. The initial event in males appears to be testicular atrophy with low serum testosterone values. FSH and LH are not appropriately elevated after clomiphine. Hyperoestrogenaemia also occurs, but oestrogen turnover is normal. An increase in numbers of cell oestrogen receptors is a likely explanation for gynaecomastia and some vascular abnormalities. Diabetes with insulin resistance is also common in cirrhosis, and in alcoholics pseudo-Cushing's syndrome occurs. Here physical features of Cushing's syndrome with high non-suppressable levels of corticosteroids are reversed when drinking stops.

Cutaneous signs of liver disease. The major abnormalities are listed in Table 9.14.

If liver cell failure fails to respond to therapy, then hepatic transplantation may be possible.

Table 9.14. Cutaneous signs of liver disease

Nails	Clubbing
	White (opaque) nails
	White bands (hypoalbuminaemia)
Skin	Paper money skin (facial telangiectasia)
	Vascular spiders
	Palmar erythema
	Jaundice
Others	(Males)
	Gynaecomastia
	Testicular atrophy
	Loss of secondary sexual hair

CIRRHOSIS OF THE LIVER

Cirrhosis (literally meaning a tawny colour) is a chronic generalised liver disease resulting from necrosis and regeneration of liver cells. It is characterised by:

1. a variable element of liver cell (hepatocyte) dysfunction
2. increased hepatic fibrosis
3. nodule formation (nodular regeneration).

The latter is most important as nodules are functionally less effective than normal liver tissue, they have an abnormal blood supply and they constrict hepatic venous outflow to produce portal hypertension. Further, malignant, change (hepatoma) may occur within them.

Causes

1. Viral hepatitis (viruses B, D and C)
2. Non-viral (autoimmune) chronic active hepatitis
3. Alcohol excess
4. Haemochromatosis (primary genetic iron overload)
5. Wilson's disease (excessive copper retention)
6. Cystic fibrosis
7. Alpha-1-antitrypsin deficiency
8. Primary biliary cirrhosis

Cirrhosis is sometimes classified by nodular size, i.e. micronodular (<1 cm), macronodular (≥1–10 cm) and mixed with a variable pattern.

Although alcohol is classically associated with micronodular cirrhosis and previous viral hepatitis with macronodular change, there are exceptions to these rules.

Symptoms and signs

Patients can be asymptomatic and present with abnormalities found on clinical examination, e.g. hepatomegaly or with abnormal investigations. Presenting symptoms may include:

1. intestinal bleeding, often severe from oesophageal varices caused by portal hypertension
2. jaundice from liver cell failure
3. fluid retention, either as ascites with abdominal distension and dyspnoea, or with ankle oedema
4. hepatic encephalopathy with confusion, tremor and coma
5. excessive bleeding, purpura, bruising and nose bleeds
6. fever, confusion and abdominal pain from *E. coli* infection of ascitic fluid with resultant septicaemia
7. weightloss, abdominal pain, ascites and bleeding from a complicating hepatoma.

The signs are variable; any or none of the following can be present:

1. The skin is pigmented and or/jaundiced.
2. There may be purpura and bruising due to a bleeding tendency.
3. The patient's palms may be warm and reddened (palmar erythema).

4. There may be finger clubbing and white (opaque) nails.
5. There may be spider naevi, i.e. dilated arterioles usually seen on the face, arms, shoulders and trunk. There may be facial telangiectasia (paper money skin).
6. The liver may be enlarged, firm and nodular, or may be smaller than normal, by percussion.
7. There may be splenomegaly.
8. There may be ascites, often with an umbilical hernia and, due to portal hypertension, enlarged abdominal veins around the umbilicus.
9. There may be peripheral oedema.
10. Signs of hepatic encephalopathy may be found.
11. Male patients may show feminisation (see p. 298).

Investigations

Mild anaemia, leukopenia and thrombocytopenia are caused by hypersplenism. The prothrombin time may be prolonged.

An ultrasonic scan of the liver confirms that it is enlarged or small, diffusely abnormal and nodular.

Tests of previous and continuing virus B, D and C infection may be positive. LFTs are usually abnormal, but in compensated cases abnormalities are minimal. A raised serum bilirubin level, moderately raised transaminases and alkaline phosphatase, reduced serum albumin and increased serum globulins, particularly the gammaglobulins, all occur.

Liver biopsy, which should be routinely stained for iron, alpha-1-antitrypsin and copper, shows fibrosis, nodule formation, liver cell damage and fragmentation. There is invariably a portal cell infiltrate.

Table 9.15 gives the major features of the various types of cirrhosis.

PRIMARY LIVER CANCER

Cancer derived from hepatocytes is a hepatoma. In 70–80% of cases it complicates cirrhosis and is most commonly seen in Africa, the Middle East and the Far East, where cirrhosis is widespread. The type of cirrhosis is variable, but preceding virus B and C infection are particularly important and incorporation of virus B into hepatocyte DNA seems a common consequence of virus B infection. Whether this mechanism or the cellular hyperactivity of the cirrhotic process is responsible for hepatoma is uncertain. Males who have well-compensated cirrhosis, e.g. haemochromatosis, may have a risk as high as 15%. Aflatoxin, a carcinogenic product of the mould *Aspergillus flavus* which contaminates stored cereals in some countries, is a further risk factor.

Hepatoma in a cirrhotic liver is commonly multiple, but in non-cirrhotic patients a single neoplasm is usual.

Symptoms and signs

These include vague ill health, weightloss and hepatic pain in a patient with previously diagnosed cirrhosis, bleeding from oesophageal varices (hepatomas tend to invade portal venous radicles), ascites, often bloodstained, and/or of high protein content, and rupture of the tumour into the peritoneal cavity with shock and pain.

The liver may be nodular, tender and perhaps increasing in size. LFTs show no specific change, but a rising alkaline phosphatase may be suggestive. In 60% of patients the serum alpha-1-fetoprotein level is raised—this is negative, however, in non-cirrhotic (fibro lamellar) growths and in cholangiocarcinoma.

Tissue diagnosis is by guided needle biopsy under ultrasound. Arteriography shows the tumour circulation and gives an idea of size as well as number of tumours.

Hepatomas can produce erythropoietin (polycythaemia), lipids (hyperlipidaemia) insulin (hypoglycaemia) or parathormone-like protein (hypercalcaemia), thus widening the clinical features. Secondary spread to neighbouring structures such as bone, lymph nodes and other abdominal viscera occurs early.

Differential diagnosis is from decompensated cirrhosis and secondary hepatic cancer.

Treatment
Resection by hepatic lobectomy may be possible with a single tumour in one lobe in a non-cirrhotic liver. Otherwise chemotherapy, e.g. adriamycin, or embolisation of the tumour via its arterial blood supply lessen pain. Hepatic transplantation is a further possibility but secondary tumour recurrence is common.

Cholangiocarcinoma
This is another form of primary hepatic cancer with growth from bile duct cells. Obstructive jaundice results. There is an association with ulcerative colitis.

PORTAL HYPERTENSION

A raised pressure within the portal circulation (Fig. 9.12) of > 10 mmHg

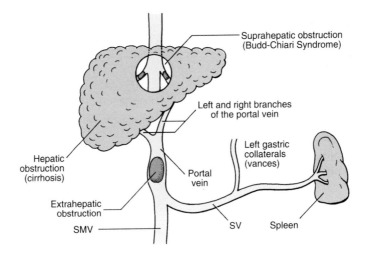

Fig. 9.12 Portal circulation and portal hypertension.

9.15. Cirrhosis of the liver

Type	Cause	Diagnosis
Cryptogenic F>M (macronodular)	Unknown ? virus C	Elimination of other causes
Primary biliary cirrhosis F>M++ 9:1 (micronodular)	Autoimmune destruction of septal bile ducts	M antibodies in blood Granulomata around bile ducts on biopsy ERCP shows patent non-dilated biliary tree
Chronic active Hepatitis (macronodular) F>M (usually young)	Autoimmune liver disease 60% HLA-B8+ve	Usually grossly deranged LFTs Hypergammaglobulinaemia Biopsy shows piecemeal necrosis, plasma cell infiltration +ve DNAds antibodies +ve Smooth muscle antibodies
Wilson's disease (macronodular/ variable) F>M (usually young)	Genetic Autosomal recessive Disorder of copper metabolism Tissue copper overload	Kaiser-Fleischer rings in eyes Serum caeruloplasmin usually low Urinary copper increased Increased copper content in liver biopsy
Haemochromatosis M>F (micronodular)	Genetic Autosomal recessive Link with HLA-A3	Raised serum iron Raised hepatic tissue iron
Alcoholic M>F (micronodular but variable)	? due to toxicity of acetaldehyde	History Liver biopsy may show fat, central hyaline sclerosis or acute alcoholic hepatitis with polymorph infiltrate and Mallory's alcoholic hyaline, etc.
Post virus B	Virus B	+ve tests for virus B Often from countries with high HBV risk or immunosupressed, or homosexual, or have been transfused
Alpha-1-antitrypsin (AT) deficiency	Genetic Autosomal recessive AT is a protease inhibitor	Suspect in young and adults with liver disease ± emphysema PAS +ve granules in periportal hepatocytes Confirmation by immuno- precipitation and phenotyping

Effects	Treatment
Bleeding varices	
Liver cell failure	
Mild obstructive jaundice	Fat-soluble vitamin
Bone disease	supplements,
Other autoimmune isorders,	ursodeoxycholate
e.g. renal tubular acidosis	? Transplantation
CREST syndrome	
(scleroderma)	
Liver cell dysfunction	Corticosteroids and
Part of multisystem disase, e.g.	azathioprine
ulcerative colitis, skin rashes,	
arthralgia (c.f. SLE)	
Liver failure	Oral D-penicillamine
Haemolysis	to remove copper
Bone disease	
CNS involuntary/movements	
Personality deterioration	
Hepatomegaly	Venesection
Skin pigmentation	to remove iron
Diabetes	
Cardiomyopathy	
Gonadal failure	
Arthralgia	
Hepatoma risk ++	
May be deeply jaundiced	Forbid alcohol;
Fever	treat liver cell failure
Hepatomegaly	
Liver cell failure	
Delirium tremens	
Peripheral neuropathy	
Dupuytren's contractures	
Mild liver cell failure or portal	May be suitable for
hypertension	antiviral treatment
May be silent	(alpha-interferon)
Neonatal hepatitis with	AT can be given
cholestasis	therapeutically for
Childhood and adult cirrhosis	lung disease
Panacinar emphysema	

results in changes which include splenomegaly, the formation of oesophageal and gastric varices and the opening up of venous connections between the portal and systemic circulation. The three major types of portal hypertension are:

1. suprahepatic, resulting from obstruction of sinusoidal outflow, e.g. thrombosis of hepatic veins or a vena caval web;
2. hepatic, resulting from sinusoidal distortion due to hepatic disease, e.g. cirrhosis;
3. prehepatic, resulting from portal vein obstruction, usually thrombosis. Portal hypertension causes:

1. splenomegaly, sometimes accompanied by pancytopenia, i.e. hypersplenism;
2. bleeding from oesophageal and gastric varices, either as haematemesis and/or melaena, or chronic anaemia;
3. the shunting of protein blood products through the portosystemic collaterals around rather than through the liver resulting in hepatic encephalopathy;
4. shunting of gut bacteria through similar collaterals, causing *E. coli* septicaemia and endotoxemia.

Hypersplenism

Usually, there are no symptoms, and splenomegaly may be the only sign.

A blood count shows panycytopenia, although not severe enough to be associated with spontaneous infection or bleeding.

Splenectomy is not recommended.

Bleeding from oesophageal varices

This is an important condition because bleeding can be massive and repeated, and bleeding in those whose portal hypertension is caused by liver disease may develop liver cell failure with jaundice, ascites and hepatic encephalopathy.

The mortality is high, about 50% of those bleeding from oesophageal varices complicating liver disease die as a result of their first bleed.

Differences between portal hypertension caused by suprahepatic and by extrahepatic portal hypertension (Fig. 9.12)

Suprahepatic portal hypertension (the Budd–Chiari syndrome) causes blockage of hepatic venous outflow, variceal bleeding, tender hepatomegaly and the rapid onset of ascites and liver cell failure. Unless obstruction of hepatic veins is partial, the mortality is > 80%. It has many causes, e.g. polycythaemia, membranous obstruction of the inferior vena cava, the contraceptive pill use, etc.

In extrahepatic portal hypertension the prognosis from bleeding varices is better because there is no liver cell disease or liver cell failure. The cause is usually a septic portal endophlebitis, arising in childhood from an infected appendix, or in adults from septicaemia or septic diverticulitis. Occasionally a clotting disease like polycythaemia or antithrobin-3 deficiency is the cause.

Symptoms and signs

Symptoms include haematemesis, melaena and those of acute or chronic anaemia.

There may be tachycardia and hypotension; if there is liver disease the cutaneous signs such as spider naevi may be present but are difficult to detect in hypovolaemic subjects. Fluid retention, particularly ascites and signs of hepatic encephalopathy, i.e. fetor, stupor, confusion, etc., develop quickly. There may be splenomegaly.

Investigations

A blood count confirms the effects of bleeding and may show a pancytopenia. LFTs are abnormal where there is hepatic disease.

Prothrombin time and other coagulation tests are prolonged where there is hepatic disease.

Endoscopy is vital to diagnose the presence of varices and to commence sclerotherapy. Hepatic ultrasound may be helpful, if feasible, to diagnose chronic liver disease.

Treatment

1. Blood volume must be restored by adequate transfusion.
2. Sedative drugs must be avoided.
3. Impending hepatic encephalopathy is treated by stopping oral protein and giving oral neomycin to prevent intestinal bacterial protein breakdown. This can be supplemented with oral lactulose (see p. 298).
4. Injection sclerotherapy is performed through the endoscope. A sclerosant such as phenylethanolamine is injected directly into the varices, 5 ml into each of those demonstrated at the oesophagogastric junction using about 15 ml in total. Injections are repeated every 3–4 weeks until all varices have been thrombosed. In those with active bleeding, cessation can usually be achieved with a Sengstaken–Blakemore tube (Fig. 9.13) and intravenous

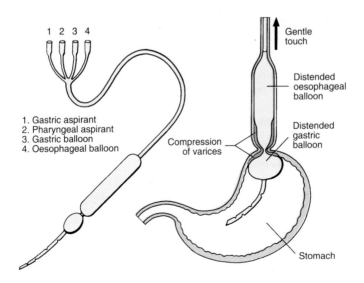

Fig. 9.13 The Sengstaken-Blakemore tube.

vasopressin or glypressin which constricts arterial flow into the portal circulation. Somatostatin is a possible but expensive alternative drug. Beta-blockers prevent recurrent variceal bleeding in the long term.

5. Surgery for those fit enough may be required if bleeding continues. The usual operation is a transection of the oesophagus and re-stapling using a staple gun, although some surgeons favour an emergency portocaval shunt. In patients with extrahepatic portal hypertension, variceal sclerotherapy is preferable as surgery does not produce lasting benefit.

DISEASES OF THE LIVER IN CHILDHOOD ALSO OCCURRING IN ADULTS

Neonatal hepatitis

Neonatal hepatitis causes neonatal jaundice and may be due to viruses, protozoa or be 'idiopathic' (75%) or familial. The long-term prognosis is fairly good although cirrhosis may develop.

Biliary Atresia

This results from failure of development or damage to the biliary tree in utero. It may be variable in completeness and causes progressive obstructive jaundice. The prognosis is poor but a Kasai operation (hepatic porto-enterostomy) performed early can prevent disease progression. For others transplantation may be possible. Prophylactic fat-soluble vitamins A, D, E and K are given.

Reye's syndrome

A fine fatty infiltration of the liver of childhood occurs following a viral infection. Cerebral oedema develops with vomiting and coma in severe cases. It can also follow aspirin administration in children.

Indian childhood cirrhosis

This is seen in middle-class Indian children. There is often a family history. The prognosis is poor. Copper overload may be a factor in the aetiology.

Fibrocystic disease (See Table 9.17).

Wilson's disease (See Table 9.15).

Cystic fibrosis (See p.183)

DISEASES OF THE LIVER SPECIFIC TO PREGNANCY

Idiopathic cholestasis

Obstructive jaundice develops in the third trimester with pruritus and disappears with delivery. It reappears with subsequent pregnancy and with oral contraceptives. It is probable that cholestasis is induced by oestrogens.

Acute fatty liver

Microvesicular fatty infiltration of the liver of uncertain cause is seen in the last trimester. It causes vomiting and liver cell failure. The white cell count and normoblasts in peripheral blood are raised. There is severe bleeding. Treatment is of liver failure and/or renal failure. Caesarean section may be necessary.

DRUG-INDUCED LIVER DISEASE

Drugs may cause any type of hepatic disease, including benign and malignant tumours. In some patients there is a known (allergic) hypersensitivity, whilst others probably depend on the production of reactive metabolites. The most important drug-induced lesions produce cholestasis, hepatocellular damage or a mixed picture (cholestatic hepatitis) (Table 9.16).

Table 9.16. Some examples of drug-induced liver disease

Cholestatic	Oral contraceptives 17-alpha alkyl substituted testosterones and nortestosterones Chlorpropamide
Hepatocellular	Paracetamol Ketoconazole Carbon tetrachloride Amiodarone Methotrexate
Cholestatic hepatitis	Chlorpromazine Erythromycin
Fatty infiltration	Sodium valproate Tetracycline
Chronic active hepatitis	Alpha methyl dopa (Aldomet) Nitrofurantoin

Hepatic tumours
  Adenoma
  Carcinoma
	
	Oral contraceptives
	Oral contraceptives
	Androgens
	Vinyl chloride

Peliosis (dilatation of sinusoids)	Oral contraceptives Androgens

OTHER IMPORTANT DISEASES OF THE LIVER

Table 9.17. Other diseases of the liver

Cause	Effect	Investigation/treatment
Non-viral infections		
Schistosomiasis		
Migration of ova from S. *mansoni* and S. *japonicum* (adult worms) in mesenteric veins	Portal hypertension due to portal fibrosis around ova No true cirrhosis	Diagnosis: ova in rectal snip or stools Prazipquantel 40—75 mg/kg or oxaminquine but needs control of water supply (snails) Sclerosis of varices
Hydatid disease		
Cystic stage of dog tapeworm (Echinococcus granulosa) — intermediate host sheep	One or several hepatic cysts May be visible and palpable Usually right lobe Cysts also possible in lung, kidney, etc.	Ultrasound confirms cystic nature Eosinophilia and +ve antibody tests Surgery required for complete cyst removal following cyst sterilisation Mebendazole and derivatives may help
Metabolic disease		
Fatty infiltration		
(a) Macrovesicular (large fat droplets due to alcohol, diabetes (b) Microvesicular(fine fat droplets) due to drugs like tetracycline and in pregnancy and in Reye's syndrome	Smooth non-tender	LFTs mildly abnormal generalised—sometimes localised—change Biopsy diagnostic Treatment is of the cause
Amyloidosis		
Fibrillar glycoprotein material either AA—due to chronic suppuration (rare) or rheumatoid arthritis (common) or familial Mediterranean fever AL— associated with myelomaor no underlying disease	Firm hepatomegaly Often proteinuria/renal failure and evidence of splenomegaly	Biopsy of liver diagnostic Biopsy of rectal mucosa helpful and of kidneys for renal involvement Treatment nil or of the cause

Table 9.17 *continued.* **Other diseases of the liver**

Cause	Effect	Investigation/treatment
Polycystic liver disease A genetic disorder with either multiple hepatic cysts, extensive fibrosis or dilatation of biliary tree	Multiple cysts—nodular liver Extensive (congenital hepatic) fibrosis— portal hypertension Dilatation of biliary tree —recurrent cholangitis and possible carcinoma	Ultrasound shows all three Biopsy helpful for fibrosis and ERCP for congenital bile duct dilatation LFTs abnormal except in presence of multiple cysts Portal hyper-tension requires sclerotherapy Resectionfor bile duct dilatation

10

NUTRITION AND OBESITY

Kenneth W. Heaton, Ralph E. Barry

DIET AND HEALTH

Rising public concern and awareness of diet–health interactions demands that tomorrow's doctors know more about nutrition than most of their teachers. Regrettably, doctors must be able to counter disinformation from vested interests, excitable reporters and cranks of all sorts.

Features of a health-preserving diet

Many official bodies have issued guidelines to healthy eating and there is a worldwide consensus, summarised in Table 10.1.

Table 10.1. Characteristics of a health-preserving diet

Desirable feature	Main problem(s) in Britain
Enough energy for normal physiological processes but no more	Most people fail to limit their intake Overnutrition fosters many diseases
Enough micronutrients (vitamins, minerals, trace elements) and essential fatty acids	Possibility of subclinical deficiencies fostering chronic disease
Saturated fat not more than 10% of calories	Excess is common, raises serum LDL cholesterol
Enough fibre (cell-wall material) to allow easy defecation and stool weight > 150 g per 24 hours	Deficiency is common, may lead to symptomatic constipation, bowel cancer
Not too much rapidly digested carbohydrate, esp. extracellular sugars ('refined carbohydrates')	Dental disease, obesity, ?hyperinsulinaemia
Salt limited to 6 g per 24 hours, preferably less	Excess fosters hypertension in susceptible people

Practical implications

1. Minimise intake of intermeal snacks, of puddings, especially sugar–fat mixtures, and of sugary drinks.
2. Fill up on unprocessed or lightly processed starch foods, especially bread (preferably wholemeal), rice, pasta, legume seeds or pulses (peas, beans, lentils), root vegetables and potatoes.
3. Minimise fried food, pastry, cold prepared meats; use vegetable oils, especially olive oil.
4. Use lean cuts of meat, poultry and fish freely. Milk, cheese and yoghurt should be consumed in moderation.
5. Eat several helpings of fruit and vegetables a day.
6. Eat breakfast.
7. Use salt sparingly in the kitchen and at the table.

MALNUTRITION IN DEVELOPED COUNTRIES

Diet-related diseases are caused by incorrect food choices or eating practices (or infected food). Overnutrition is much more common than undernutrition in terms of energy balance but suboptimal intake of protective factors in fruit, seeds and vegetables is common, especially fibre (cell-wall material) and, perhaps, anti-oxidant vitamins and essential fatty acids.

OVERNUTRITION

Besides obvious obesity, lesser degrees of excess body fat are almost universal. With age, muscle mass and bone mass tend to decrease so people whose weight stays the same may be laying down fat. Excess fat has many metabolic consequences, especially if the fat is intra-abdominal. In fact, 85% of people in Britain gain weight during adult life. Among the serious consequences of changed body composition are 'essential' hypertension, hyperlipidaemia, insulin resistance resulting in hyperinsulinaemia or hyperglycaemia, and gallstones. Furthermore, several common cancers are linked with overnutrition, especially carcinomas of the colon, breast, uterus (endometrium) and ovary. It is for these reasons that the World Health Organization and many other bodies begin their guidelines to healthy eating with 'maintain desirable body weight'. Unfortunately such advice is too vague to be helpful. More practical and effective would be 'keep your waist measurement unchanged from early adulthood'.

Avoiding overnutrition is difficult in a society where food is abundant and relatively cheap and many manufactured foods and drinks are laced with extra calories in the form of sugars or fats. Such foods and drinks are inherently attractive, heavily promoted and associated with positive emotions like affection and gratitude. Much eating and drinking occurs for social reasons and some for emotional reasons rather than physiological ones.

Success in the battle of the bulge always requires self-discipline and is aided by peer pressure and vigorous exercise.

UNDERNUTRITION

In a welfare state, chronic undernutrition (a low total food intake) has psychological causes or is secondary to organic disease. Aversion to food occurs in some teenagers (anorexia nervosa, see p. 505) and in some depressed people, especially the lonely and old. The latter may maintain an adequate energy intake but, because they live mainly on white bread, biscuits and sweetened tea, they develop deficiencies of ascorbic acid, folic acid and iron. Substance abuse is often associated with neglect of food. Alcoholics are especially prone to folic acid and thiamine deficiency.

Acute undernutrition

Acute undernutrition especially of protein, is liable to occur with any major illness or trauma, including burns and surgical operations. Not only is food intake reduced but catabolism of protein is increased. Recovery from major illness or trauma is aided by adequate diet. This may require enteral or parenteral nutrition using nutritionally complete liquid feeds. The expertise of a dietitian or, better, a nutrition team is very desirable here.

FOOD INTOLERANCE

Adverse reactions to food are uncommon (other than infected food and psychological food aversion) but can be serious. There are three main types:
1. reactions to pharmacologically active substances in foods, such as caffeine, causing tachycardia and tremor, and tyramine in certain cheeses, causing vascular headaches
2. idiosyncratic reactions due to lack of enzymes, e.g. deficiency of lactase in small bowel mucosa resulting in osmotic diarrhoea when milk is ingested
3. true allergy with immunological hypersensitivity, usually acute and IgE-mediated but occasionally delayed as in coeliac disease (gluten enteropathy).

Table 10.2 shows the main recognised syndromes of food allergy.

UNDERNUTRITION IN POOR COUNTRIES

Starvation

When food intake stops the body lives on its energy reserves. These are mostly triglycerides (fat) in the adipose tissue but protein is also utilised. In a normal,

Table 10.2. Syndromes of true food allergy

Systemic	Anaphylaxis
Gastrointestinal	Lip swelling, vomiting, diarrhoea, malabsorption (coeliac disease)
Skin	Urticaria, eczema
Respiratory	Rhinitis, asthma

non-obese man it take 40 days on average for the available energy stores to be exhausted and death to occur. Women tend to last longer because their fat stores are twice as large (26% of bodyweight in a healthy young woman). The very young and the very old are most vulnerable. During starvation all tissues and organs shrink except the brain. The heart can shrink to a third of its normal weight before it fails. The small intestine becomes paper-thin and inefficient at absorption. Unfortunately, this counteracts the benefits of re-feeding and can prejudice recovery. Re-feeding must be cautious and gradual.

With partial starvation, as in famines, symptoms include feeling cold, nocturia, amenorrhoea and impotence. People become irritable, apathetic or vicious. The pulse is slow and blood pressure low, the ECG low voltage. Oedema is common and is not just the result of hypoalbuminaemia. The abdomen distends. Terminally there is diarrhoea, and intercurrent infections of various kinds are common. Treatment is simply provision of food but this should be done gradually, restricting salt. Severely underweight people (weight for height <70% of standard; weight in kg/height in m^2 <15.7) need hospital-type treatment. Most starvation is political and social rather than medical in origin.

MALNUTRITION IN CHILDREN

Because growing children have higher protein requirements per calorie and are more at risk of being given a low-protein diet than adults, they are more liable to protein deficiency. This is common in poor countries. The World Health Organization has estimated that about 100 million children are suffering from it at any one time (up to a quarter of Third World children). The commonest and most regrettable form which is called marasmus is simply starvation of babies. It is usually caused by ignorant, very poor mothers weaning their babies on to too-dilute formula feeds. Poor hygiene leads to gastroenteritis and a vicious circle starts as the ill baby loses its appetite. Losing more weight, its small intestine atrophies and malabsorption exacerbates the diarrhoea.

KWASHIORKOR

Kwashiorkor ('first-second' in the Ga language of Ghana) is the sickness of a child which is displaced from its mother's breast by the arrival of a new baby and is weaned on to a gruel which is relatively adequate in energy but too low in protein. Such gruels or porridges are based on cassava, plantain, maize, rice or banana which are the staple foods of villagers in Africa, West Indies, Indonesia etc.

The biochemistry is complex but seems to involve preservation of insulin secretion (unlike marasmus) and, perhaps, zinc deficiency. Because hypoalbuminaemia and oedema are prominent features the child may not look thin or be underweight, but reduced circumference of the upper arm is always present (e.g. under 12 cm at 1–5 years). Mild to moderate cases are 7–10 times more common than the severe, classical ones (Table 10.3); their most obvious manifestations are failure to grow and frequent infections, learning problems and

Table 10.3. The physical signs of Kwashiorkor

Failure to grow	Muscle wasting
Unhappy, apathetic	Skin peeling
Sparse, thin hair	Depigmentation or patchy pigmentation
Anaemia	Enlarged liver
Smooth tongue	Watery diarrohoea
Angular stomatitis	Oedema of legs

Table 10.4. Nomenclature and daily requirements of vitamins for healthy non-pregnant adults

Recommended name	Alternative name	Usual pharmaceutical preparation	Daily requirements for adults
Water-soluble			
Thiamine	Vitamin B_1	Thiamine hydrochloride	1 mg
Riboflavin	Vitamin B_2	Riboflavin	1.5 mg
Niacin	Nicotinic acid Nicotinamide	Nicotinamide	15–20 mg
Vitamin B_6	Pyridoxine	Pyridoxine hydrochloride	3 mg
Folate	Folacin	Folic acid	200 μg
Vitamin B_{12}	Cobalamin	Hydroxo-cobalamin	3μg
Vitamin C	Ascorbic acid	Ascorbic acid	30–60 mg
Fat-soluble			
Vitamin A	Retinol	Vitamin A	1 mg
Vitamin D	Vitamin D2, Vitamin D3	Calciferol, alfacalcidol, calcitriol	3 μg*
Vitamin E	Tocopherols	Alpha tocopheryl acetate	10 mg
Vitamin K	—	Menadiol sodium phosphate, phytomenadione	100 μg

* No dietary requirement when adequate exposure to sunlight

slow motor development. Subclinical cases lead to nutritional dwarfism. Treatment of severe cases is difficult, involving rehydration, repletion of electrolytes, correction of acidosis, hypothermia and hypoglycaemia, and treatment of acute and chronic infections and infestations. Gradual re-feeding is essential, as is nutritional education of the mother.

VITAMIN DEFICIENCIES AND EXCESSES

Required in mg or µg quantities, vitamins are all cofactors for the enzymes of metabolic step(s) in the human body. The variety of names may confuse, so they are set out in Table 10.4 together with their daily requirements. Vitamins have caught the popular imagination and are now big business. In the West, deficiencies are rare and unwise selfmedication can lead to overdosage.

Table 10.5 summarises the effects of deficiency and overdosage and the metabolic roles of vitamins. Lists of foods which provide vitamins are not given because a sensible mixed diet provides enough of all of them. Most highly processed foods are deficient in vitamins, especially those rich in sugars and fats.

There is particular interest at the moment in the antioxidant vitamins A, C and E and their possible role in preventing certain chronic diseases mediated by oxygen radicals and other free radicals, such as atherosclerosis and cancer.

NUTRITIONAL SUPPORT

In patients who are seriously malnourished, perhaps 10–15% or more below ideal weight, supplementary feeding may be required. These subjects have other hallmarks of malnutrition, including anthropometric abnormalities such as reduced skinfold thickness measures at standard sites and reduced concentrations of some serum proteins such as albumin, transferrin and retinal binding protein (RBP).

The possible ways of giving increased nutrition will depend on:
1. whether the small bowel is accessible (e.g. not obstructed) and with a normal absorptive mucosa
2. whether the intention is to 'rest' the bowel as for an intestinal fistula or Crohn's disease
3. how long extra nutrition will be required, e.g. over the span of a corrective operation, or recovery from, for example, burns or permanently because of small bowel resection.

METHODS

Oral carbohydrate protein and whole food liquid formulas can be used to supplement a nutritious diet. Preparations include Isocal or Ensure (complete feeds), Caloreen or Fortical (carbohydrate preparations) or Casilan (whole protein).

Oral elemental/peptide diets

These low-residue preparations contain amino acids, peptides, triglycerides and glucose. They may be of value when it is required to 'rest' the small bowel, e.g. Crohn's disease. Preparations include Pepti 2000 and EO 28 which is amino acid containing.

Enteral feeding

A fine-bore nasal tube (2 mm diameter) is passed into the stomach or even positioned endoscopically and is used together with a pump to allow

Table 10.5. Effects of deficiency and excess of the major vitamins

Vitamin	Chief metabolic role	Effects of edeficiency	Effects of excess
Thiamine	Metabolism of carbohydrate (esp. pyruvate)	Beri-beri (heart failure) Wernicke-Korsakoff syndrome Peripheral neuropathy	—
Riboflavin	Cellular oxidation (FAD)	Angular stomatitis, cheilosis Facial erythema Oro-genital syndrome	—
Niacin	Cellular oxidation (NAD, NADP)	Pellagra (maize eaters) Scaly dermatitis Glossitis, stomatitis, dementia	Flushing. Lowers plasma cholesterol
Vit B_6	Transamination, decarboxylation	Not a problem Prevents isoniazid neuropathy	Peripheral neuropathy
Folate	Haemopoiesis	Megaloblastic anaemia	None except with B_{12} deficiency
Vit B_{12}	Haemopoiesis	Megaloblastic anaemia	—
Vit C	Collagen synthesis, antioxidant	Impaired healing Scurvy and bleeding into tissues and joints Perifollicular haemorrhages Swollen bleeding gums, loose teeth	Increased urinary oxalate and urate
Vit A	Night vision, epithelial function, antioxidant	Night blindness, xerophthalmia (major cause of blindness in SE Asia) Perifollicular hyperkeratosis	Raised intracranial pressure, liver damage, skin changes
Vit D	Calcium metabolism	Rickets and osteomalacia (associated with sunlight deprivation, malabsorption)	Hypercalcaemia
Vit E	Red cell function, antioxidant	Mild haemolytic anaemia Neuropathy in children	—
Vit K	Synthesis of clotting factors (II, VII, IX, X)	Bleeding diathesis	—

continuous feeding. Whole protein and glucose polymer feeds, e.g. Neutrison, are used.

Complications include tube displacement, gastro-oesophageal reflux, abdominal discomfort and diarrhoea.

Parenteral nutrition

This is a major procedure and is used when the gastrointestinal tract is either unavailable or inadequate. A silicone catheter is passed into the superior vena cava using strict aseptic technique. A single 3-litre container of amino acids, glucose and other sugars, and lipid is given each 24 hours, supplemented with vitamins and minerals.

The major complication is sepsis (septicaemia), hyperglycaemia and cholestasis possibly caused by gallbladder immobility and bile sludging. However, trained patients can with help manage this technique at home, long term, for example, for the short bowel syndrome.

OBESITY

Obesity is best measured by the body mass index (BMI).

$$BMI = \frac{weight\ (kg)}{height^2(m)}$$

The Normal BMI is approximately 24, obesity = 25–30 and gross obesity > 30. Prevalence varies with culture and social class but is high in the UK—35% in men, greater in women and lower socioeconomic groups. There is a familial tendency which may be genetic or cultural.

Obese patients may not be eating large amounts but their energy intake, however small, exceeds their energy expenditure if they are gaining weight. An understanding of this simple principle is critical to the management of obesity.

Obesity is most usefully classified as simple (static) or progressive, where patients usually gain approximately 5 kg per year. Patients with gross ('morbid') obesity, BMI 35 and over, usually have progressive obesity.

Other causes of obesity are rare, but include endocrine disease (myxoedema, Cushing's syndrome, Fröhlich's syndrome, hypogonadism etc.). Genetic disorders (Prader-Willi and Laurence-Moon-Biedl syndromes, Von Gierke's disease etc.), and hypothalamic disease/trauma.

Symptoms and signs

By far the most common symptomatology in obesity results from emotional morbidity. Depression, poor self-esteem, marital or sexual dissatisfaction, unemployment, inactivity, social and financial deprivation may be directly caused by obesity itself or the attitudes of society and the medical profession to obesity and its management.

There are no physical symptoms specific to obesity. The most common presenting complaints are joint pains (ligamentous strain rather than arthritis) and exertional dyspnoea. Other symptoms arise from the multiple pathology associated with or caused by obesity. These include accidents, suicide, diabetes mellitus, gallstones, obstructive sleep apnoea, cardiovascular disease (sudden cardiac death, hypertension), respiratory infections and insufficiency, appendicitis, hyperuricaemia, and hepatic cirrhosis.

Table 10.6. Disorders associated with obesity

Stroke	Hernia
Respiratory failure	Arthritis
Coronary heart disease	Varicose veins and
Hypertension	thrombo-embolism
Gallstones	Clumsiness hence accidents
Diabetes	Increased risk of suicide

Mortality (Table 10.6)

Mortality ratio plotted against increasing BMI produces a J-shaped curve with nadir at approximately BMI 20–24, i.e. increasing weight is associated with increasing mortality.

Investigations

Electrocardiogram to measure the QTc interval for pretreatment baseline. Fasting blood glucose, lipids and serum uric acid.

Treatment

The risk/benefit/cost ratios must be considered. Unsuccessful treatment reinforces depression and poor self-esteem. Mild to moderate static obesity of middle-age or long standing has very poor prognosis for success. The younger the patient and the more severe the obesity, the greater the urgency for treatment.

Associated conditions, e.g. depression, diabetes, hypertension, chronic venous insufficiency, should be concurrently treated.

The patient must be motivated. Obesity is a chronic condition requiring life long management, the major burden of which falls on the patient, not the doctor. It also requires sensitive, sensible, practical support from family, friends, partner etc.

The patient's expectations must be taken into account. Are they realistic with respect to expected weightloss and time scale? What about the prevention of post-treatment weight gain?

The doctor and patient should agree a 'contract' indicating the target weight in a realistic time scale.

Conservative treatment options

Reducing diet. Energy intake is kept consistently below energy expenditure. The major problem is compliance but this can be maximised by visible success, regular realistic support and counselling and abdominal banding.

Diet plus anorectic drugs. Anorectic drugs produce additional weightloss which is rarely of clinical significance. These drugs are rarely justified. Almost all are modified amphetamines with greater or lesser undesirable CNS effects, including habituation.

Behaviour modification. An individualised programme supervised by a clinical psychologist helps the patient to recognise and avoid 'triggers' which precipitate eating. However, prolonged individualised 1 : 1 therapy is expensive.

Very low calorie and starvation diets. These are suitable for short-term use only. There is an increased incidence of sudden cardiac death.

Radical treatment options
These are suitable only for highly selected young grossly obese patients.

Vertical banded gastroplasty. Weightloss can be large and permanent but there may be problems with vomiting, tolerance and patient selection.

Jejunoileal bypass. Weightloss can be large and permanent but there is a high incidence of both long- and short-term metabolic complications. Diarrhoea may also be present. These patients require high quality long-term postoperative follow-up.

Jaw wiring. Weightloss can be large but it is only a short-term measure. It can be highly dangerous (e.g. with vomiting) and the long-term results are poor.

All successful regimens lose adipose and lean body mass in the short term, therefore the QTc interval on the ECG should be monitored.

11

HAEMATOLOGY

Geoffrey L. Scott

Diseases of the blood and the blood-forming organs are prevalent throughout the world. In industrialised countries anaemia occurs in children, the poor, the elderly and in pregnancy while in Third World nations infection, e.g. with intestinal worms, adds to the problem. Some diseases such as sickle cell disease (Africa) and thalassaemia (The Mediterranean) are found in certain ethnic groups or specific areas.

Childhood leukaemia seems to be a problem of advanced nations.
This chapter describes these diseases in detail.

ANAEMIA

In the adult, haemopoiesis occurs in the bone marrow, ribs, sternum, pelvis, vertebral bodies and ends of the long bones. Exceptionally, the liver and spleen may be involved (extramedullary haemopoiesis). Haemopoiesis depends on the presence of stem cells which generate functional cells (Fig. 11.1) and is

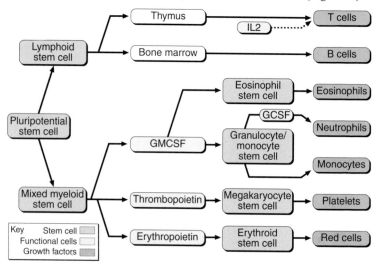

Fig. 11.1 Haemopoiesis.

Table 11.1. Normal red cell values

	Haemoglobin (g/dl)	Red cell count ($\times 10^{12}$/l)	PCV ratio	MCV (fl)	MCH (pg)
Adult male	13–18	4.5–6.5	0.40–0.54	80–96	27–32
Adult female	11.5–16.5	3.8–5.8	0.37–0.47	80–96	26–31
Children (10–12 years)	11.5–14.5	4.0–5.2	0.38–0.45	79–93	24–30

Reticulocytes 0.2–2.0% assuming normal red cell count.
Absolute numbers 0.025–0.085 $\times 10^{12}$/l.

Note: modern analytical techniques suggest that these ranges may be too wide.

governed by growth factors which control the production of the major cell lines. Manipulation of growth factors has exciting therapeutic potential in the treatment of haematological malignancies.

Normal red cell values are shown in Table 11.1. The use of modern, automated, cell counters, has simplified the diagnosis of anaemia. Mild abnormalities may be detected before they are visible on a blood film. Morphologically, anaemia may be divided into three types:

1. *Normochromic, normocytic* (normal mean cell volume (MCV), normal mean cell haemoglobin (MCH)), e.g. anaemia of chronic disease, malignancy, renal failure, aplastic anaemia.
2. *Hypochromic, microcytic* (low MCV, low MCH), e.g. iron deficiency, thalassaemia, sideroblastic anaemia, anaemia of chronic disease (severe).
3. *Macrocytic* (raised MCV), megaloblastic anaemia but also reticulocytosis (haemolysis or haemorrhage), liver disease, alcoholism, sideroblastic anaemia, cytotoxic therapy, aplastic anaemia, hypothyroidism.

The main causes of anaemia are shown in Table 11.2.

IRON DEFICIENCY ANAEMIA

Iron deficiency is the commonest cause of anaemia in the world. It usually results from a combination of inadequate intake and excessive loss; acute erosions, gastritis, duodenal ulcers and iron malabsorption are other causes. Premenopausal women and children are particularly susceptible and in some underdeveloped countries, it is almost universal from a combination of poor diet and chronic blood loss from parasitic infestation.

The normal iron requirements are approximately 1 mg per day for men and 2 m mg per day for premenopausal women. Pregnancy and lactation cause an average net loss of 500 mg. The average Western diet contains 15–20 mg of iron per day but only about 10% of this can be absorbed. The principal site of iron absorption is the duodenum and factors which promote absorption include acidity, iron deficiency and active erythropoiesis. Absorption is impaired following partial gastrectomy and by the presence of dietary phosphates and phytates.

Table 11.2. Causes of anaemia

Decreased red cell production (low reticulocyte count)

Failure of haemoglobin synthesis (hypochromic, microcytic)
Iron deficiency
Thalassaemia
Sideroblastic anaemia
Anaemia of chronic disease (severe)

Failure of DNA synthesis (macrocytic)
Megaloblastic anaemia from vitamin B_{12} or folate deficiency
Cytotoxic drug therapy
Other rare causes (congenital enzyme deficiency)

Bone marrow failure or replacement (usually normocytic but may be macrocytic)
Aplastic anaemia
Infiltration caused by leukaemia, myeloma, lymphoma, carcinoma or
myelofibrosis (usually leukoerythroblastic)

Miscellaneous (usually normocytic)
Hormone deficiency
Hypothyroidism (sometimes macrocytic)
Erythropoietin lack
Chronic renal failure
Lack of raw material, e.g. vitamin B_{12}, iron, folic acid etc.

Decreased red cell survival (increased reticulocyte count)

Haemolysis
Chronic blood loss (usually leads to iron deficiency) e.g. ulcers, menorrhagia,
haemorrhoids

In women, the commonest causes of iron deficiency are menorrhagia and pregnancy. In men, it is chronic intestinal blood loss.

Pathology

Severe iron deficiency causes tissue changes as well as anaemia. These include atrophy of the oral and gastric mucosa, changes in the nails (koilonychia) and the formation of an oesophageal web (Patterson-Kelly-Brown syndrome).

Symptoms

Iron deficiency is often symptomless. In severe cases, symptoms may be due to anaemia, i.e. lassitude, dyspnoea and even cardiac failure, or to tissue deficiency, i.e. angular stomatitis or dysphagia caused by an oesophageal web.

Investigations

The majority of cases do not require proof of iron deficiency. The haematological findings alone are sufficient. It is, however, essential to establish the cause; in men and postmenopausal women this usually means investigation of the gastrointestinal tract if occult bleeding has been proved.

Differential diagnosis

Iron deficiency anaemia which is not responsive to treatment with iron must be distinguished from other causes of hypochromic anaemia.

The anaemia of chronic disease. This is the most important and occurs in chronic infection, chronic inflammatory disease, e.g. rheumatoid arthritis, and malignancy. The most useful parameter is the serum ferritin level which is invariably low in iron deficiency and normal or raised in chronic disease. In addition, the plasma viscosity or erythrocyte sedimentation rate (ESR) is usually raised in chronic disease.

Thalassaemia minor. See Thalassaemia, p. 334.

Sideroblastic anaemia. This may also be hypochromic. It is usually associated with dimorphic red cells. The serum ferritin level is high and the diagnosis is confirmed by the presence of ring sideroblasts in the bone marrow. It is predominantly a disease of the elderly.

Treatment

The majority of cases of iron deficiency will respond to oral iron therapy. Ferrous sulphate 200 mg 8-hourly after meals is the cheapest and most effective. Ferrous gluconate may be used as an alternative. The haemoglobin level should rise at the rate of around 1 g per week. Only where there is genuine iron intolerance or failure of compliance, should parenteral iron be used; intramuscular iron is much safer than intravenous which should rarely be used. The most common reason for failure of iron therapy is patient non-compliance.

MEGALOBLASTIC ANAEMIA

Megaloblastic anaemia is the result of defective DNA synthesis and is caused by deficiency of vitamin B_{12} or folate or both. Vitamin B_{12} is one of the cobalamins, the physiological form being hydroxy cobalomin. It is contained in most animal produce. The average daily intake is 30 μg and the average daily need is 2 μg. Body stores in the liver are around 3 mg. For absorption, vitamin B_{12} must combine with intrinsic factor secreted by the gastric parietal cells. Absorption occurs via specific receptors in the terminal ileum.

Folic acid is one of the glutamates. It is present in most green vegetables, yeast and liver, in the form of polyglutamates. These are split to monoglutamates for absorption throughout the small intestine. The average daily requirement is about 100 μg. Folate needs are increased where there is rapid cell proliferation, e.g. haemolysis, malignancy and pregnancy. The body stores, mainly in the liver, are about 10–15 mg.

The principles of vitamin B_{12} and folate metabolism are shown in Figure 11.2. The main causes of vitamin B_{12} and folate deficiency are shown in Tables 11.3 and 11.4.

Pathology

Both vitamin B_{12} and folate deficiency affect all rapidly proliferating tissue, including epithelial cells and the gonads as well as the bone marrow. The nuclei show a characteristic open chromatin pattern.

The main cause of vitamin B_{12} deficiency is pernicious anaemia which is an autoimmune disease leading to gastric atrophy.

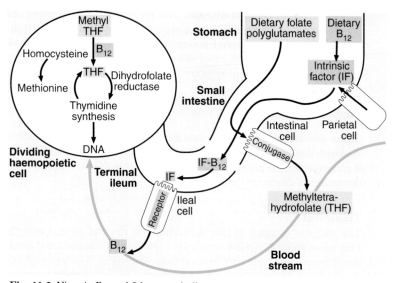

Fig. 11.2 Vitamin B$_{12}$ and folate metabolism.

Table 11.3. Causes of vitamin B$_{12}$ deficiency

Inadequate intake (Normal Schilling test)*	Strict vegetarianism—vegans, extreme malnutrition, food faddism
Gastric lesions (Abnormal part 1 Schilling test, without intrinsic factor)	Pernicious anaemia, partial or total gastrectomy, congenital intrinsic factor deficiency (very rare)
Intestinal lesions (Abnormal parts 1 and 2 Schilling test, with and without intrinsic factor)	Blind loop syndrome, tropical sprue (indicate bacterial overgrowth), Crohn's disease, coeliac disease, ileal resection (absence of specific receptors), fish tapeworm (rare except in Scandinavia), congenital B$_{12}$ malabsorption (very rare)

* Vitamin B$_{12}$ absorbtion test measures absorbtion of a small dose of radioactive B$_{12}$.

Symptoms and signs

Early megaloblastic anaemia is asymptomatic and may be discovered accidentally by finding a raised MCV.

Symptoms of more advanced disease include those of anaemia, jaundice from ineffective erythropoiesis and painful glossitis.

Vitamin B$_{12}$ deficiency can also cause neurological complications such as peripheral neuritis, spastic paraplegia, posterior column signs, confusion, dementia and optic atrophy.

In pernicious anaemia, associated autoimmune diseases are common and include hypothyroidism, vitiligo and, rarely, Addison's disease.

Table 11.4. Causes of folate deficiency

Inadequate intake	Malnutrition, old age ('tea and toast' diet), poverty, psychiatric disturbance, alcoholism (other factors, cirrhosis, haemolysis)
Malabsorption	Coeliac disease (may be only manifestation), tropical sprue, dermatitis herpetiformis enteropathy
Excess demands	Pregnancy, lactation, prematurity, chronic haemolysis, malignancy (widespread carcinoma, leukaemia and lymphoma, myeloproliferative disorders, e.g. myelofibrosis, polycythaemia), exfoliative skin disorders, inflammatory diseases, e.g. rheumatoid arthritis
Drugs	Anticonvulsants (often combined with inadequate intake), alcohol (several actions), oral contraceptives (rare, mainly high oestrogen), folate antagonists (methotrexate, pyrimethamine, cotrimoxazole)

Investigations

Megaloblastic anaemia must be distinguished from other causes of macrocytosis. Serum vitamin B_{12} and red cell folate levels must be measured prior to treatment in all cases of macrocytosis.

In severe cases, other haematological findings include oval macrocytes, hypersegmented polymorphs and reduced white cell and platelet counts. Characteristic changes are found in the bone marrow but this is rarely needed as a routine procedure.

The presence of gastric parietal cell antibodies is of little value unlike intrinsic factor antibodies which are present in about 60% of cases of pernicious anaemia.

Most cases of megaloblastic anaemia in older patients are caused by pernicious anaemia and a vitamin B_{12} absorption tests (Schilling test) is rarely required; however, it is useful in problem cases or in younger patients.

Further investigations of the GI tract are often needed in younger patients and all patients with unexplained folate deficiency should have a small intestinal biopsy to exclude coeliac disease.

Differential diagnosis

Other causes of macrocytosis (see above).

Treatment

Treatment is of the cause if possible; otherwise, replacement therapy is needed. Vitamin B_{12} deficiency is treated with hydroxycobalamin. In acute cases, particularly with neurological complications, six intramuscular injections of 1 mg are given over a 2-week period, followed by 1 mg in alternate months. Patients with pernicious anaemia should be kept under surveillance because of the risk of the development of hypothyroidism or gastric carcinoma.

Folic acid deficiency is treated by oral folic acid 5 mg daily.

If there is any doubt, treatment should not be with folic acid alone because of the risk of precipitating subacute combined degeneration (see p. 142). Vitamin B_{12} and folate should be administered together.

Table 11.5. Causes of pancytopenia

Cellular bone marrow

Normal maturation
  Excess destruction
  Hypersplenism
  Felty's syndrome (rheumatoid arthritis)
  Systemic lupus erythematosus (SLE) (antibody formation)

Abnormal maturation
  Megaloblastic anaemia
  Myelodysplasia

Infiltration
  Carcinoma (usually leukoerythroblastic picture)
  Myelofibrosis (splenomegaly tear drop poikilocytes)
  Acute leukaemia
  Myeloma

Hypocellular bone marrow

Aplastic anaemia
Paroxysmal nocturnal haemoglobinuria

Note: bone marrow examination (usually a trephine) is essential in all cases.

ANAEMIA FROM BONE MARROW FAILURE

This form of anaemia is caused by either the failure of haemopoietic stem cells or their replacement by other tissue, usually malignant. It results in a reduction of all haemopoietic cell lines, i.e. pancytopenia (Table 11.5).

Aplastic anaemia

Aplastic anaemia is caused by the reduction in the number of haemopoietic stem cells in the presence of all the essential factors required for normal haemopoiesis. Usually, all haemopoietic cell lines are involved but selective reduction may occur.

Many cases of aplastic anaemia are the result of damage to marrow from drugs, chemicals or viruses although some cases appear to be idiopathic. Individual susceptibility is very important. The known causes of aplastic anaemia can be classified as follows:

1. Marrow-suppressant drugs, e.g. cytotoxic drugs, especially alkylating agents. Their effect is dose related.

2. Other drugs, reaction to which is unpredictable. Only a small percentage of patients receiving them will react adversely. Usually several courses rather than continuous treatment are needed although the total dose received may be small. At present, there is no known way in which the susceptible subject may be identified by laboratory tests. A large number of drugs have been suspected of causing aplastic anaemia although there is difficulty in establishing a causal relationship. Known high-risk drugs include chloramphenicol, phenylbutazone and derivatives, gold, penicillamine, anticonvulsants, oral hypoglycaemic agents.

The incidence of aplastic anaemia in the UK has fallen since the withdrawal of phenylbutazone.

3. Chemicals, the high-risk ones being benzene, toluene, DDT, gammabenzene and hexochloride.

   All chemicals, particularly solvents, insecticides and weed killers, are capable of producing aplastic anaemia and should be handled with extreme caution.

4. Viruses: aplasia following viral hepatitis is well recognised. The hepatitis is often mild and aplastic anaemia develops several months after recovery. The fatality rate is high.

   Parvo virus is known to be a cause of aplasia in patients with haemolytic anaemia.

5. Excessive radiation.

6. Miscellaneous, including:
   a. *Congenital aplastic anaemia.* Several rare varieties exist, e.g. Diamond Blackfan syndrome (red cell aplasia).
   b. *Pure red cell aplasia.* Red cell series alone are affected. It may have an immunological basis as it is often associated with autoimmune disease and a thymoma.

Symptoms and signs

The symptoms and signs are those of anaemia: neutropenia, causing infection, especially of the throat and tonsils; thrombocytopenia, causing bruising and bleeding from mucous membranes.

Investigations

Anaemia is invariable and may be severe. It is usually normocytic although macrocytosis may occur. Reticulocytes are low or absent. Granulocytes and platelets are variable although usually low.

Bad prognostic features are platelets $<20 \times 10^9/l$, neutrophils $<0.5 \times 10^9/l$, reticulocytes $<0.010 \times 10^{12}/l$.

It is usually impossible to aspirate bone marrow and a *trephine is mandatory* in all cases. This shows hypoplasia with the marrow replaced by fat spaces.

A Ham's test to exclude paroxysmal nocturnal haemoglobinuria (PNH) should be done.

Treatment

1. An exhaustive search should be made for a toxic cause and any drugs suspected should be withdrawn immediately. Chelating agents are of use in gold or heavy metal poisoning.

2. The basis of treatment is supportive therapy to prevent death from anaemia, haemorrhage or infection until spontaneous recovery occurs, usually, if at all, within 6 weeks.

3. Patients in whom anaemia is a major problem may be maintained for many years by regular blood transfusions although difficulty may arise from lack of veins, antibody production and haemosiderosis.

4. Haemorrhage may be prevented by platelet transfusions but antibody formation may lead to resistance. Infections should be treated vigorously with broad-spectrum antibiotics.

5. Androgenic steroids may have a beneficial effect on anaemia. Oxymethalone is the most widely used because of its low androgenic effect. It must be used in a high dose (2–5 mg per kg per 24 hours) and treatment may be needed for several months before any effect is seen. Regular liver function tests (LFTs) are needed to detect impending liver damage.
6. Some patients, particularly where an immunological mechanism is involved, may respond to antilymphocyte globulin (expensive).
7. For those who do not respond, bone marrow transplantation offers the only hope of a permanent cure. For this reason, exposure to blood products should be limited as far as possible to avoid sensitisation.

Prognosis
Aplastic anaemia is a serious disease. For those with bad prognostic features, the mortality rate at 5 years is 90% in the absence of bone marrow transplantation.

Anaema from bone marrow infiltration

Carcinoma and other malignancies may infiltrate the bone marrow and cause anaemia. The blood picture is usually leukoerythroblastic, i.e. both immature white cells and normoblasts are seen. Although lymphomatous infiltration may respond to cytotoxic therapy, the prognosis in carcinoma is usually very poor.

ANAEMIA FROM MISCELLANEOUS CAUSES

In uraemia, bone marrow function is depressed partly because of a direct toxic effect and partly from a lack of erythropoietin.

The anaemia of liver disease is complicated and includes marrow depression as well as haemolysis, hypersplenism and iron and folate deficiency.

In hypothyroidism, a normocytic anaemia is commonly seen although it may be macrocytic. The main factor is diminished tissue needs for oxygen.

HAEMOLYTIC ANAEMIA

Haemolytic anaemia occurs when the red cell lifespan (normally 100–120 days) is shortened by premature destruction and the capacity of the bone marrow to compensate is exceeded. Premature destruction of red cells may be caused by intrinsic abnormalities of the red cells or by extracorpuscular factors, e.g. antibodies (Table 11.6).

Pathology
Increased haemolysis leads to expansion of the marrow into the shafts of the long bones. In children with severe congenital haemolytic anaemia, expansion of the marrow cavity may lead to changes in the cortical bone, producing clinical and radiological evidence of bone expansion. Hyperbilirubinaemia occurs because of increased haemoglobin breakdown. Pigment gallstones are commonly found in chronic haemolysis and splenomegaly occurs in many types of haemolytic anaemia.

Table 11.6. Causes of haemolytic anaemia

Congenital red cell defects

Membrane defects
  Hereditary spherocytosis
  Hereditary elliptocytosis (severe haemolysis rare)

Enzyme defects
  Pyruvate kinase (PK) deficiency
  Glucose-6-phosphate dehydrogenase (G6PD) deficiency

Haemoglobin defects
  Structural abnormalities: sickle cell disease
  Abnormal chain synthesis: thalassaemia

Acquired haemolytic anaemia

Immune
  Autoimmune haemolytic anaemia (AIHA)
  Isoimmune—incompatible blood transfusions
  Haemolytic disease of the newborn

Infections
  Malaria
  Septicaemia (especially *Staphylococcus, Clostridum welchii*)

Drugs and chemicals
  (Usually overdose or industrial exposure)

Membrane disorders
  Paroxysmal nocturnal haemoglobinuria (PNH)

Mechanical
  Microangiopathic haemolytic anaemia
  Cardiac valve prosthesis (majority aortic)
  March haemoglobinuria

Hypersplenism

Miscellaneous (usually several causes for anaemia)
  Liver disease
  Malignancy
  Uraemia

Symptoms and signs

Usually the only symptoms are those of anaemia. Upper abdominal pain may be caused by gallstones.

The principal signs are of anaemia and jaundice. Splenomegaly is common and, rarely, leg ulcers may be present. Anaemia may result in bony abnormalities and infantilism.

Investigations

See Table 11.7.

Treatment

Treatment should be directed at the elimination of the cause, if possible. Folic acid should be given to all patients with chronic haemolysis. Splenectomy may be indicated in some cases.

Table 11.7. Investigation of haemolytic anaemia

Peripheral blood (increased red cell production)

Anaemia	Depends on the degree of compensation
Reticulocytosis	Raised—absolute number best. Normal 0.02–0.085 x 10^{12}
Red cells	Polychromasia (reticulocytosis) Macrocytosis (reticulocytosis) Nucleated red cells Spherocytosis, fragmented cells (non-specific but always indicative of haemolysis)

Bile pigments (increased haemoglobin breakdown)

	Serum bilirubin increased (unconjugated) Urine and faecal uro- and stercobilinogen increased (Note: bilirubin not normally found in urine)
Haemoglobin pigments (intravascular haemolysis)	Haemoglobinaemia (plasma pink) Haemoglobinuria (urine pink) Methaemalbuminaemia Haemosiderinuria Reduced haptoglobins (Hb transport protein)

Red cell survival (^{51}Cr labelled red cells)

	Decreased Surface scanning may show selective splenic sequestration

---

Specific causes of haemolysis

Hereditary spherocytosis

This disorder, inherited as an autosomal dominant of incomplete penetrance, is a membrane defect causing the formation of spherocytic red cells which are abnormally sequestered in the spleen.

Many patients are asymptomatic and only detected by chance. The commonest clinical picture is of recurrent episodes of anaemia and jaundice in childhood caused by a temporarily increased rate of haemolysis and/or bone marrow suppression, usually caused by infection.

Severe cases may present at birth as haemolytic disease of the newborn. Other modes of presentation include gallstones and intractable leg ulcers.

The diagnosis is readily made clinically and from family and blood studies.

The important differential diagnosis is autoimmune haemolytic anaemia where the direct Coomb's test (DCT) is positive.

The only treatment is splenectomy if there are recurrent crises or gallstones.

Glucose-6-phosphate dehydrogenase (G6PD) deficiency

This is a widespread sex-linked abnormality occurring in Blacks and certain Mediterranean and Oriental groups. The red cells are unusually susceptible to oxidative stress, usually caused by drugs, particularly antimalarials (primaquine), phenacitin, sulphonamides, dapsone, nitrofurantoin and vitamin K in the new-born. Severe self-limiting haemolysis may occur following exposure to these drugs.

Patients with the Mediterranean variety of G6PD deficiency may also be susceptible to the broad bean (*Vicia faba*), the condition known as Favism, usually seen in childhood and adolescence.

Diagnosis is made by G6PD assay.

Autoimmune haemolytic anaemia (AIHA)

AIHA results from the destruction of red cells by autoantibodies. The two main types depend on the nature of the antibody, i.e. IgG (warm) and IgM (cold) antibodies.

The causes of AIHA are shown in Table 11.8.

Warm-antibody AIHA causes extravascular haemolysis and the symptoms are principally those of anaemia. The blood film shows spherocytosis and the diagnosis is confirmed by a positive DCT. A search for a primary cause, particularly systemic lupus erythematosus (SLE) or lymphoma, should be made.

Treatment is with steroids starting at a high dose, e.g. prednisolone 60 mg per 24 hours, reduced as the haemolysis comes under control. Most cases of idiopathic AIHA become chronic. If the disease cannot be controlled by a minimal dose of steroids, then splenectomy is the next choice.

Cold-antibody AIHA causes intravascular haemolysis. The symptoms are due to cold-induced red cell agglutination causing Raynaud's phenomena and to intravascular haemolysis causing haemoglobinuria. Most cases respond to avoidance of cold but if this is ineffective, chlorambucil should be used. Steroids have no place in the treatment of cold-antibody AIHA.

Microangiopathic haemolytic anaemia

Microangiopathic haemolytic anaemia is caused by the destruction of red cells by a fibrin meshwork laid down within small blood vessels. It is characterised by the presence of fragmented red cells of bizarre shapes in the blood film.

Table 11.8. Causes of autoimmune haemolytic anaemia

'Warm' antibody	IgG, occasionally with complement, DCT positive
Primary	Idiopathic
Secondary	Lymphoma, e.g. chronic lymphatic leukaemia (CLL)
	Autoimmune disease, e.g. systemic lupus erythematosus (SLE)
	Viral infections, e.g. infectious mononucleosis
	Drugs, e.g. methyldopa
'Cold' antibody	IgM, usually with complement, DCT weak positive or negative
Primary	The cold haemagglutination syndrome (CHAD)
Secondary	Lymphoma
	Infections—mycoplasma, infectious mononucleosis
	Paroxysmal cold haemoglobinuria (PCH)

It may occur in a wide variety of conditions as a result of either disease of the vessels themselves or as a part of the disseminated intravascular coagulation (DIC) syndrome, e.g. malignant hypertension, glomerulonephritis and malignant invasion of small vessels, especially by mucin-secreting carcinomas. It is usually associated with thrombocytopenia.

Haemolytic–uraemic syndrome (HUS). This occurs in children, usually after infection.

Thrombotic thrombocytopenic purpura (TTP). This is a rare disease in adults and the features are anaemia, thrombocytopenic purpura and bizarre disseminated neurological signs caused by multiple small thrombotic lesions.

Miscellaneous causes of haemolysis
See Table 11.9.

Disorders of haemoglobin

Haemoglobin is a tetramer of four chains. In the normal adult, most of the haemoglobin is haemoglobin A (alpha 2, beta 2) and the remainder haemoglobin A2 (alpha 2, delta 2). In the fetus, most of the haemoglobin is haemoglobin F (alpha 2, gamma 2). Disorders of haemoglobin are of two types. The structural variants in which an abnormal form of haemoglobin is produced and the thalassaemias, in which there is failure to produce haemoglobin chains at the required rate. (Table 11.10).

Table 11.9. Miscellaneous causes of haemolysis

Type	Cause	Effects/diagnosis	Therapy
Hereditary elliptocytosis	Membrane defect	Elliptocytes Variable haemolytic anaemia	Usually none
Pyruvate kinase deficiency	Enzyme defect	'Prickle cells' Haemolytic anaemia, may be severe	Splenectomy
Paroxysmal nocturnal haemoglobinuria	Acquired membrane defect Sensitivity to complement	Haemolytic episodes Haemoglobinuria Thrombotic episodes Positive Ham's test	Blood transfusion (washed red cells) Anticoagulants if thromboses
March haemoglobinuria	Mechanical damage to red cells caused by running	Haemoglobinuria following exercise	Run in trainers with spongy soles
Paroxysmal cold haemoglobinuria	Cold antibody usually related to viral infection, especially in children	Acute intravascular haemolysis with haemoglobinuria	Usually self limiting. Keep patient warm

Table 11.10. Disorders of haemoglobin

	Haemoglobin	Haematology	Clinical effects
Normal adult	A 97%, A_2 3%		
Fetus	F 85%		
Sickle cell disease	S 80–100%	Sickle cells Target cells	Sickle crises, anaemia
Sickle cell trait	S 40%, A 60%	Target cells	Usually none
Hb SC disease	S C	Target cells	Mild anaemia, sickle crises
Hb C disease	C 90%	Target cells +	Mild anaemia, Splenomegaly
Sickle thalassaemia	$ß^0$ S 85–90% ß+ 55–75%	Hypochromic Microcytic Target cells	Sickle crises, anaemia Usually asymptomatic
ß Thalassaemia major	F 70–100% A_2	Hypochromic Microcytic + Target cells	Severe anaemia
ß Thalassaemia minor	A_2 3.5–7%	Hypochromic Microcytic Target cells	Normal or mild anaemia, asymptomatic
∝ Thalassaemia	Barts (Fetus)	Hypochromic	
Hb H disease	H 5–40%	Microcytic 'H' bodies Target cells	Moderate anaemia, splenomegaly
Trait	H trace	Mild hypochromia 'H' bodies	None
Unstable haemoglobins	e.g. Hb Köln	Heinz bodies Heat-unstable haemoglobin	Mild haemolytic anaemia, often precipitated by oxidant drugs

Sickle cell disease

Sickle cell disease is the presence of an abnormal beta haemoglobin chain, haemoglobin S. In the homozygous state (SS), virtually all the haemoglobin is in the form of haemoglobin S. In the heterozygous state, sickle cell trait (SA), only about 40% is haemoglobin S, the remainder being haemoglobin A.

In the deoxygenated state, haemoglobin S molecules can link to form chains which distort the red cell, making it inflexible, leading to entrapment of the red cells in small vessels causing infarction and haemolysis. Infarction occurs in many tissues including bones, muscles, the gut, the spleen, the kidney and the retina. Precipitating factors are *hypoxia, infection, dehydration and cold*.

Sickle cell disease occurs principally in Blacks of African origin and is therefore common in Afro-Caribbeans. Amongst this population, 10% carry the haemoglibin S gene and 0.25% have sickle cell disease. There are smaller pockets in Greece, the Middle East and India.

Symptoms and signs. The symptoms are mainly due to infarction which causes acute pain—sickle cell 'crisis.' Gut infarcts may mimic an acute abdomen and bone infarcts may be confused with acute arthritis or osteomyelitis.

Two particularly dangerous complications are the acute chest syndrome, which presents with dyspnoea and severe chest pain, and acute splenic sequestration, which occurs in children causing rapid splenic enlargement and severe anaemia.

Patients with sickle cell trait are usually asymptomatic.

Investigations. Patients with sickle cell disease are invariably anaemic (haemoglobin 8–9 g/dl). Sickle cells are usually present in the blood film, especially in crises.

Simple screening tests are available to detect the presence of haemoglobin S but the definitive diagnosis is made by haemoglobin electrophoresis.

Patients with sickle cell trait are usually not anaemic.

Treatment. Prevention of sickle crises is important. The management of a crisis depends on ensuring adequate oxygenation, rehydration and treatment of infection. *Sickle crises are extremely painful and adequate analgesia is essential.* Severe crises, particularly the acute chest syndrome, may require exchange transfusion.

Other Sickling Syndromes

Another form of abnormal haemoglobin also found in Africa is haemoglobin C. Homozygous C disease (CC) gives rise to mild anaemia and splenomegaly but without crises. The combination of haemoglobin S and C disease causes mild anaemia and also sickle crises, particularly affecting the retina and kidney. In some populations where the genes for sickle cell disease and thalassaemia co-exist, sickle thalassaemia may occur. In most cases, this is asymptomatic, although in some, where the level of haemoglobin S is high, sickle crises may occur.

Thalassaemia

Background. In the thalassaemias, there is defective synthesis of one of the chains needed to form adult haemoglobin. The commonest variety is *beta thalassaemia* in which there is restriction of beta chain synthesis resulting in defective formation of haemoglobin A. In the homozygous condition, *thalassaemia major*, there is little or no haemoglobin A synthesis resulting in severe anaemia. In the heterozygous condition, *thalassaemia trait*, although there is restriction of haemoglobin A synthesis, the degree of anaemia is not severe.

In *alpha thalassaemia*, there is a restriction of alpha chain synthesis. As a compensation, tetramers are formed of gamma chains (haemoglobin Barts) in the fetus, and beta chains (haemoglobin H) in the adult.

Thalassaemia is widespread, occurring around the Mediterranean and into the Middle East, India and the Far East, where alpha thalassaemia predominates.

Symptoms and signs. Beta thalassaemia major causes severe anaemia a few months after birth. It is associated with skeletal abnormalities and gross hepatosplenomegaly due to ineffective erythropoiesis.

The severest form of alpha thalassaemia is not compatible with life, and death occurs in utero. An intermediate form, known as haemoglobin H disease causes moderate anaemia and splenomegaly. Less severe forms resemble thalassaemia minor and are symptomless.

Investigations. Beta thalassaemia major causes gross anaemia with microcytosis and hypochromia. Electrophoresis shows the almost complete absence of haemoglobin A.

In beta thalassaemia minor, there is a microcytic, hypochromic blood picture with a normal or slightly reduced haemoglobin which has to be distinguished from iron deficiency. This is achieved by demonstrating a normal ferritin level and an increased level of haemoglobin A_2.

Alpha thalassaemia is diagnosed by finding the presence of haemoglobin Barts in the fetus and haemoglobin H in the adult. Haemoglobin H can be detected by a special stain which shows inclusions in the red cells (H bodies).

Treatment. Children with thalassaemia major will die unless regularly transfused. Hypertransfusion prevents the development of skeletal abnormalities and hepatosplenomegaly. Nevertheless, death will occur in adolescence unless chelation therapy with desferrioxamine is started early to prevent iron overload. This must be given by slow subcutaneous infusion on at least 5 days per week. Oral iron chelators may be available shortly. Bone marrow transplantation offers the chance of permanent cure for a small number of patients.

Patients with thalassaemia minor require no treatment. It is important that the condition is diagnosed so that repeated investigation and treatment of nonexistent iron deficiency is avoided.

Other abnormal haemoglobins

Many of these are known but most produce no clinical effects. One important group are the unstable haemoglobins, e.g., haemoglobin Koln in which haemolytic anaemia can be precipitated by oxidant drugs as in G6PD deficiency.

DISORDERS OF WHITE CELLS

The normal distribution of white blood cells is shown in Table 11.11. Variations in the number and distribution of white cells occurs in many diseases and is a useful aid to diagnosis.

MAJOR VARIATIONS IN WHITE CELLS

Neutrophil leukocytosis ($>7.5 \times 10^9/l$)

An increased neutrophil count may be seen in
1. physiological states. Considerable variation in neutrophil count occurs in an individual during the day, the influencing factors being exercise, food and stress

Table 11.11. Normal white cell values (x 10⁹/1)

	Adults (Whites)	Adults (Blacks)	Children (8–12 years)
Total WBC	4.0–11.0	2.6–9.0	4.5–13.0
Neutrophils	2.5–7.5	1.0–4.0	2.5–8.0
Lymphocytes	1.5–4.0	1.0–4.0	2.0–4.5
Monocytes	0.2–0.8	0.2–0.8	0.5–1.0
Eosinophils	0.04–0.4		0.1–0.6
Basophils	<0.01–0.1		

2. late pregnancy
3. infections (especially pyogenic infections)
4. tissue necrosis
5. haemorrhage
6. malignant neoplasms
7. metabolic disorders (e.g. diabetic ketosis)
8. myeloproliferative disorders (e.g., primary polycythaemia, chronic granulocytic leukaemia).

Eosinophilia (>0.4 × 10⁹/l)

An increased eosinophil count occurs with:
1. allergy, asthma, drug sensitivity
2. parasitic infestation (usually tissue invasion is required), e.g. filaria, toxocara
3. pulmonary eosinophilia (Löffler's syndrome), probably parasitic in origin
4. skin diseases, e.g. pemphigus, exfoliative dermatitis
5. infections—usually in the convalescent period
6. polyarteritis nodosa
7. malignant disease (particularly Hodgkin's disease)
8. other rare conditions, e.g. eosinophilic granuloma, eosinophilic leukaemia (a doubtful syndrome).

Lymphocytosis (>3.5 × 10⁹/l)

An increased lymphocyte count is seen in:
1. viral infections, especially in children—infectious hepatitis and infectious mononucleosis
2. leukaemia—acute and especially chronic lymphatic leukaemia
3. 'atypical lymphocytosis' in many viral diseases, especially infectious mononucleosis.

Monocytosis (>0.8 × 10⁹/l)

An increased monocyte count occurs with:

1. infections, especially chronic (e.g. tuberculosis, subacute bacterial endo-carditis), protozoal infections, and infectious mononucleosis
2. malignant disease—monocytic leukaemia, carcinoma
3. chronic inflammatory intestinal disease, e.g. Crohn's disease.

Neutropenia (<2.5×10^9/l)

A decreased neutrophil count occurs with:
1. aplastic anaemia
2. bone marrow infiltration, e.g. leukaemia, carcinoma etc.
3. viral or overwhelming bacterial infections
4. hypersplenism, particularly Felty's syndrome (depression of neutrophil production may be a factor in this condition)
5. immune disorders, e.g. SLE
7. chronic idiopathic neutropenia and 'cyclic neutropenia', a rare condition with a cyclic change in the neutrophil count.

Drug-induced agranulocytosis

A number of drugs are known to cause agranulocytosis either as part of the aplastic anaemia syndrome or else selectively, e.g. gold and the antithyroid drugs.

Great care should be taken over the prescription of all drugs known to cause agranulocytosis and regular blood counts should be performed.

MALIGNANT AND PROLIFERATIVE DISEASES OF HAEMOPOIETIC TISSUE

These diseases are confusing because they are difficult to classify and overlap occurs between them. A number of basic concepts need to be borne in mind.
1. Most of these diseases are clonal, i.e. they arise from an abnormality affecting one cell line which has the biological advantage to outgrow normal marrow cells.
2. Most affect stem cells and the transformation may cause either uncontrolled but orderly proliferation of end cells, as in polycythaemia, or uncontrolled proliferation of stem cells without differentiation, as in acute leukaemia.
3. It is likely that a series of events occurs which transforms a normal cell into a malignant one. Consequently, the disease may show evolution from a benign proliferative process to an aggressive malignant one.
4. The nature of the events which cause transformation is unknown but postulated factors include viruses, drugs and radiation.
5. Improved technology has helped to recognise the cell or origin by analysis of surface markers. This has led to a greater understanding of these diseases.

A simple division may be made between diseases of the *myeloid cells*, i.e. those giving rise to red cells, granulocytes and platelets, and diseases of the *lymphoid system*.

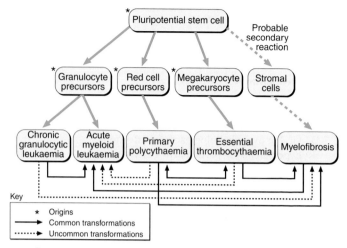

Fig. 11.3 The myeloproliferative disorders showing origins and inter-relationship between diseases.

Clinically, it is convenient to consider these diseases under the following headings:

1. myeloproliferative disease
2. acute leukaemia and myelodysplasia
3. lymphoproliferative disease.

THE MYELOPROLIFERATIVE DISORDERS (Fig. 11.3)

This group of disorders is thought to arise from an aberration of myeloid stem cells, characterised by an initial benign phase, sometimes followed by transformation to a more aggressive malignant phase. There are common features and transition from one form to another may occur. All may terminate as acute myeloid leukaemia. The diseases involved are primary polycythaemia (polycythaemia rubra vera), essential thrombocythaemia, myelofibrosis and chronic granulocytic leukaemia.

Primary polycythaemia

Polycythaemia, i.e. an increase in haemoglobin and haematocrit, may be either true or relative (Fig. 11.4) and true polycythaemia may be either primary or secondary.

Secondary polycythaemia is caused by increased erythropoietin which may be either appropriate, e.g. as in hypoxia, or inappropriate, as in erythropoietin-secreting tumours.

Symptoms and signs

These may be due to:

1. raised blood viscosity—headache, confusion, arterial and venous thromboses, congestive cardiac failure, stroke

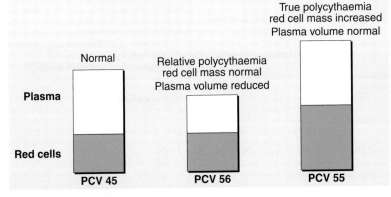

Fig. 11.4 True and relative polycythaemia.

2. abnormal bleeding, particularly gastrointestinal, often leading to iron deficiency because of abnormal platelet function
3. pruritus (especially after hot baths), possibly caused by histamine overproduction
4. gout because of hyperuricaemia from increased cell turnover.

These patients often show a ruddy cyanosis and 70% of cases have splenomegaly.

Investigations
The haemoglobin level and haematocrit are above the upper limit of normal. In 70% of cases, the white cell count and platelet count are elevated. The absolute red cell mass is increased.

Differential diagnosis
Secondary and relative polycythaemia (Table 11.12).

Treatment
The cardinal rule of treatment is to keep the haematocrit within the normal range. The simplest method is venesection. If this is unacceptable or if there is thrombocytosis, a myelosuppressive agent must be used. ^{32}P is simple but leukaemogenic and should be reserved for older patients. In younger patients, hydroxyurea is the treatment of choice.

Provided that thrombosis is avoided, the prognosis is very good. Transition to myelofibrosis or acute leukaemia may occur but usually only after several decades.

Essential thrombocythaemia

This is a myelproliferative disorder principally affecting the committed platelet stem cell causing a high platelet count. Overlap with polycythaemia occurs. It is principally seen in middle aged or elderly patients but may occur in younger ones.

Symptoms and signs
Essential thrombocythaemia may be asymptomatic, especially in younger patients.

Table 11.12. Differential diagnosis

Type	Primary	Anoxic	Renal	Other secondary causes	'Pseudopolycythaemia' (relative polycythaemies)
PCV	↑	↑	↑	↑	↑
WBC	N or ↑	N	N	N	N
Platelets	N or ↑	N	N	N	N
Red cell mass	↑	↑	↑	↑	N
Plasma volume	N or ↑	N	N	N	↓
PO$_2$	N	↓	N	N	N
IVP	N	N	abnormal	N	N
Erythropoietin	N or ↑	↑	↑	↑	N

PCV = packed cell volume; WBC = white blood cells; IVP = intravenous pyelogram.

Micro-thrombotic lesions, particularly in digital vessels in the feet, are caused by abnormal platelet aggregation. There may be digital ischaemia. Defective platelet function leads to abnormal bruising and bleeding.

Splenomegaly may become marked as the disease progresses to myelofibrosis.

Investigations
The platelet count is usually markedly raised, often in excess of $1000 \times 10^9/l$. Abnormal platelet morphology and function may be present.

Differential diagnosis
Other causes of reactive thrombocytosis are haemorrhage, infection, malignant disease, chronic inflammatory disease. (Platelet function and morphology may help to discriminate.)

Treatment
The aim is to reduce the platelet count to normal using hydroxyurea, busulphan or ^{32}P. Younger patients may require no treatment.

Prognosis is usually excellent. Long remissions may occur following treatment although eventual transition to myelofibrosis or acute leukaemia may be seen.

Myelofibrosis

Replacement of bone marrow by fibrous tissue and new bone formation is often the terminal stage of polycythaemia or thrombocythaemia but may be seen de novo. Extramedullary haemopoiesis with massive splenomegaly occurs.

Symptoms and signs

These are caused by anaemia. Splenomegaly (often massive) leads to abdominal discomfort and splenic infarction to acute pain (see Table 11.13). Sweating and weightloss result from a raised metabolic rate.

Investigations

The blood film usually shows a leukoerythroblastic anaemia with immature red and white cells. Tear drop poikilocytes are characteristic.

White cell and platelet counts are variable, usually normal or low but they may be high.

Bone marrow aspiration yields a dry tap. Trephine biopsy shows increased fibrosis and new bone formation.

Differential diagnosis

From other causes of leukoerythroblastic anaemia, principally infiltration by carcinoma.

Treatment

There is no effective treatment other than blood transfusion if indicated symptomatically. Splenectomy may be helpful in reducing transfusion requirements, and should preferably be performed before the spleen becomes massive. Patients usually survive several years from diagnosis although termination as acute leukaemia is common.

Chronic granulocytic leukaemia (CGL)

CGL is a malignant disease of either a totipotential or a committed myeloid stem cell. Peak incidence is in middle age and a juvenile form exists. It characteristically progresses through three stages:
1. a benign phase which is responsive to treatment
2. an accelerated phase unresponsive to treatment
3. a terminal phase resembling acute leukaemia.

Exposure to irradiation is a known aetiological factor. A unique feature is the presence of a specific chromosomal abnormality, the Philadelphia chromosome, in the majority of cases. This is a reciprocal translocation between chromosomes 9 and 22, resulting in the activation of the oncogene, c-abl.

Symptoms and signs

CGL is usually of insidious onset with weakness and weightloss or symptoms of anaemia. Splenomegaly may be massive. Gout is caused by hyperuricaemia.

Investigations

The white cell count is invariably raised and is usually over 100×10^9/l. Some asymptomatic cases may be picked up before this on routine blood count. The

Table 11.13. Causes of splenomegaly

Haematological malignancy

Myeloproliferative disease	Primary polycythaemia Myelofibrosis* Chronic myeloid leukaemia*
Acute leukaemia—mainly ALL in children	
Lymphoproliferative disease	Hodgkin's disease Non-Hodgkin's lymphoma* Chronic lymphatic leukaemia Hairy cell leukaemia*
Anaemia (usually only minor enlargement)	Iron deficiency Megaloblastic anaemia
Idiopathic	Primary hypersplenism (? lymphoma)
Congestive	Portal hypertension Cirrhosis Splenic or portal vein thrombosis
Connective tissue disease	Systemic lupus erythematosus (SLE) Rheumatoid arthritis (Felty's syndrome)
Storage Disease	Gaucher's* Niemann-Pick disease Histiocytosis X (children usually)
Miscellaneous	Amyloid (often associated with hyposplenic blood picture) Sarcoid Cysts Tumours (rare)

Infections

Bacterial	Septicaemia Subacute bacterial endocarditis (SBE) Typhoid Tuberculosis (TB) Brucellosis
Viral	Acute viral illness, especially in children Infectious mononucleosis HIV
Parasitic	Acute malaria Chronic malaria (tropical splenomegaly)* Leishmaniasis (kala-azar)* Schistosomiasis (portal hypertension)

Haemolytic anaemia

	Hereditary spherocytosis Autoimmune haemolytic anaemia Sickle cell disease (children; in adults, often splenic atrophy) Other haemoglobinopathies Thalassaemia*

* Enlargement may be massive

differential white cell count shows a neutrophilia with immature form, i.e. bands, metamyelocytes, myelocytes (left shift). There may be a basophilia.

Anaemia is usual. The platelet count is usually normal or raised with abnormal forms. It often falls as the disease progresses.

The neutrophil alkaline phosphatase (NAP), is low or absent. Cytogenetic studies usually show the Philadelphia chromosome.

Differential diagnosis

Advanced cases present little difficulty but cases detected by chance with a white cell count of around $50 \times 10^9/l$ need to be distinguished from a myeloid leukaemoid reaction, e.g. severe infection, malignancy. The NAP and cytogenetic studies are useful in these cases.

Treatment

This remains disappointing. In the benign phase, the disease is readily controllable with hydroxyurea or busulphan. More complicated regimens have little to offer.

No form of chemotherapy succeeds in eliminating the Philadelphia clone. Recent work suggests that alpha-interferon may eliminate the clone in some cases and prolong the duration of the benign phase.

Once transformation to the accelerated phase or acute leukaemia has occurred, treatment is usually very unsuccessful.

For younger patients with an HLA-compatible sibling, bone marrow transplantation may offer the hope of a permanent cure.

ACUTE LEUKAEMIA

The acute leukaemias are disorders of primitive stem cells which proliferate showing little or no differentiation. Two main varieties are recognised, *myeloid* and *lymphoid*, each being further subdivided into a number of types (Table 11.14). Correct diagnosis depends on analysis of surface markers and, increasingly, on DNA studies. Chromosome abnormalities are common and some have predictive value. Correct diagnosis is important because treatment and prognosis may depend on it. Acute lymphoblastic leukaemia (ALL) has its peak incidence in early childhood. Acute myeloid leukaemia (AML) is predominantly a disease of the elderly.

The aetiology is unknown but a number of factors have been postulated. These include viruses, genetic abnormalities, e.g. Down's syndrome, drugs and ionising irradiation. The importance of exposure to naturally occurring radiation, particularly radon, is becoming increasingly recognised.

Symptoms and signs

Acute leukaemia usually has a short history although some cases, particularly in the elderly, may have a more gradual onset.

The symptoms and signs are principally due to bone marrow failure from replacement of normal haemopoietic tissue by leukaemic blast cells. They include anaemia, infection (due to neutropenia), shock (due to septicaemia), mouth ulceration (neutropenia) and gingival overgrowth (especially in monocytic leukaemia). Skin lesions (infection, infiltration or miscellaneous, e.g. pyoderma gangrenosum) are seen. Bleeding into skin and mucous membranes is caused by thrombocytopenia.

Table 11.14. Classification of acute leukaemia and myelodysplasia

Acute leukaemia

Lymphoblastic (ALL)
    Common ALL (Calla pos), mainly children
    T cell ALL (poor prognosis)
    B cell ALL (resembles Burkitt's lymphoma)
    'Lymphosarcoma' leukaemia (elderly)
Myeloblastic (AML)
    Myeloid (with or without differentiation)
    Promyelocytic (often associated with DIC)
    Myelomonocytic
    Monocytic
    Erythroleukaemia
    Megakaryocytic

Myelodysplasia

    Refractory anaemia (RA)
    Refractory anaemia with ring sideroblasts (RAS)
    Refractory anaemia with excess blasts (RAEB)
    RAEB in transformation (RAEB-t)
    Chronic myelomonocytic leukaemia (CMMoL)

Other symptoms include bone pain, particularly in children, and joint pain due to hyperuricaemia.

Signs include tonsillar enlargement or splenomegaly (usually ALL).

Investigations

Most patients are anaemic, neutropenic and thrombocytopenic, often severely so. The white cell count is variable but is usually raised with a predominance of blast cells. Some cases have a low white cell count with no blast cells (aleukaemic leukaemia). In these cases, diagnosis depends on bone marrow examination.

Accurate typing of the blast cells and cytogenetic studies, should be carried out in all younger patients.

Treatment

The treatment of acute leukaemia is complicated, usually unpleasant for the patient and expensive. It should only be practised in specialist centres. The mainstay of treatment is chemotherapy but equally important is supportive therapy with platelet transfusions and antibiotics.

The principal of therapy is to induce remission with cytotoxic drugs, that is, elimination of all visible leukaemic cells and restoration of normal marrow function. This is followed by more intensive chemotherapy aimed at eliminating any residual leukaemic cells.

In ALL, maintenance therapy is usually given for several years. There is no evidence that maintenance therapy is beneficial in AML. Also, in ALL, CNS prophylaxis is essential to prevent meningeal relapse.

Bone marrow transplantation, particularly if there is an HLA-compatible sibling, should be considered in all younger patients with AML in first remission and in patients with ALL with poor prognostic features.

The role of autotransplantation is still to be established.

Treatment of AML in the over 60 age group is very unrewarding. Even though remissions may be obtained, they are usually short lived. It is doubtful whether most of these patients should be subjected to intensive chemotherapy.

Prognosis

The prognosis in common ALL in childhood has improved dramatically with over 90% achieving remission and over 50% having long-term survival and probable cure.

The prognosis of AML and ALL in adults remains poor. Although remission rates of over 80% can be expected, the problem of relapse remains and 5-year survival is around 30% with conventional chemotherapy. The results are particularly poor in the elderly with the majority relapsing within 2 years. In some elderly patients, the disease runs a chronic course and reasonable quality survival for several years may be achieved with supportive therapy only.

At the moment, allogeneic bone marrow transplantation seems to offer the best hope for younger patients.

Myelodysplastic syndromes (MDS) (See Table 11.14)

This term is applied to a miscellaneous group of disorders characterised by progressive cytopenias with a cellular marrow and characteristic morphological changes affecting all cell lines. At the most benign end of the spectrum is refractory anaemia which affects red cells only. In many cases, all three cells lines are affected, giving rise to pancytopenia. Other cases show a progressive increase in the number of blast cells and eventually terminate as acute leukaemia. The interest in MDS is that it provides a model for the development of acute leukaemia. Many cases are associated with chromosomal abnormalities and most are thought to be clonal in origin.

There is no effective treatment other than blood transfusion and the prognosis is variable. Patients with refractory anaemia may survive for 5 years or more with regular transfusions. Those who have an excess of blasts rarely survive longer than 1 year.

LYMPHOPROLIFERATIVE DISEASE

These diseases arise from malignant transformation of lymphoid cells at some stage of their development (Fig. 11.5). Clinically, they may be divided into the following groups:
1. chronic lymphatic leukaemia
2. lymphoma
   a. Hodgkin's disease
   b. non-Hodgkin's lymphoma
   c. T cell lymphoma
3. immunoproliferative disease
   a. myeloma
   b. macroglobulinaemia.

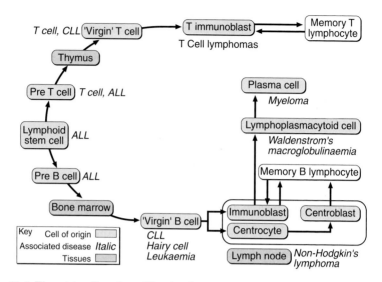

Fig. 11.5 The origin of lymphoproliferative disorders. ALL = acute lymphoblastic leukaemia; CLL = chronic lymphatic leukaemia.

Chronic lymphatic leukaemia (CLL)

CLL is a common form of leukaemia occurring principally in elderly patients. There is progressive proliferation of lymphocytes (usually B cell) with infiltration of the bone marrow causing a peripheral blood lymphocytosis. It may be accompanied by enlargement of the lymph nodes and/or splenomegaly.

Normal lymphocyte function is impaired and immune paresis develops. Autoimmune phenomena, i.e. anaemia and thrombocytopenia, may occur.

Symptoms and signs

Often there are no symptoms and the disease is discovered by chance. Anaemia and thrombocytopenia may be due to marrow infiltration or auto-immunity. There is lymph node enlargement and splenomegaly. Occasionally, there is skin infiltration or salivary gland enlargement. Recurrent infection, particularly chest infection due to hypogammaglobulinaemia, occurs.

Investigations

Lymphocytosis ($>5 \times 10^9/l$), is invariable. The lymphocyte count may exceed $500 \times 10^9/l$. 'Smear cells' (disintegrated lymphocytes) are seen in the blood film.

The bone marrow is infiltrated by lymphocytes with variable reduction in normal haemopoietic tissue.

Lymph node biopsy is rarely needed but shows replacement of normal structure by small lymphocytes. Reduction of serum immunoglobulin is common. The Coombs' test may be positive.

Differential diagnosis

CLL has to be distinguished from hairy cell leukaemia, prolymphocytic leukaemia and exfoliative lymphoma.

Treatment

Patients with lymphocytosis only require no treatment.

Indications for treatment are marrow failure, progressive lymph node enlargement or autoimmune phenomena. Intermittent chlorambucil and prednisolone are the mainstays of treatment. Localised lymph node masses may be treated with deep X-ray therapy (DXR). Vigorous treatment of infection is needed and patients with recurrent infection may benefit from immunoglobulin replacement.

Many patients with CLL survive for many years without treatment but marrow failure is a bad sign and the survival is usually under 5 years.

Lymphoma

Hodgkin's disease

This form of lymphoma is separated from the others because of its histology and natural history. In the Western World, it has a peak incidence in early adulthood and another peak in the elderly. Epidemiological evidence suggests that it has an infective origin and there is increasing evidence to link it with Epstein–Barr virus (EBV) infection.

Pathology. The hallmark of the disease is the Reed-Sternberg cell which is a large cell with two or more nuclei with prominent nucleoli. It is accompanied by reactive cells, lymphocytes, histiocytes and eosinophils. It is unusual amongst tumours in that the malignant cell is in the minority. The origin of the Reed-Sternberg cell is uncertain but it is now thought that it can be of either B or T cell origin. Various histological grades are recognised. The greater the lymphocyte proliferation, the better the prognosis.

The disease spreads in an orderly fashion from one group of lymph nodes to another. Extranodal involvement is rare. Characteristically there is early loss of cellular immunity, leading to infections with opportunistic organisms.

Symptoms and signs. The commonest presentation is painless enlargement of cervical nodes. In more advanced disease, other lymph node areas may be involved.

Systemic symptoms (B symptoms) include undulating fever (Pel Ebstein), night sweats and weightloss. Pruritus and alcohol-induced pain are uncommon symptoms of uncertain aetiology. Splenomegaly may occur.

Investigations. Lymph node biopsy is essential for histological diagnosis.

The blood count is usually normal although anaemia, eosinophilia and raised plasma viscosity or ESR may occur. Bone marrow involvement is uncommon.

It is important to delineate the extent of the disease. This is most easily done by CT scanning.

Table 11.15. Causes of lymphadenopathy

Generalised	Localised
Infectious mononucleosis	Local infection (pyogenic, tuberculosis, pediculosis)
HIV infection, AIDS	
Chronic lymphatic leukaemia	Cat scratch fever
Acute lymphoblastic leukaemia	Rubella (occipital)
Lymphoma	Lymphoma—non-Hodgkin's lymphoma or Hodgkin's disease
Rheumatoid arthritis (and Still's disease)	
	Secondary carcinoma
Sarcoidosis	
Tuberculosis	
Toxoplasmosis—cytomegalovirus	
Toxoplasmosis	
Drug therapy, e.g. Epanutin, PAS	
Secondary syphilis	

PAS = para-aminosalicylic acid.

Differential diagnosis. Other causes of lymphadenopathy (Table 11.15) should be excluded.

Treatment. Stage 1 disease, i.e. that limited to one group of lymph glands, is treatable by radiotherapy. All other stages, particularly if B symptoms are present, should be treated with combination chemotherapy. With modern treatment, the prognosis is excellent. With localised disease, the cure rate is in the order of 80%. Even advanced disease with extranodal spread has the possibility of long remission and even cure.

Non-Hodgkin's lymphoma (NHL)

This is a heterogeneous group of disorders which may affect any age group although the commonest incidence is in the elderly. The aetiology is unknown but a viral cause is suspected in some cases, notably Burkitt's lymphoma (EBV) and T cell leukaemia lymphoma syndrome (HTLV1).

Pathology. The majority of NHLS are of B cell origin, particularly the follicular centre cells. Some are of T cell origin. True histiocytic lymphomas are exceedingly rare.

Modern classifications try to identify the cell of origin but clinically, they can be divided into three groups:
1. low grade—predominantly small lymphocytes or cells arranged in a follicular pattern
2. intermediate grade—usually a mixture of follicular cells, centrocytes and centroblasts
3. high grade—predominance of centroblasts or immunoblasts with total destruction of nodal architecture.

Unlike Hodgkin's disease, blood-borne spread is common and the disease may be widespread at presentation even if only microscopically. Extranodal involvement is much more common.

T cell diseases frequently involve the skin and the CNS. Two cutaneous T cell lymphomas are *mycosis fungoides* and *Sezary's syndrome.*

Symptoms and signs. Lymphadenopathy, either localised or generalised, is the commonest presentation. Splenomegaly, often massive, may occur and in some cases, the disease may be localised to the spleen.

B symptoms are as for Hodgkin's disease. Lymphoma should be suspected in any case of pyrexia of unknown origin (PUO). The presentation of NHL may be very varied and almost every organ may be affected. Marrow involvement may cause pancytopenia.

Investigations. Histological diagnosis is essential. Staging is less important as treatment depends more on histological grade.

Differential diagnosis. Other causes of lymphadenopathy and other causes of PUO. Marrow and blood involvement may resemble leukaemia.

Treatment. Low grade disease, particularly in the elderly, may require no treatment for a number of years. Localised disease may be treated with radiotherapy. Low grade NHL is not curable and eventually transforms to aggressive disease. The mean survival is approximately 7 years.

High grade disease, particularly in younger patients, requires intensive combination chemotherapy and usually responds well to treatment but relapse is frequent. Long-term survival is around 30%, most of these cases being permanently cured. The role of autotransplantation still needs to be defined.

Myeloma

This disease is the result of malignant proliferation of plasma cells. It is a not uncommon disorder and occurs principally in the elderly.

Pathology

Plasma cells proliferate in the bone marrow and secrete an osteoclast activating factor causing bone destruction. This can result in osteolytic lesions and osteopenia.

The plasma cells secrete an identical immunoglobulin molecule (paraprotein) which forms a discrete band on electrophoresis. The production of heavy and light chains may be asynchronous leading to an excess of light chains with appear in the urine (Bence-Jones protein) and which can damage renal tubular cells, causing renal failure. Excess light chains may also cause amyloid deposition in skin, mucous membranes, nerves, kidneys, spleen, liver and heart.

Normal immunoglobulin production is suppressed leading to hypogammaglobulinaemia.

Symptoms and signs

Bone pain, particularly back pain, is the commonest symptom and is caused by vertebral collapse and nerve entrapment. Pathological fractures of ribs or long bones are common as is bone tenderness. Spinal cord compression may also lead to neurological complications.

Symptoms of hypercalcaemia are caused by excessive bone destruction and those of renal failure are due to hypercalcaemia, myeloma kidney or amyloid. Amyloid may cause extensive bruising, neuropathy or cardiac failure. It may infiltrate the skin, joints, mucous membranes and the tongue (causing macroglossia).

Infections are frequent because of immune paresis.

Occasionally, excess of paraprotein may result in the hyperviscosity syndrome which is characterised by weakness, visual disturbance, bleeding and, in severe cases, coma.

Investigations

Anaemia is common. In advanced disease pancytopenia may occur. The plasma viscosity or ESR is usually raised but not invariably so, especially in light chain disease. Plasma cells are increased in the bone marrow.

A monoclonal protein, usually IgG or IgA, can be detected in the serum in 80% of cases. In the remainder, light chains (Bence-Jones protein) can be detected in the urine. There is usually suppression of normal immunoglobulins.

Biochemical tests for hypercalcaemia and renal function are essential. The alkaline phosphatase is usually normal, distinguishing it from secondary carcinoma.

Radiology usually shows punched-out osteolytic lesions in the long bones and the skull. Diffuse osteopenia may also be a feature.

Differential diagnosis

Distinguishing features of other causes of paraproteinaemia, particularly benign monoclonal gammopathy, are absence of immunosuppression, lack of plasmacytosis and skeletal changes. Follow-up shows little change in the paraprotein level with time.

Treatment

Treatment is generally unsatisfactory. Melphalan and prednisolone are the mainstay of treatment, particularly in the elderly. Younger patients may benefit by combination chemotherapy. Localised bone lesions causing pain can be treated with radiotherapy.

Correction of metabolic abnormalities, e.g. hypercalcaemia, is essential. Occasionally, the hyperviscosity syndrome may require plasmapheresis.

Prognosis

For most patients, the mean survival is around 3 years. For patients presenting with advanced renal failure, the survival is usually under 1 year.

Waldenstrom's macroglobulinaemia

This is an uncommon disorder in which the paraprotein is IgM. Unlike myeloma, bone lesions do not occur but lymphadenopathy and splenomegaly may. The main symptoms are due to hyperviscosity or marrow failure.

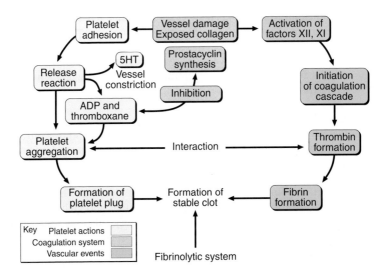

Fig. 11.6 Mechanism of haemostasis.

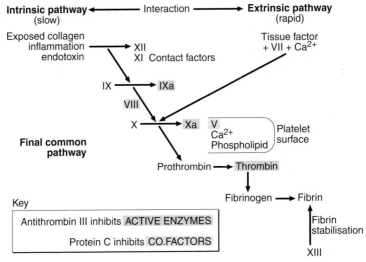

Fig. 11.7 The coagulation system.

Plasmapheresis may be needed, otherwise the treatment is with chlorambucil.

BLEEDING DISORDERS

The arrest of haemorrhage is a complicated process and depends on the interaction between the vessel wall, the platelets, the coagulation system and the fibrinolytic system (Fig 11.6 and 11.7). The key factor is damage to vascular endothelium which causes platelet adhesion and activation of the coagulation mechanism. These result in the formation of a platelet plug which is reinforced by a fibrin clot.

Failure of haemostasis results from vascular disorders, thrombocytopenia, platelet functional disorders (thrombocytopathy), coagulation disorders and excessive fibrinolysis.

Symptoms
Platelet disorders give rise to bleeding into the skin and mucous membranes whereas coagulation disorders cause bleeding into joints and muscles.

Investigations
Important points are the type and extent of bleeding. The onset of bleeding and past history, particularly surgical operations and including dental extraction. Other points to be noted are family history, other medical conditions and drug therapy.

The Hess test is of little value and the bleeding time is useful only if platelet dysfunction is suspected. It must be performed in a standard fashion.

Diagnosis depends upon laboratory investigation. Essential investigations are a full blood count and screening test of blood coagulation. The most useful are (Fig. 11.8):

1. *The prothrombin time* (PT), a test of the extrinsic system, is useful in the diagnosis of coagulation defects secondary to liver disease, or to monitor anticoagulant therapy.
2. *Activated partial thromboplastin time* (APTT), a test of the intrinsic system, is used for the diagnosis of haemophilia A and B and also to monitor heparin therapy.

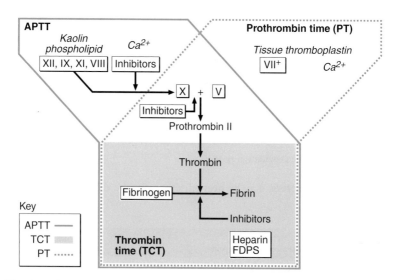

Fig. 11.8 Screening tests for coagulation showing inter-relationships between TCT, APTT and PT.

3. *Thrombin clotting time (TCT)* detects fibrinogen deficiency and inhibitors including heparin and fibrin degradation products (FDPs). Its main use is in the diagnosis of DIC.

Other useful investigations include factor assays and platelet function tests. Tests of fibrinolytic activity are difficult and rarely useful clinically.

VASCULAR DISORDERS

These may be congenital or acquired and are characterised by bleeding into the skin and bleeding from mucous membranes. They are caused by inflammatory damage to small vessels or changes in the supporting matrix (Table 11.16).

Hereditary haemorrhagic telangiectasia (Osler-Rendu-Weber disease)

This is inherited as an autosomal dominant and is characterised by multiple telangiectases in the skin and mucous membranes, particularly in the nose and GI tract. Arteriovenous shunts may develop in the lungs and elsewhere.

Symptoms and signs
Epistaxis, haemoptysis and GI tract bleeding, leading to anaemia, are more noticeable with ageing.

Table 11.16. Vascular causes of abnormal bleeding

Congenital
Hereditary haemorrhagic telangiectasia (Osler-Rendu-Weber disease)
Ehlers-Danlos disease (loose skin, joint hypermobility)

Acquired
Easy bruising
    Simple, easy bruising (young women, normal clotting studies)
    Autoerythrocyte sensitisation (crops of painful nodules, psychological disturbance)
    Atrophic (geographic lesions on extensor surface),
    e.g. senile purpura, steroids, Cushing's syndrome
    Scurvy (perifollicular haemorrhage)

Vasculitis (non-thrombocytopenic purpura)
    Drugs—penicillin, sulphonamides
    Infections
    Henoch–Schönlein purpura
    Systemic lupus erythematosus
    Rheumatoid arthritis
    Amyloid

Dysglobulinaemia
    Benign hyperglobulinaemia
    Cryoglobulinaemia
    Macroglobulinaemia

There are multiple telangiectases in the mouth, lips and finger tips. Bruits are present over the skull, chest or abdomen if there are arteriovenous fistulae.

Investigations
Essentially, the diagnosis is clinical although endoscopy may be necessary.

Differential diagnosis
Other vascular abnormalities include Campbell De Morgan's spots and purpura. Note: telangiectasies blanche on pressure.

Treatment
Repeated bleeding usually requires iron. Repeated epistaxis may be helped by oestrogen therapy and antifibrinolytic agents, e.g. tranexamic acid.

GI lesions may respond to endoscopic laser therapy.

Henoch-Schönlein purpura (HSP)

This is an example of vasculitis, i.e. damage to small blood vessels, usually due to an immunological or inflammatory mechanism, leading to increased capillary permeability.

HSP occurs mostly in children and is often preceded by streptococcal infection or drug therapy. It is probably caused by immune complex deposition and affects vessels in the intestine, joints and kidneys.

Symptoms and signs
Purpura occurs especially over the lower buttocks and lower limbs. Arthritis affects the knees, ankles and hands. There is colicky abdominal pain associated with diarrhoea (there may be intussusception). Haematuria and sometimes oedema are seen.

Investigations
Platelets and coagulation tests are normal. Skin biopsy (not usually necessary) shows perivascular inflammation.

Differential diagnosis
HSP must be distinguished from thrombocytopenic purpura and other causes of vasculitis, particularly drugs.

Treatment
No treatment is necessary unless progressive renal failure develops. Corticosteroids are of doubtful value and immunosuppressive agents may be more helpful. Prognosis is excellent unless chronic renal failure develops.

THROMBOCYTOPENIA
See Table 11.17.

Idiopathic thrombocytopenic purpura (ITP)

This is an autoimmune disease, although in children it may be post viral. There is bleeding into skin and mucous membranes. The most serious compli-

Table 11.17. Causes of thrombocytopenia

A Impaired platelet production (decreased megakaryocytes in bone marrow)

Hereditary congenital hypoplasia (rare), e.g.Wiskott-Aldrich syndrome, May-Hegglin anomaly

Megaloblastic anaemia

Marrow replacement, e.g. carcinoma, leukaemia.

Viral infections

Aplastic anaemia caused by drugs, chemicals, alcohol, radiation

B Excessive platelet destruction or use (increased megakaryocytes in bone marrow)

Immune mediated
  Autoimmune idiopathic thrombocytopenic purpura, systemic lupus erythematosus, lymphoproliferative diseases
  Drug induced (thiazides, quinine)
  AIHA (Evans syndrome)
  AIDS, other viral infections

Excessive consumption
  Disseminated intravascular coagulation (DIC)
  Giant haemangioma
  Hypersplenism
  Cardiac bypass operations
  Haemodialysis
  Massive transfusion (dilution effect and possible DIC)

cation is CNS haemorrhage. Splenomegaly does not occur; if it is present, an alternative diagnosis should be considered.

Investigations
The blood count is normal other than the thrombocytopenia. Increased megakaryocytes are seen in the bone marrow. Antiplatelet antibodies are rarely demonstrable in the serum. Platelet-associated IgG is diagnostic but the test is not readily available.

Screening tests for SLE should be performed.

Differential diagnosis
ITP must be distinguished from drug-induced thrombocytopenia, SLE, and immune thrombocytopenia complicating lymphoproliferative disease.

Treatment
The basis of treatment is steroids starting at a high dose, e.g. prednisolone 60 mg per 24 hours. Relapse usually occurs when steroids are withdrawn and a small maintenance dose may be needed. If a high maintenance dose of steroids is necessary to control the platelet count, splenectomy may be needed.

Immunosuppressive agents such as azathioprine or vincristine may help to reduce steroid dosage.

High-dose intravenous immunoglobulin will raise the platelet count quickly in an emergency although its effect is temporary and it is very expensive.

Table 11.18. Coagulation disorders

Inherited factor deficiencies
  VIII Haemophilia A
  IX Haemophilia B (Christmas disease)
  VIII Related antigen Von Willebrand's disease
  Other rare deficiencies: I, II, V, VII, X, XI, XII, XIII.

Acquired factor deficiencies
  Prothrombin complex deficiency (II, VII, IX, X)
  Prolonged PT and APTT
  Oral anticoagulants
  Severe vitamin K deficiency

Liver disease
  Prothrombin complex plus V and fibrinogen
  deficiency
  PT and APTT prolonged

Intravascular coagulation syndrome (DIC)
  Fibrinogen, V, VIII and platelet deficiency
  PT and APTT and TCT may be prolonged
  Fibrin degradation products (FDPs) raised

Factor VIII inhibitor
  Haemophiliacs (mostly severe)
  Pregnancy
  Malignancy
  Autoimmune disease

Lupus inhibitor
  (Prolonged APTT, an in vivo phenomena, often
  associated with thrombosis)

  SLE and other conditions, e.g. recurrent abortion, recurrent thrombosis

In children, the disease is usually self limiting but in adults it is usually chronic.

FUNCTIONAL PLATELET DEFECTS (THROMBOCYTOPATHY)

The clinical picture is similar to that of thrombocytopenia but the platelet count is normal. Congenital platelet defects are extremely rare. The commonest causes are drugs, particularly aspirin and non-steroidal anti-inflammatory agents (NSAIDs). Other causes include uraemia, paraproteinaemia and myeloproliferative disease.

COAGULATION DISORDERS (See Table 11.18).

Haemophilia

There are two main types, haemophilia A (factor VIII deficiency) and haemophilia B (factor IX deficiency). Both are inherited as sex-linked characters and have a similar clinical picture. An abnormal protein which retains some functional activity is produced. The severity depends upon the level of functional activity: <2% is severe, 2–10% moderate, and 10–25% mild.

Patients with severe haemophilia suffer spontaneous bleeds into joints, muscles and soft tissues. Repeated haemarthroses lead to synovial overgrowth and eventually to joint destruction (haemophiliac arthropathy). Bleeding from mucous membranes is rare and purpura does not occur. Mild haemophilia only leads to bleeds in response to trauma or surgery.

Symptoms and signs

Acute, painful joints are caused by haemarthrosis. There is chronic arthropathy. Retroperitoneal haemorrhage may mimic an acute abdomen.

Severe bleeding post surgery, particularly dental extraction, may be the first manifestation in mild haemophilia.

Investigations

In the clotting screen, only the APTT is prolonged. Specific factor assays confirm the diagnosis, and DNA studies are useful in detecting carriers.

Differential diagnosis

Other congenital bleeding disorders.

Mild haemophilia must be distinguished from Von Willebrand's disease.

In older patients, acquired haemophilia, caused by inhibitor formation, must be considered.

Treatment

The treatment of acute episodes is by factor replacement, given as freeze-dried concentrate. It is usually necessary to raise the factor level to around 30% for spontaneous haemarthroses, and to maintain a level above 50% for surgery until healing has occurred.

Most haemophiliacs can now be taught to treat themselves.

DDAVP (vasopressin) raises the factor VIII level. It may be all that is required for treatment in mild haemophilia. A test dose should be given first.

The management of the haemophiliac patient as a whole, is very important. A team approach, consisting of physician, orthopaedic surgeon, dentist, physiotherapist, geneticist and social worker, is best and all haemophiliacs should be under the care of a haemophilia centre.

Modern factor concentrates are virtually free of the risk of viral contamination, but in the past HIV infection and virus B and C hepatitis have been serious side-effects of infused factor VIII.

With proper care and treatment, there is no reason why haemophiliacs should not have a normal lifestyle and life expectancy.

Von Willebrand's disease

This disease may be confused with mild haemophilia. It is inherited as an autosomal character and therefore women may be affected. There is defective synthesis of the carrier part of the factor VIII molecule, resulting in defective platelet function as well as a reduction in factor VIII activity. Von Willebrand's disease varies widely in severity. Common symptoms include epistaxis, menorrhagia or abnormal bleeding following surgery or dental extraction. Haemarthrosis is uncommon.

Most patients can be treated with DDAVP although more severely affected patients may need factor VIII concentrate.

Bleeding caused by multiple factor deficiency

This is usually caused by defective synthesis of factors in the liver, particularly those which are vitamin K dependent (factors II, VII, IX and X).

Aetiological conditions include liver disease, obstructive jaundice, severe malabsorption and oral anticoagulant overdose. Excessive bruising, GI tract bleeding and haematuria may occur and treatment is with fresh frozen plasma 10–15 ml per kg.

Disseminated intravascular coagulation (DIC)

Intravascular coagulation occurs in many conditions (Table 11.19). The clinical picture and laboratory findings vary widely depending upon the cause, the extent and the speed of the onset and, as a consequence, a number of seemingly different syndromes exist. They all have in common the formation of fibrin within the vascular tree, the consumption of clotting factors (including platelets) to a variable degree and the stimulation of fibrinolysis.

Table 11.19. The intravascular coagulation syndromes

Acute

Obstetric complications
  Abruptio placentae
  Amniotic fluid embolism
  Eclampsia
  Retained products of dead fetus
  Septic abortion

Infections
  Septicaemia, especially gram-negative, meningoccal
  Malaria

Surgery
  Especially on the lungs and prostate
  Extracorporeal circulation

Trauma and burns

Shock

Snake bites, e.g. vipers

Incompatible blood transfusions, especially ABO

Chronic

Neoplasms, e.g. lung, stomach, colon

Leukaemia, especially promyelocytic

Thrombotic thrombocytopenic purpura

Haemolytic–uraemic syndrome

Giant haemangiomas

Miscellaneous causes, e.g. collagen disorders, amyloid, allergic vasculitis

Factors which may trigger DIC include:

1. The release of thromboplastin into the blood stream, e.g. obstetric accidents, carcinoma and leukaemia.
2. Activation of factor XII by contact with foreign surfaces, endotoxin and complement components.
3. Platelet aggregation by endotoxin, immune complexes or contact with a foreign surface.
4. Endothelial damage, e.g. malignant hypertension, renal disease, acute hepatic necrosis. This activates factor XII and stimulates platelet aggregation.

As a result of activation of the clotting mechanism, fibrin formation occurs with consumption of some of the clotting factors, particularly platelets, fibrinogen and factors V and VIII. In chronic DIC, increased synthesis may balance excessive consumption and their level may be normal or even raised. DIC activates the fibrinolytic system causing breakdown of fibrin with the production of FDPs. These have an anticoagulant effect by inhibiting fibrin formation and thus may potentiate the bleeding tendency. Fibrin formation in small vessels may lead to microthrombi and micro-infarcts and these may be responsible for the clinical picture. They may also cause microangiopathic haemolytic anaemia.

Symptoms and signs

1. Acute cases, e.g. obstetric complications, cause severe bleeding because of the rapid depletion of clotting factors.
2. In chronic DIC, e.g. that associated with disseminated malignancy, thrombocytopenia is the principal manifestation.
3. Where microthrombus formation predominates, widespread symptoms affecting many organs may occur. This is particularly so in TTP, where bizarre neurological complications are prominent.

Investigations

Full blood count. Results are variable and depend upon the cause. Thrombocytopenia is usual. Features of microangiopathic haemolytic anaemia may be present.

Clotting tests. Again the picture is variable. In severe cases, depletion of fibrinogen and factors V and VIII leads to prolongation of the TCT, PT and APTT.

Prolongation of the TCT may be caused by hypofibrinogenaemia or the presence of FDPs. Fibrinogen assay and tests for FDPs are essential.

In chronic cases, the clotting tests may be normal or even shortened because of circulating activated clotting factors. In such cases, the presence of raised FDPs is diagnostic.

Treatment

The cardinal rules of the treatment of DIC are to treat the cause, if possible, and to replace missing factors and platelets.

There is little place for heparin except in some chronic conditions where it may block the process and stop microangiopathic haemolytic anaemia.

Antifibrinolytic drugs may give rise to a Schwartzmann type reaction and are therefore not suitable.

DIC is often a marker of serious disease and the prognosis reflects the underlying state. TTP has a high mortality.

Bleeding caused by excessive fibrinolysis

Primary fibrinolytic disorders are very rare; usually, excessive fibrinolysis is secondary to intravascular coagulation. Primary fibrinolysis may occur in some neoplasms, especially prostatic carcinoma, and during some operations, especially prostatic and pulmonary.

Excessive fibrinolysis may be blocked by antifibrinolytic drugs such as tranexamic acid. These should be used with care but have a part to play in the management of postoperative bleeding.

12

RHEUMATOLOGY

Peter Hollingworth

Many rheumatic disorders are mediated through the immune system, so a better understanding of their pathogenesis and major advances in therapy are promised by pharmacological manipulation of the immune system.

Contrary to popular misconceptions, the more serious rheumatic diseases commonly begin in young adults and they become chronic as the joint has little capacity for repair. Much can be done to alleviate pain and maintain function, although cure is still rarely possible.

Rheumatic diseases are a major health burden; they account for one-fifth of consultations with family doctors and for one-third of the disabled population.

The principal rheumatic diseases are listed in Table 12.1. Connective tissue diseases are described in Chapter 13. Many general medical diseases have rheumatological manifestations and many rheumatic diseases have extra-articular manifestations that may present to other specialists.

Table 12.1. The principal rheumatic diseases

Rheumatoid arthritis
Spondarthritis
    Ankylosing spondylitis
    Reiter's disease
    Arthritis of inflammatory bowel disease
    Psoriatic arthritis
Osteoarthritis
Back pain
Crystal deposition diseases
Septic arthritis
Shoulder pain
Polymyalgia rheumatica

Terminology

'Arthritis' applies specifically to joint inflammation, and 'arthrosis' or 'arthropathy' apply to non-inflammatory joint diseases. 'Arthralgia' indicates joint pain with no particular connotations. 'Rheumatism' and 'rheumatic' have no medical use except in general terms such as 'soft tissue rheumatism' or 'rheumatic disorders'.

SYMPTOMS OF JOINT DISEASE

Pain

This is the most common presenting symptom. Joint pain worse after rest suggests joint inflammation. Joint pain better after rest, or worsening with activity and as the day goes on, suggests osteoarthritis. Night pain which prevents sleep is a major burden. By enhancing pain perception, depression and anxiety make management difficult.

As pain fibres arising from central joints enter the spinal cord at several levels, pain from these joints is perceived over a wide and often misleading area: glenohumeral pain radiates down the outer upper arm to the elbow; lumbar spinal pain to the buttock and posterior thigh; hip pain from the groin to the anterior thigh and, sometimes exclusively, the knee. In contrast, the patient accurately localises pain arising from a distal interphalangeal joint (DIPJ).

It should never be assumed that pain felt in a joint arises from that joint, and pain arising from juxta-articular or distant structures should always be excluded (Table 12.2).

Table 12.2. Joint pain arising from juxta-articular structures

Structures	Signs
Bone destruction: stress fracture, sepsis, metastases	Tenderness away from the joint line, abnormal radiograph
Sprain of ligament or tendon	Point tenderness away from joint line Worse on passive stretching—ligamentous Worse on resisted movement—tendinous
Bursa	Tenderness or swelling
Referred pain, e.g. shoulder pain may arise from cervical nerve irritation, thoracic or abdominal structures	Joint clinically normal, signs of distant disease
Diffuse limb pains	Consider—radiculopathy, spinal stenosis, peripheral neuropathy, polymyalgia rheumatica, bone disease, arterial or venous claudication, Parkinson's disease, depression

Immobility stiffness

A cardinal sign of joint inflammation is prolonged joint stiffness, lasting from half-an-hour to several hours, on getting up in the morning. It improves with activity and returns on rest and in the evening.

Loss of function

The consequences of unremitting inflammatory joint disease may be loss of leisure pursuits, loss of employment and, finally, loss of independence.

When assessing function, questions should be directed to practical difficulties relating to the patient's life—ambulation, personal toilet, housework, cooking, employment, sexual function etc.

Each impaired joint brings its own particular functional problem (Table 12.3).

SIGNS OF JOINT DISEASE

Examination can indicate the joint pathology (Table 12.4) and diagnosis. Pain felt in a clinically normal joint suggests that either it is referred pain or it has a psychological cause.

A general examination is necessary, paying particular attention to the hands, skin, eyes, and mucous membranes, looking for diagnostic clues (Table 12.5 and Figs 12.1 and 12.2).

DIAGNOSIS OF RHEUMATIC DISORDERS

Often the diagnosis is given by the history and examination alone, while investigations merely confirm it and assess the extent of joint damage. Additional clues are given by the age, sex and race of the patient, the family history, the time course of the disease, and the distribution of joints affected.

Table 12.3. Functional problems peculiar to particular joints

Joint	Functional problems
Cervical spine	Reversing car
Shoulder	Reaching nape of the neck, perineal toilet, fastening brassiere or reaching back pocket
Elbow	Fastening top shirt button, reaching face-drinking, eating, blowing nose
Wrist	Supination to receive change, weakness of the hand from collapse of the carpus slackening the flexor tendons
Hip	Lifting the leg high to climb stairs, alight a bus, get into a car, get out of a bath, dress lower half, sexual intercourse in women
Subtalar joint	Walking on uneven or sloping ground

Table 12.4 Signs of joint disease

Sign	Pathology	Diagnosis
Swelling		
Fluctuation (i.e. fluid)	Non-inflammatory synovial effusion: high viscosity, low WBC count	Osteoarthritis
	Inflammatory synovial effusion: low viscosity, high WBC count	Inflammatory joint disease
	Blood	Trauma, anticoagulants, haemophilia
	Pus: green or yellow	Septic arthritis
Bony	Osteophytes	Osteoarthritis
Synovial thickening	Synovitis	Inflammatory joint disease
Deformity		
Flexion	Periarticular contracture	Mainly inflammatory joint disease
Later: valgus/varus deformity	Cartilage or ligament damage	Any destructive joint disease
Restricted movement	As above	As above
Redness	Intense synovitis	Acute crystal arthritis, septic arthritis, periarthritis
Crepitus	Cartilage damage	Usually osteoarthritis

Non-specific signs: muscle wasting, warmth, pain on movement, tenderness at the joint line

Age, sex and race

Certain diseases tend to strike specific groups. Rheumatoid arthritis and connective tissue diseases chiefly affect women while ankylosing spondylitis and primary gout affect men. Pyrophosphate arthropathy and polymyalgia rheumatica are diseases of the elderly, while Reiter's disease and gonococcal arthritis present in the young. Systemic lupus erythematosus (SLE) is more common in Blacks and Asians.

Family history

Spondarthropathies, primary gout and psoriatic arthritis tend to run in families.

Time-course of the disease

Inflammatory joint disease may begin dramatically and fluctuate in severity, while osteoarthritis tends to progress slowly. Recurrent bouts of brief severe

Table 12.5. Skin and mucous membrane findings in rheumatic diseases

Clinical features	Diagnosis
Psoriasis	Psoriatic arthritis
Butterfly rash	Systemic lupus erythematosus (SLE)
Gottron's papules	Dermatomyositis
Vasculitis	Vasculitic syndromes
Erythema nodosum	Acute sarcoidosis and inflammatory bowel disease
Pustular psoriasis	Reiter's disease
Livedo reticularis	Antiphospholipid syndrome
Raynaud's syndrome or acrocyanosis	Rheumatoid arthritis and connective tissue diseases, especially scleroderma, (SLE) and mixed connective tissue disease
Subcutaneous tophi	Tophaceous gout
Rheumatoid nodules	Rheumatoid arthritis
Thickened tethered skin	Scleroderma
Diffuse or scarring alopecia	SLE
Mouth and genitourinary ulceration	Painless: Reiter's disease; painful: Behçet's disease
Dry eyes and mouth	Sjögren's syndrome

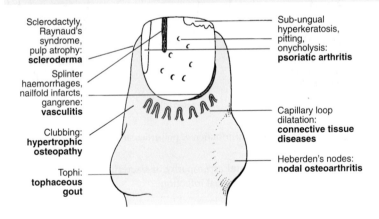

Fig. 12.1 The fingertips in rheumatic diseases.

arthritis affecting one or a few joints at a time and resolving in hours or days is called palindromic arthritis. It occurs in gout, early rheumatoid arthritis, SLE and spondarthropathies.

The distribution of joints affected

This is a most important diagnostic indicator (Fig. 12.3). The differential diagnosis of a monoarthritis is wholly different from a polyarthritis. When

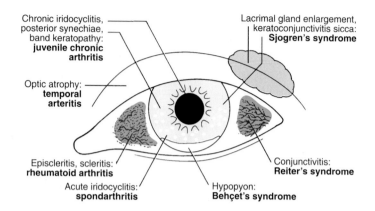

Fig. 12.2 The eye in rheumatic diseases.

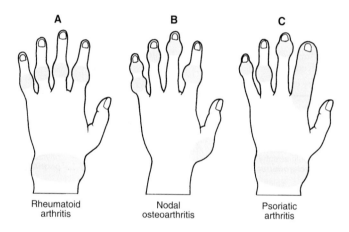

Fig. 12.3 Characteristic distribution of polyarticular disease.

acute, it suggests a crystal arthropathy or bacterial sepsis, and when chronic, osteoarthritis or mycobacterial infection.

INVESTIGATIONS

Imaging techniques

Plain radiographs are most important in the investigation and monitoring of joint disease. Single views only of appropriate sites no more frequently than 6-monthly may be indicated.

Bone scintigraphy scanning soon after injection of radiolabelled technetium diphosphonate detects synovitis; late scans detect bone disease—metastases, Paget's disease and osteomyelitis.

Computerised axial tomography is useful in the assessment of spinal stenosis. Magnetic resonance imaging is used in the detection of spinal and disc disease, osteonecrosis and internal joint derangement.

Blood investigations

Non-specific indices of inflammation are elevation of the ESR, plasma viscosity, C-reactive protein and complement levels.

IgM rheumatoid factor is found in high titre in rheumatoid arthritis. The latex test for rheumatoid factor (RF) is so sensitive it tends to give false positive results. The Rose Waaler test is less sensitive but more specific.

Some antinuclear and extractable nuclear antibodies are strongly associated with certain disease features in connective tissue disease (Ch. 13).

Complement consumption occurs in active connective tissue diseases, notably SLE and systemic rheumatoid arthritis.

Immune complexes are usually elevated in rheumatoid arthritis and connective tissue diseases but only crudely reflect disease activity.

Analysis of synovial fluid detects infection or crystal arthropathies.

Other investigations include arthroscopy, synovial biopsy and arthrography and are used in the diagnosis of monoarticular disease.

PRINCIPLES OF MANAGEMENT OF JOINT DISEASE

Arthritis may disrupt all aspects of the patient's life, so management is of the whole person, not just of the joints and involves the combined facilities of physiotherapy, occupational therapy, surgery, drugs, psychological and social support. With regular evaluation, problems are anticipated and corrected early.

Explanation of the probable disease course, self-help and the use of drugs allay unnecessary fears.

Bedrest is indicated only for severe, acute polyarthritis. Individual joints should be rested with splinting. Special shoes accommodate deformed feet. Shoe inserts correct or support painful foot deformities.

Physiotherapy

A combination of active, passive and resisted exercises maintain or correct joint position, joint movement and muscle strength. Various techniques for applying cold or heat to deep structures help relieve pain.

Occupational therapy

Functional problems are overcome by exploitation of residual function, mechanical devices, or altering the patient's environment.

Drugs

The principles are:
1. prescribe the minimum number,
2. use the least toxic first, in the minimum therapeutically effective dose.

Several groups of drugs are available. Some drugs for specific conditions are mentioned later.

Analgesics. Paracetamol and co-proxamol.

Non-steroidal anti-inflammatory drugs (NSAIDs). Used principally for inflammatory joint disease to alleviate pain, stiffness and swelling, many are available and the response individualistic. Side-effects are common, particularly in the elderly, and include gastrointestinal ulceration, fluid retention etc.

Slow-acting antirheumatic drugs (SAARDs). These appear to actually modify the course of rheumatoid arthritis and other inflammatory joint diseases. Indications for use include failure to respond to NSAIDs, progressive joint damage, serious extra-articular complications, reduction of steroid dosage. The disease may appear to remit and the rate of joint destruction decrease, at least temporarily.

The dosage is slowly increased. No benefit is seen for weeks or months. Regular monitoring detects side-effects early which are common but rarely irreversible.

The principal SAARDs and their side-effects are seen in Table 12.6.

Prednisolone. This is reserved for severe synovitis in inflammatory joint diseases or serious extra-articular complications. A dose lower than 7.5 mg per 24 hours carries minimal risk, perhaps less than that for NSAIDs in the elderly.

Intra-articular steroids. These are used for relieving symptoms from synovitis, where one or a few joints are particularly affected. The benefit may last weeks. Post-injection 'flares' are common. The risk of infection is small but multiple injections might damage cartilage.

Intra-articular radioactive colloids. These give longer relief than steroid injections by giving a 'chemical synovectomy'.

Surgery

The inflamed synovium may be removed, sometimes arthroscopically, and destroyed joints excised, fused, realigned or replaced by prostheses.

RHEUMATOID ARTHRITIS

Rheumatoid arthritis (RA) is the most common serious rheumatic disorder and affects 1% of people worldwide. The six-fold greater prevalence in women

Table 12.6. Slow-acting anti-rheumatic drugs and their side-effects

Penicillamine	Rashes, thrombocytopenia, renal protein leak
Gold salts (oral and injectible)	As above
Hydroxychloroquine	Retinopathy
Sulphasalazine	Neutropenia, headaches, intestinal disturbance, male subfertility
Azathioprine	Marrow suppression, hepatitis
Methotrexate	Marrow suppression, pulmonary and hepatic fibrosis

halves after the menopause. All ages after puberty are affected, it is rare in adolescence, peaks between the third and fifth decades and tends to be more severe in the elderly.

Its exact cause is unknown. Reports implicating various triggering infectious agents remain unconfirmed. The risk is increased with HLA-DR4 (four-fold), particularly for severe disease, with female sex and with multiparity. Oral contraceptives may be protective. Remission occurs in pregnancy.

Pathology

The disease starts in the synovium, but all organs except the brain may eventually be affected.

The immunopathology commences with antigen-presenting cells in the synovium activating T helper cells to induce B cell production of RF. This spills out from the synovium and forms immune complexes with IgG in the synovial fluid, cartilage and the blood. Activation of the complement and other inflammatory mediators causes the synovitis and some of the extra-articular complications. In an attempt to eradicate immune complexes in cartilage, the pluripotential cells at the chondrosynovial junction metamorphose to granulation tissue which creeps centripetally over the cartilage, secreting enzymes that destroy the underlying cartilage and bone.

Symptoms

The onset of RA is usually subacute with a symmetrical arthritis of the hands and feet causing pain, prolonged morning stiffness, and swelling. Involvement of more proximal joints follows, potentially affecting all synovial structures—joints, bursae and tendon sheaths.

Less common presentations include systemic onset (fever, weightloss, anaemia), palindromic, monoarthritis and polymyalgic, particularly in the elderly.

Extra-articular features
These occur in 75% of patients. The most common are the least severe.
1. Subcutaneous nodules over pressure points, notably the olecranon and in the finger pulp.
2. Eye problems: episcleritis, scleritis (painful red eye) and keratoconjunctivitis sicca (dry eye).
3. Vasculitis: this underlies many extra-articular complications. Nailfold infarcts are common. Fevers, weightloss, night sweats and falling haemoglobin, associated with complement consumption and high levels of immune complexes, suggests systemic (widespread) vasculitis. Vasculitic leg ulcers are large, deep and develop rapidly. Rarely, digital vasculitis causes gangrene of toes.
4. Neurological complications: erosion of the odontoid peg or cruciate ligament causes atlantoaxial subluxation which can compress the cervical cord and result in a quadriparesis. Pressure by deformed or swollen joints on peripheral nerves can cause an entrapment neuropathy, such as carpal

tunnel syndrome (see p. 164). A mild sensory neuropathy is common. Mononeuritis multiplex is a serious complication of systemic vasculitis.

5. Kidney: amyloidosis.
6. Felty's syndrome: neutropenia, splenomegaly, recurrent sepsis and leg ulcers.

Signs

In the early stages there is symmetrical synovitis of the metacarpophalangeal joints (MCPJs), proximal interphalangeal joints (PIPJs) and the wrists, notably over the ulnar styloid. A complete fist cannot be made. The late deformities are: ulnar deviation of the fingers at the MCPJs; hyperextension of the PIPJs (Boutonnière deformity); hyperextension of the PIPJs (swan-necking); a Z-shaped thumb (hyperflexion of the MCPJ and hyperextension of the interphalangeal joint); subluxation of the wrist (Figs. 12.4 and 12.5). Shoulders lose abduction and external rotation. Elbows and knees flex. Hind-feet slip into valgus. The toes deviate laterally and cock-up, pulling the fibrous fatty cushion forwards from under the metatarsal heads.

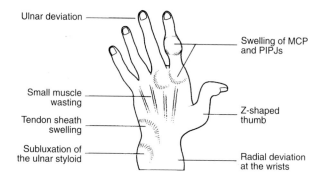

Ulnar deviation —

Swelling of MCP and PIPJs

Small muscle wasting

Tendon sheath swelling

Subluxation of the ulnar styloid

Z-shaped thumb

Radial deviation at the wrists

Fig. 12.4 The hand in rheumatoid arthritis.

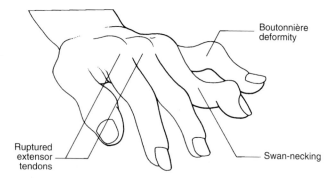

Boutonnière deformity

Ruptured extensor tendons

Swan-necking

Fig. 12.5 Finger deformities in rheumatoid arthritis.

Investigations

Blood shows normochromic and normocytic anaemia, and elevation of the ESR or plasma viscosity. RF is present in 80%.

Early radiographs show juxta-articular osteoporosis and soft tissue swelling. Later, marginal erosions, loss of joint space and deformity are seen, and eventually there is complete joint destruction with secondary osteoarthritis.

Before anaesthesia or where there is an unexplained functional decline, a lateral radiograph of the cervical spine in flexion should be examined for atlantoaxial subluxation.

Differential diagnosis

The diagnosis of RA is definite with the combination of a peripheral symmetrical arthritis, serum RF, radiographic erosions and extra-articular features, particularly nodules.

When the diagnosis is not definite, Reiter's disease, psoriatic arthritis, SLE, nodal osteoarthritis, crystal arthropathies and viral arthritis should be considered.

Treatment

Treatment should be tailored to the state of the disease: paracetamol for mild disease; NSAIDs for relief of pain and stiffness; SAARDs where NSAIDs fail, erosions or deformities develop, for troublesome extra-articular features, or to reduce steroid requirements; prednisolone for severe resistant synovitis or major extra-articular complications; surgery for destroyed joints.

Prognosis

10% of patients remit altogether, 10% run a remittent course, and the remainder have a persistent, fluctuating disease with slow deterioration. The presence of RF, early marginal erosions, and late age of onset suggest a worse prognosis. Most joint damage occurs in the first 2 years with a slower deterioration subsequently.

10% of patients become severely disabled and the remainder have mild or moderate disability. Mortality is increased, particularly in older patients, from infection, extra-articular disease and complications of therapy, notably NSAID-induced peptic ulceration.

SERONEGATIVE SPONDARTHROPATHIES

The principal members of this group are ankylosing sponylitis, Reiter's disease/reactive arthritis, arthritis of chronic inflammatory bowel disease, psoriatic arthritis. These are considered together as they share characteristics that suggest a similar pathogenesis, notably a strong association with HLA-B27 and the implication of infection as a trigger (Table 12.7). The term seronegative spondarthritis (spondyloarthritis, spondyloarthropathy) emphasises the distinction from RA (negative serum test for RF), the spinal (spondylos = vertebra) and peripheral joint involvement.

Table 12.7. Characteristic features of the spondarthritides

- Strong association with HLA B27: family history common
- Infection implicated as a triggering factor
- Primary lesion at the enthesis (the site of insertion of ligament, joint capsule tendon or fascia into bone
- Peripheral arthritis: often asymmetrical and lower limb
- Mucocutaneous manifestations: psoriasis, genital and mouth ulcers, conjunctivitis
- Actue iritis: independently associated with HLA B27
- Absent rheumatoid factor

Infection is a proven trigger in Reiter's disease and suspected in the others. The immune response against the infecting organism appears to be misdirected against structures bearing the HLA-B27 molecule. Why the enthesis is attacked is unknown. The spine is particularly involved as it is rich in entheses (hence spondylitis) notably in the sacroiliac joint (hence sacroiliitis) which is bridged by a massive ligament. Involvement of the entheses of the plantar fascia and Achilles tendon into the calcaneum commonly causes heel pain.

The early enthesopathy is tender and may show radiographically as an erosion. It heals with a spur of new bone, so forming a new enthesis at its tip. If the process continues the ligament may be entirely replaced by bone and fuse the joint it bridges, leaving a rigid painless joint.

The peripheral arthritis is a synovitis, perhaps mediated by immune complex deposition, and is often asymmetrical.

Mucocutaneous manifestations are psoriasis, genital and mouth ulcers and conjunctivitis.

ANKYLOSING SPONDYLITIS (AS)

95% of patients carry HLA-B27. The geographic distribution reflects the racial gene frequency of HLA-B27, which is found in 10% of Whites, 0.5% of whom develop AS, rarely in Blacks or Japanese, and up to 50% of certain North American Indian tribes.

Males predominate eight-fold with the classical disease, but when atypical disease is included the sex ratio equalises. The age of onset is usually about 20 and never over 45. One-third give a family history of a spondarthritis.

Klebsiella infections and inflammatory bowel disease (see p. 280) have been implicated.

Symptoms and signs

Presentation is with low back pain from sacroiilitis or spondylitis. Sacroiilitis causes buttock pain radiating to the posterior thigh.

Spondylitic pain is typical; it disturbs sleep, is worse in the morning, when the back is stiff and improves with activity to return with rest.

Early, the normal lumbar lordosis is flattened. If the disease progresses, a lumbar kyphosis develops, lumbar spinal movements are lost, chest expansion is diminished (from costovertebral joint involvement) and the cervical spine is craned forward and restricted.

One-fifth have large joint disease, chiefly involving the hip. Heel pain is common. 20% suffer from recurrent acute iritis. Aortic regurgitation and pulmonary fibrosis are rare complications.

Women tend to present with neck pain and peripheral arthritis.

Investigations

Radiographs show symmetrical sacroiliitis: cortical erosions, sub-articular sclerosis with fusion later. Lateral radiographs of the lumbar spine show enthesopathic new bone bridging the disc spaces (syndesmophytes).

Differential diagnosis

This includes all causes of back pain (Table 12.8).

Treatment

A daily exercise regime will maintain spinal position and movement, and chest expansion. NSAIDs, hip arthroplasty and genetic counselling will all need to be considered.

Table 12.8. Specific causes of back pain

Diagnosis	Clinical features
Spondylitis: Ankylosing spondylitis Psoriatic or Reiter's disease complicating inflammatory bowel disease	Prolonged morning stiffness, radiographic sacroiliitis
Malignancy or infection	Unremitting pain, often thoracic, unrelieved by rest, weightloss and fever, elevated ESR and alkaline phosphatase level, destructive changes on radiograph
Osteoporotic collapse	Recurrent bouts of sudden back pain in postmenopausal women, radiographic osteoporosis and vertebral collapse
Lumbar disc prolapse	Dermatomal pain radiating below the knee worse on coughing or sneezing, limited straight leg raising, motor or sensory deficit in one leg
Back pain referred from retroperitoneal structures	Spine clinically normal, evidence of abdominal disease
Psychogenic back pain	Normal spine, psychological disturbance

Prognosis

90% of patients have mild disease settling in the fourth decade; 10% have severe spinal restriction, often with hip disease, within 10 years.

REITER'S DISEASE

The 15-fold excess in young men may be an overestimate as the genitourinary features are easily missed in women. 90% of patients carry HLA-B27.

The triggering organisms are *Salmonella*, some *Shigella* species, *Yersinia* and *Helicobacter*, which present with diarrhoea, and *Chlamydia trachomatis*, contracted venereally and presenting with urethritis.

Symptoms and signs

The disease starts 1–3 weeks after the infection, which may be subclinical. Reiter's disease refers to the triad of arthritis, urethritis and conjunctivitis, but incomplete forms are common, and the term 'reactive arthritis' is used when arthritis is the sole feature.

The manifestations of Reiter's disease include:

1. arthritis (100%): lower limb, principally the foot, acute, asymmetrical and migratory
2. conjunctivitis (60%): usually bilateral and often severe
3. urethritis (90%): dysuria and urethral discharge distinct from chlamydial urethritis as it is sterile and an integral feature of the disease
4. enthesopathy: one-third have sacroiilitis or spondylitis at the onset and two-thirds have heel pain. Painful, red, swollen 'sausage toes' may be caused by periostitis
5. balanitis—coalescing around the corona
6. pustular psoriasis of the soles—keratoderma blennorrhagica
7. painless buccal ulceration
8. recurrent acute iritis.

Investigations

Testing for HLA-B27 is not helpful. Early, there may be evidence of the triggering infection. Later, radiographs may show sacroiilitis or spondylitis, but unlike AS, these are asymmetrical and the syndesmophytes are coarse.

Differential diagnosis

Psoriatic arthritis, RA, gout, gonococcal arthritis.

Prognosis

Half improve over several months, the remainder have repeated episodes of arthritis or mucocutaneous manifestations over many years. One-third develop spondylitis.

Treatment

The triggering infection is treated with antibiotics, both in the patient and the sexual partner, although this does not alter the course of Reiter's disease. NSAIDs usually control joint pain. Sulphasalazine, azathioprine or methotrexate may be required.

ARTHRITIS OF INFLAMMATORY BOWEL DISEASE

Spondylitis, clinically and radiographically identical to AS occurs in one-fifth of patients, two-thirds of whom carry HLA-B27, and progresses regardless of the activity of the bowel disease.

20% of patients with ulcerative colitis and 10% with Crohn's disease develop a peripheral arthritis, probably mediated by immune complex deposition and unassociated with HLA-B27. It usually affects the large joints, parallels the bowel disease and resolves completely.

PSORIATIC ARTHRITIS

5% of patients with psoriasis develop arthritis. 90% have psoriatic nail changes against 30% with the rash alone. The sex incidence is equal and the peak age of onset 30–50 years. The arthritis usually presents with or after the rash. Several forms are recognised (Table 12.9, Fig. 12.6).

Investigations

Rheumatoid factor is absent. The radiographic features are typical: predilection for DIPJs, a combination of erosions and new bone formation at the joint margins, tendency to bony fusion, heel spurs, sacroiilitis and spondylitis.

Table 12.9. Patterns of psoriatic arthritis

70% (1) Predominantly hands and feet; asymmetrical; DIPJ involvement of all the structures in one ray — DIPJ, PIPJ, MCPJ and flexor tendon, giving a 'fat finger'. Periostitis causing sausage toes. Enthesopathic heel pain	5% (3) Arthritis mutilans: Resorption of the ends of the phalanges causing flail fingers
	5% (4) Isolated DIPJ involvement in the hands: drumstick fingers
15% (2) Peripheral, symmetrical arthritis distinguished from RA only by the presence of psoriasis and the absence of rheumatoid factor or rheumatoid extra-articular features	5% (5) Spondylitis, clinically identical to AS, but radiographically resembling Reiter's syndrome – 90% carry HLA B27

One third of those with peripheral arthritis also have sacroiliitis

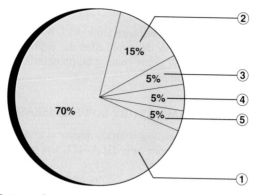

Fig. 12.6 Patterns of psoriatic arthritis.

Treatment

Treatment with NSAIDs. Methotrexate or azathioprine are indicated for the few with severe destructive disease.

OSTEOARTHRITIS

Osteoarthritis (OA, osteoarthrosis, degenerative joint disease) is a major cause of disability. Radiographically it is universally evident after the age of 60 years and symptomatic in 10% of the population.

Normal use and ageing alone do not cause OA. It is not a single disease, but a final common pathway following various insults to the cartilage. It should be regarded as an attempt at healing which becomes symptomatic only when it fails.

In the early stages, the virtually inert chondrocytes increase the turnover of cartilage matrix, which swells, fibrillates and is eventually lost. The underlying bone becomes vascular and sclerotic, and remodels at the margins (osteophyte formation).

The hips or knees are most commonly affected. Mild hip dysplasia may predispose to the former. Occasionally previous cartilage damage from joint inflammation, incongruity of joint surfaces following orthopaedic problems or metabolic abnormalities (gout, pyrophosphate arthropathy) are identifiable causes.

Nodal OA is a polyarticular variant affecting chiefly middle-aged women, often with a family history (see below).

Symptoms and signs

The main problem is pain which tends to improve with rest and worsen with activity. Exacerbations follow trauma or changes in barometric pressure. Troublesome night pain results from interosseus venous hypertension. Morning stiffness is brief. Progression is slow, and serious loss of function occurs only after many years.

Nodal OA in the hand causes bony enlargement of the DIPJs and PIPJs (Heberden's and Bouchard's nodes) and at the base of the thumb.

The hip loses rotation, flexes up and may develop an adduction deformity.

The knee develops effusions, periarticular thickening with tender points, crepitus, a flexion deformity with loss of free flexion, quadriceps wasting and, later, varus deformity, as the medial tibiofemoral compartment is affected first.

Investigations

Blood tests are normal. Radiographs show loss of joint space, marginal osteophyte formation with remodelling, and subchondral sclerosis with cysts.

Differential diagnosis

Symptoms must not be attributed to radiographically evident OA, which is a common incidental finding. Mono-articular onset of a polyarthritis, pyrophosphate arthropathy or chronic infection must be considered. Gouty tophi and psoriatic arthritis of the DIPJs may mimic Heberden's nodes.

Treatment

Nothing alters the disease progression. Pain may be alleviated by strengthening the quadriceps, weight reduction and walking aids. NSAIDs should be avoided in the elderly. Peri- or intra-articular steroid injections help acute exacerbations. Prosthetic replacement is needed for incapacitating symptoms.

BACK PAIN

Few escape back pain. 4% of the adult population consult their family doctors for it annually, half are better within 1 week. Two-thirds have 'non-specific' back pain which is postural or occupational, and no specific cause can be found: lumbar osteoarthrosis is a common incidental finding.

One-fifth of the cases of back pain have a specific cause, requiring a specific treatment (Table 12.8). A prolapsed lumbar disc accounts for the majority of these. Warnings of a specific cause of back pain are onset before age 20 or after age 55, symptoms persisting beyond 2 months, thoracic pain, restriction of spinal movements.

CRYSTAL ARTHROPATHIES

Joints and periarticular tissue are susceptible to crystal deposition. Several kinds occur which manifest either as a recurrent acute monoarthritis or chronic destructive arthritis (Table 12.10). The former is initiated by crystal activation of inflammatory mediators, chiefly Hageman factor and complement, and release of lysosmal enzymes from neutrophils that phagocytose the crystals. The latter results from the physical effects of the crystals and synovial release of destructive enzymes.

Table 12.10. Crystal arthropathies

Crystal	Acute arthritis	Chronic destructive arthritis
Sodium urate	Gout	Tophaceous gout
Calcium pyrophosphate	Pseudogout	Chronic pyrophosphate arthropathy
Hydroxyapatite	Acute calcific periarthritis	Apatite-associated destructive arthritis

Hydroxyapatite arthropathies are uncommon and will not be discussed.

GOUT

Hyperuricaemia predisposes to the crystallisation of sodium urate. Most of the body pool of urate derives from endogenous purine breakdown from nucleic acids, and the dietary contribution is small. Excretion is principally by the renal tubule. Obesity and excess alcohol intake accelerate urate production. Hyperuricaemia is associated with hypertension and hypertriglyceridaemia which predispose to atherosclerosis.

Urate levels are lower in women than in men until the menopause, when they equalise. Hence, gout is eight times more common in men, with a prevalence of 0.1%, and presents at a mean age of 40, compared with 70 in women.

In practice, gout in men is commonly 'primary': obese, hypertensive, middle-aged men with a high alcohol intake and a family history (one-third) who are under-secretors of urate. In women, it presents after the age of 70 and results from diuretic inhibition of urate excretion from the renal tubules. Less common is gout from overproduction from a myeloproliferative disorder, especially during treatment. Occasionally, a young man with severe gout and marked overproduction will be found to have an inherited partial deficiency of hypoxanthine-guanine-phosphoribosyl-transferase (Lesch-Nyhan syndrome).

Urate slowly crystallises on the cartilage surface. Shedding initiates acute attacks. Further accumulation of solid deposits of urate eventually damages the joints: tophaceous gout. Uric acid crystallisation within the renal collecting ducts causes stones in 10% of gout sufferers.

Symptoms and signs

Acute gout

Hyperuricaemia may be present years before the first attack. This is precipitated by trauma, including surgery, intercurrent illness, dietary or alcohol excess. Typically, the attack is monarticular in a lower limb joint, notably at the base of the great toe. Within hours the joint is very painful, swollen, red and shiny. It resolves completely within days on NSAIDs and 2 weeks if untreated, with skin desquamation. 90% of patients have recurrent attacks.

Tophaceous gout

This is rare since the advent of hypouricaemic drugs and is now usually associated with diuretic intake. After recurrent acute gout, solid deposits of urate develop around the interphalangeal joints of the fingers and great toe, the pinna and olecranon. They shine white through the overlying skin which may ulcerate or become infected. Untreated, tophi eventually destroy joints.

Diagnosis and differential diagnosis

Patients are hyperuricaemic even between attacks. Only 20% of individuals with hyperuricaemia ever develop gout, which is diagnosed too frequently. Hence, it is important to confirm the diagnosis by identification of urate crystals from synovial fluid or tophi, which have a characteristic appearance on polarised light microscopy. Early radiographs are normal. Later, tophi produce periarticular erosions with a sclerotic margin.

Other causes of acute monoarthritis are septic arthritis, pseudogout, Reiter's disease, psoriatic and palindromic arthritis. Tophi in the hands may be mistaken for nodal OA or psoriatic arthritis.

Treatment

Asymptomatic hyperuricaemia should not be treated. Gout often points to more serious problems: alcohol abuse, obesity, atherosclerosis, hypertriglyceridemia, hypertension and renal disease.

High-dose NSAIDs or colchicine are effective in acute attacks.

Further acute attacks may be prevented by reducing weight or alcoholic intake, or stopping diuretics.

The urate lowering drug allopurinol is indicated for life when there are frequent attacks, tophi, joint damage or renal calculi. Allopurinol initially triggers acute attacks which can be prevented by concomitant NSAIDs.

PYROPHOSPHATE ARTHROPATHY

Pyrophosphate is formed in many metabolic reactions and its calcium salt may be deposited in cartilage, particularly fibrocartilage, identified radiographically as chondrocalcinosis as (age 40: 1%, age 90: 40%). Pyrophosphate arthropathy is chiefly a disease of elderly women. Other associations are joint instability (hypermobility, following meniscectomy, metabolic (hypothyroidism, hyperparathyroidism) and rare inherited forms.

The distribution of joints affected reflects the presence of intra-articular fibrocartilaginous structures. In order of frequency are the knees, with particular patellofemoral joint involvement, wrists, shoulders, hips and ankles.

PSEUDOGOUT

This is the commonest cause of acute monoarthritis in the elderly.

The joint, usually knee, rapidly becomes severely inflamed and swollen, sometimes with marked systemic features. Resolution may take weeks and attacks tend to recur.

Diagnosis is by demonstration of pyrophosphate crystals in synovial fluid by polarised light microscopy.

Hypothyroidism and hyperparathyroidism should be excluded.
Treatment is with an intra-articular steroid injection or NSAIDs.

CHRONIC PYROPHOSPHATE ARTHROPATHY

The clinical picture resembles OA, affecting particularly the knees, but there are important differences: joints are involved that are rarely affected by OA— shoulders, elbows or wrists; a history suggesting pseudogout; radiographs show chondrocalcinosis, exuberant osteophyte formation, and greater joint destruction; pyrophosphate crystals are present in the synovial fluid.

Treatment is as for OA (see p. 376).

POLYMYALGIA RHEUMATICA

This is a common disease of the elderly. The onset is usually after the age of 60, and women are affected twice as frequently. It is strongly associated with temporal arteritis. The cause is unknown.

Severe, symmetrical pain, stiffness and tenderness in the muscles of the neck, shoulder and hip girdle develop, usually over weeks. Characteristically, nights are terrible with difficulty in rolling over in bed, getting up and dressing in the morning. Fever, weightloss, night sweats and anaemia may be marked. The girdle muscles may be tender. The ESR is markedly raised, and the response to prednisolone dramatic.

A similar picture may be seen in the onset of RA, bacterial endocarditis, occult malignancy and hypothyroidism.

Prednisolone is slowly withdrawn over about 3 years. Giant cell (temporal) arteritis occasionally develops (see p. 130).

RHEUMATOLOGICAL EMERGENCIES

There are five warning signs: fever, neurological symptoms, acute monoarthritis, renal impairment and collapse. The principal emergencies are:

1. Septic arthritis: a severe monoarthritis with fever. Misleadingly mild features are found in patients who are debilitated, taking immunosuppressive drugs, or who have arthritis.
2. Atlantoaxial subluxation: complicating RA, this may cause an acute quadriparesis or a general functional decline.
3. Acute cerebral lupus: fits, focal neurological signs or impaired consciousness.
4. Rapidly progressive renal failure may result form NSAIDs, SLE, polyarteritis nodosa or scleroderma.
5. Mononeuritis multiplex: RA, SLE and polyarteritis nodosa.
6. Temporal arteritis: sudden blindness.
7. Collapse: gut bleeding or perforation from NSAIDs.

13

CONNECTIVE TISSUE DISEASES AND IMMUNOLOGY

John R. Kirwan

CONNECTIVE TISSUE DISEASES

A group of disorders which share many clinical characteristics enter into the differential diagnosis in most patients presenting with multisystem inflammatory disease. These conditions are often referred to as 'collagen vascular diseases' or '(systemic) connective tissue diseases' and include those listed in Table. 13.1. There is evidence that this group of conditions share pathogenetic and even aetiological factors. Shared features include multisystem involvement, arthritis and vasculitis, the presence of antibodies against 'self' antigens and evidence of immune complex deposition. Furthermore, there are many patients who either present with a mixture of features which overlap two or more diagnostic categories, or who are clearly in one category but gradually change their clinical picture to that of another. These features all raise the possibility of a common underlying pathology which is modulated by genetic and environmental factors so as to be expressed in a particular way in each patient. Much evidence points to abnormalities in immune function as this common pathology.

Table 13.1. Systemic connective tissue diseases

Systemic lupus erythematosus (SLE)

Systemic sclerosis (Scleroderma)

Arteritis
   Polyarteritis nodosa (PAN)
   Wegener's granulomatosis

Polymyositis and dermatomyositis

Sjögren's syndrome

Raynaud's syndrome

Mixed connective tissue disease (MCTD)

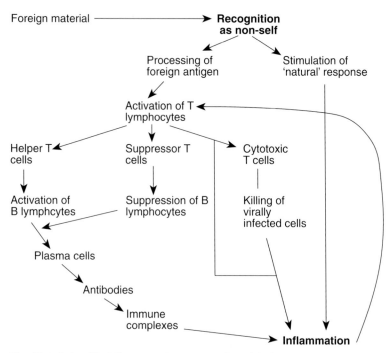

Fig. 13.1 A simplified diagrammatic representation of the immune system.

Immune system function and connective tissue disease

Immunity is usually concerned with the disposal of foreign or 'non-self' material. This involves recognition of the material, intracellular processing and stimulation of natural (usually non-specific) or adaptive (specific) responses, priming the system for future specific responses, and controlling or suppressing the response when it is no longer required (Fig. 13.1). The 'final common pathway' is the initiation of inflammation (Fig. 13.2). These processes are amplified at each step, producing an increasing cascade of response. Uncontrolled, this positive feedback system would continue to generate tissue damage after the initiating event had been dealt with, but most of the mechanisms by which the immune system 'switches off' inflammation are not understood. In connective tissue diseases immune stimulation and inflammation become chronic. This could result from a persisting stimulus from either non-self or self antigens, or from a failure in the feedback control of inflammation.

Autoantibodies

Autoantibody production is part of normal immune system function, and low levels of autoantibody are frequently found in normal individuals. In the connective tissue diseases, autoantibodies reach high titres and account for a large proportion of the circulating immunoglobulin. Of all the possible antibodies which might be produced, only a few are synthesised in excess in any one con-

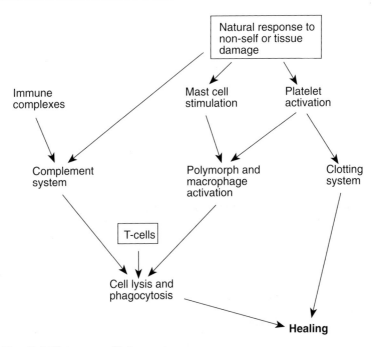

Fig. 13.2 The process of inflammation.

dition. In rheumatoid arthritis the autoantibodies are directed against the Fc portion of IgG molecules and are called rheumatoid factors. The IgM autoantibodies produced can be readily detected by their ability to stick together sheep red blood cells coated with human IgG (the sheep cell agglutination test, SCAT) or similarly coated latex beads (the latex test). IgG and IgA rheumatoid factors and other autoantibodies may be detected by an enzyme linked immunosorbant assay (ELISA) while antibodies against tissue components are frequently identified by immunofluorescent staining or immunodiffussion.

Many of the antigens have been identified. A few are nucleic acids but most are proteins, often ones which form macromolecular complexes with other proteins and nucleic acids. Scl-70, for example, is the enzyme topoisomerase I, which unwinds the supercoiled structure of DNA prior to replication or transcription.

It may be that the function of each antigen is not relevant to the pathogenesis of autoimmune disease because there is little evidence that antibodies enter cells, but these functions may throw light on aetiology. One current hypothesis is that the autoantibodies are made to react with bacterial or viral material and, almost by chance, cross-react also with various cellular components. Another postulates viral infection which renders cellular replication systems antigenic when they are complexed with viral, 'non-self' material.

SYSTEMIC LUPUS ERYTHEMATOSUS (SLE)

SLE is a relatively uncommon disorder (Table 13.2) affecting especially females during childbearing years. The pathogenesis includes the deposition

Table 13.2. Characteristics of some connective tissue diseases

	Approximate prevalence (per 1000)	Sex ratio (F: M)	Peak age of onset	Common autoantibodies*
Rheumatoid arthritis	20	3 : 1	30–50	RF 75%, ANA 10%
Systemic lupus erythematosus	1†	10 : 1	15–30	ANA 90%, dsDNA 30%, Others 25%
Systemic sclerosis	0.1	3 : 1	30–50	Scl-70 20%
Wegener's granulomatosis	<0.1	2 : 1	40–50	ANCA 80%
Sjögren's syndrome	10	9 : 1	40–50	Anti-Ro 85%, Anti-La 60%
Mixed connective tissue disease	?			RNP 100%

* RF = Rheumatoid factor;
ANA = antinuclear antibody; dsDNA = double-stranded DNA antibodies;
ANCA = anti-neutrophil cytoplasmic antibodies; RNP = Ribonucleoprotein antibodies.
†More prevalent in black and Chinese people.

Table 13.3. Systemic effects of SLE

Organ System Effects

Joints	Flitting arthralgia Persistent arthralgia Synovitis Joint destruction	Blood	Leucopenia Anaemia Thrombocytopenia Autoimmune haemolytic anaemia
Skin	Photosensitivity Hair loss Cutaneous vasculitis Nailfold capillary changes Butterfly rash	CVS	Raynaud's phenomenon Vasculitis Myocarditis Endocarditis
Kidney	Proteinuria Microscopic haematuria Hypertension Chronic renal failure Acute renal failure Nephrotic syndrome	RS	Pleurisy Pulmonary effusion Pulmonary fibrosis
		Muscles	Myositis Myopathy
CNS	Headache Psychosis Epilepsy Hemiplegia Peripheral or cranial anaemia		

of circulating immune complexes in almost any tissue, resulting in a very wide range of clinical presentations (Table 13.3). Nephritis occurs when immune complexes in the glomerular basement membrane activate complement and initiate inflammation. Deposition in blood vessel walls leads to vasculitis, which may underlie most manifestations of the disease. SLE is episodic and may be life-threatening at times. Because any organ or tissue may be involved, SLE may mimic many other diseases.

Symptoms and signs

Joint involvement (pain and/or inflammation) occurs in over 90% of cases, although joint destruction is rare. A wide variety of skin rashes and photosensitivity are common. Raynaud's phenomenon (intermittent digital artery spasm) and hair loss are also characteristic.

One of the important clinical complications is renal disease, manifest by proteinuria and microscopic haematuria. This may progress to hypertension, renal failure or nephrotic syndrome.

Other serious developments which warrant urgent treatment include cerebral vasculitis, retinal vasculitis and autoimmune haemolytic anaemia.

Investigations

The diagnosis of SLE usually requires identification of antinuclear antibodies and clinical differentiation from other connective tissue diseases. During active episodes serum complement may be reduced because of complement consumption at inflammatory sites, and complement breakdown products may be increased. Skin vasculitis may be confirmed by biopsy. Plasma viscosity or ESR will indicate an acute phase response, but C-reactive protein (CRP) levels are often not markedly elevated unless there are added complications such as infection.

Treatment

Treatment of acute episodes hinges on the use of large doses (perhaps 80 mg per 24 hours) of prednisolone and sometimes immunosuppressive drugs such as cyclophosphamide or azathioprine. In between acute episodes patients may require only analgesics or anti-inflammatory drugs, although some who have evidence of persisting disease activity may require low doses of steroids.

Prognosis

Immunosuppressive therapy has transformed the prognosis of patients with renal and widespread systemic disease and about 90% of patients seen in hospitals survive more than 10 years after diagnosis. As increasingly milder cases are now being identified this figure may increase.

SYSTEMIC SCLEROSIS (SCLERODERMA)

Systemic sclerosis (SS) is a rare disease in which there is excessive collagen deposition and fibrosis of interstitial tissues, particularly in the skin and in small arterioles where vasculitis may also develop. The nature of the underlying stimulus for excessive fibrosis is unknown. Skin lesions may be localised ('morphea'), confined to the extremities (especially when SS overlaps with other conditions), or generalised.

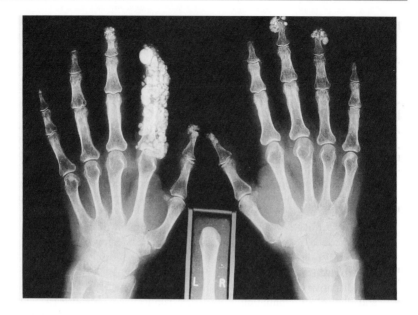

Fig. 13.3 Severe digital calcinosis. (Photograph courtesy P A Dieppe).

Symptoms and signs

Skin changes vary from a mild thickening and induration of the fingertips (sclerodactyly) to extensive involvement of the arms, face, trunk and sometimes the legs with taut, hidebound thickened skin (scleroderma), loss of skin appendages, telangiectasia, oedema, altered pigmentation, atrophy of the finger pulps and calcinosis (calcification within soft tissues) (Fig. 13.3).

Facial involvement may produce microstomia. Loss of oesophageal motility may cause difficulty in swallowing or symptoms of heartburn while pulmonary fibrosis may lead to slowly progressive dyspnoea.

Raynaud's phenomenon (Fig. 13.4), which may occur with any of the connective tissue diseases, is particularly common in SS. Sclerosis of renal arterioles may lead to hypertension and renal failure. Small bowel bacterial invasion in the immobile gut leads to malabsorption.

Investigations

There are no specific diagnostic tests for systemic sclerosis but it is often accompanied by a positive antinuclear antibody known as Scl-70.

Treatment and prognosis

There is no treatment available which can halt this process, although long periods with little deterioration or even some improvement may occur. Complications (Raynaud's, hypertension, organ failure) are managed as they occur. About half of the patients survive more than 5 years after diagnosis. Renal lesions are the most common cause of death.

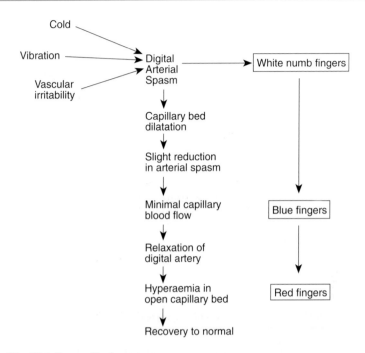

Fig. 13.4 Raynaud's phenomenon.

POLYARTERITIS NODOSA (PAN) AND WEGENER'S GRANULOMATOSIS

Inflammation in and around the blood vessel walls, particularly in arteries, can occur in all connective tissue diseases and is the main histological feature in a few. Small vessel vasculitis produces a variety of skin changes and is generally benign. Nodular areas of inflammation in medium sized arteries in PAN may cause peripheral tissue necrosis and life-threatening organ dysfunction, alleviated by high doses of steroids. The cellular inflammatory response may be so great that granulomata develop. In Wegener's granulomatosis massive tissue damage may occur in the upper or lower respiratory tract. Lesions may be confused with carcinoma on a chest X-ray. Cyclophosphamide is effective treatment. Table 13.4 indicates the usual clinical manifestations.

POLYMYOSITIS (Table 13.5)

Diffuse skeletal muscle inflammation causing weakness and pain may occur in many of the connective tissue diseases. When it predominates (which is rare) it is called 'pure' polymyositis and this may occur with particular skin changes (dermatomyositis). The pattern of progress is extremely variable ranging from rapid deterioration producing myoglobinuria and death within a few weeks to such gradual development that the patient may not notice the weakness coming on.

Diagnosis is based on muscle weakness, increased serum levels of muscle breakdown enzymes (especially creatine phosphokinase), electromyographical

Table 13.4. Systemic effects of polyarteritis nodosa (PAN) and Wegener's granulomatosis

	PAN	Wegener's granulomatosis
Joints	Joint pains	PAN plus granulomatous
Muscles	Muscle pain and tenderness	infiltration of:
Skin	Subcutaneous nodules, livideo reticularis, skin ulcers	Orbits: exophthalmos Sinuses: sinusitis
Kidney	Haematuria, proteinuria, acute and chronic renal failure, hypertension	Nose: epistaxis, saddle nose Pharynx ulceration etc. Lungs: pneumonic nodular shadowing, pleurisy, pleural effusion etc.
CNS	Peripheral neuropathy, stroke	
Blood	Anaemia, leukocytosis, raised ESR	
Heart	Aneurysm formation	
Lungs	Pulmonary infiltrates, pleurisy ± effusion	

Table 13.5. Systemic effects of polymyositis (dermatomyositis)

Skin	Various skin rashes Characteristically violaceous rash and oedema of eyelids and over heads of metacarpals 'Gottrons patches' Nail dystrophy Erythema over affected muscles
Muscles	Proximal muscle weakness and tenderness Bulbar neck and respiratory weakness Atrophy of muscles/calcification
Lungs	Aspiration pneumonia Fibrosing alveolitis
Heart	Heart failure/cardiac arrythmias
General	In older patients there may be complicating cancer(s)

evidence of muscle cell destruction and muscle biopsy. There is an increased frequency of polymyositis in patients with malignancy but most cases will not suffer from neoplasia and investigations should depend upon and be guided by other clinical evidence of malignancy.

SJÖGREN'S SYNDROME

Defective tear secretion (xerophthalmia) and salivary secretion (xerostomia) are the most obvious signs of a more general exocrine failure in some patients with a connective tissue disease or rheumatoid arthritis. This condition is called Sjögren's syndrome and is mediated by cellular inflammatory infiltrates which invade and destroy exocrine glands.

'NEW' DISEASES

Mixed connective tissue disease (MCTD). This 'overlap' syndrome combines features of SLE, scleroderma and polymyositis and has been proposed as a separate entity because of the very frequent occurrence of a particular autoantibody (against ribonulcleoprotein) which is relatively rare in other conditions. It is not yet clear whether this really does represent a separate disease.

Antiphospholipid syndrome. The identification of a circulating anticoagulant in patients with SLE (the 'lupus anticoagulant') was linked to an apparently paradoxical increase in venous and arterial thromboses and repeated abortions caused by placental infarcts. The in vitro anticoagulant effect appears to be related to a small group of antiphospholipid autoantibodies which may occur independently of SLE.

HIV infection. Some patients with AIDS (acquired immunodeficiency syndrome) develop a variety of rheumatological conditions, but it is not yet clear if HIV is directly responsible or if they represent the chance occurrence of AIDS and arthritis.

FURTHER DEVELOPMENTS IN THE IMMUNOLOGY OF CONNECTIVE TISSUE DISEASES

Enormous increases in our understanding of the cellular and molecular basis of immune system function have occurred over the last 20 years. Inhibitors and modifiers of cell interactions are now being developed as potential treatments for many illnesses which are driven by the immune system. (See Table 13.6). Basic biological investigations of immune system function will continue and their impact on connective tissue diseases in the next 10 years is likely to be through the introduction of these new therapeutic agents.

Table 13.6. Immune deficiency syndromes
These may be either primary (of unknown cause) or secondary (owing to factors like cancer, drugs, X-ray therapy or AIDS). Only the primary causes are included.

Syndrome	Clinical effects	Cause
I Hypogammaglobulinaemia Selective IgA deficiency, IgM deficiency Brutons disease (X-linked) (congenital)	Bacterial infections	Deficient antibody production
II Di George' syndrome Ataxia telangiectasia Wiscott-Aldrich syndrome	Viral infections	T cell deficiency
III Common variable immune deficiency	Childhood infections	T and B cell deficiency
IV Chronic granulomatous disease	Abscesses Chronic granulomatous infections	Myeloid cell dysfunction
Chediack-Higashi syndrome	Pneumonia	

14

INFECTIOUS DISEASES AND HIV

Stuart Glover

The pattern of infectious diseases has changed dramatically over the last 40 years in parallel with improvements in social and biomedical standards. Antibiotics have allowed better control of infection and immunisation has eradicated or reduced many common viral diseases. However, the 1980s have brought new diseases in the form of acquired immune deficiency syndrome (AIDS) while widespread international travel has introduced exotic infections.

GASTROINTESTINAL INFECTIONS

'Gastroenteritis' is a common cause of infant mortality in underdeveloped countries and a frequent cause of morbidity in the developed world. There are three clinical types:

1. food poisoning caused by the ingestion of preformed bacterial toxins and organic and inorganic chemicals
2. enteritis and enterocolitis caused by the multiplication of pathogenic microbes in the large and small bowel
3. dysentery caused by infection and mucosal invasion of the colon and rectum.

FOOD POISONING

There is rapid onset of vomiting, profuse watery diarrhoea and abdominal pain after eating contaminated food. It is often epidemic or institutional. Toxins may affect other organs, e.g. botulinum and the central nervous system (CNS); mycotoxins (mushrooms) and the liver.

The principal causative organisms are *Staphylococcus aureus*, *Clostridium perfringens* type A and *Bacillus cereus*.

Staphylococcus aureus

Heat-stable enterotoxins, types A, D and E. Infection arises from human nasal carriers. The onset is sudden after 1–6 hours' incubation with profuse salivation, vomiting, abdominal pain, and diarrhoea but no fever. It may result in severe dehydration and hypovolaemia. Treatment is supportive.

Clostridium perfringens type A

Heat-labile enterotoxin. The incubation period is 6–24 hours and there is cramping abdominal pain and diarrhoea but no fever. It is associated with reheated, previously cooked meat in institutional outbreaks.

Bacillus cereus

Two distinct toxins produce sudden onset of vomiting or a slightly delayed diarrhoea. It is associated with reheated rice.

Other causes of food poisoning include enterotoxogenic *Escherichia coli*. Other, non-microbial, causes of food poisoning include paralytic shellfish, neurotoxic shellfish, green potatoes (solanine), uncooked red kidney beans and monosodium glutamate (Chinese restaurant syndrome).

ENTERITIS/ENTEROCOLITIS

There are two major mechanisms of disease production:

1. Enteroinvasive: bacteria invade and damage the mucosa of the small intestine, e.g. *Shigella* spp, *Campylobacter jejuni*, *Salmonella* spp, enteroinvasive *E. coli* and *Yersinia enterocolitica*.
2. Damage to enterocytes and brush border, e.g. viruses (Rotavirus, Norwalk, SRSV), protozoa (*Giardia intestinalis*, *Cryptosporidium* spp).

Enteritis caused by invasive micro-organisms can be complicated by bacteraemia if the inoculum of micro-organisms is large, in patients with impaired gastric acid secretion (pernicious anaemia, post gastrectomy, H_2-blocker therapy) and in neutropenia.

Symptoms

Enteroinvasive
The incubation period is 1–5 days. The patient is febrile and has colicky abdominal pain with diarrhoea containing blood and pus. The duration of the illness is 5–7 days.

Surface damage
1. Viral gastroenteritis occurs in children under 2 years of age with a winter onset. There is fever, vomiting, diarrhoea and upper respiratory tract symptoms.
2. Protozoal infestation leads to loose, offensive diarrhoea, steatorrhoea, anorexia, weightloss and malabsorption. Abdominal pain occurs with distension and borborygmi, flatulence and eructation but no fever.

DYSENTERY

Microbial infection of the colon and rectum is characterised by frequent, small-volume stools containing blood and pus. Causative microbes include *Shigella* spp, *Campylobacter* spp, *Salmonella* spp, *Y. enterocolitica*, *E. coli* 0157, H7, *Clostridium difficile*, *Entamoeba histolytica* and cytomegalovirus (CMV) in HIV disease.

Some of these micro-organisms also infect the small intestine and may produce enterotoxins in addition to infecting the colon and rectum.

Symptoms

There is fever, abdominal pain, small-volume but frequent stools which may contain blood, mucus and pus. Systemic invasion may occur in predisposed patients.

Investigation of gastroenteritis (See Table 14.1)

The epidemiology of gastroenteritis: type of food ingested, foreign travel, sexual orientation, occupation, animal exposure, contact history, recreational history, any predisposing medical conditions or recent antibiotic ingestion.

Differential diagnosis (See Table 14.2)

Table 14.1. Investigation of gastroenteritis

Stool sample	Leukocytes, ova, cysts, parasites, & blood	Enteritis; dysentery Protozoans—*Giardia*, *Cryptosporidium*
	Modified acid-fast stain	*Cryptosporidium*
	Culture	Bacteria
	Cold enrichment	*Yersinia*
	Electron microscopy	Rotavirus
	ELISA	Rotavirus
	Toxin detection	*Clostridium difficile*
Sigmoidoscopy	Rectal biopsy	Amoebiasis cytomegalovirus, schistosomiasis, inflammatory bowel disease
Blood cultures		Systemic disease, e.g. salmonellosis
Serial serology		*Yersinia*, schistosomiasis
Radiology	Straight abdominal films	Toxic megacolon Colonic thrumbprinting, ischaemic colitis etc.
Duodenal aspiration		Protozoans—*Giardia*, *Cryptosporidium*, *Strongyloides*
Small bowel biopsy	Per-endoscope or Crosby capsule	Coeliac disease, Whipple's disease

NB Barium enema studies are contraindicated in infective gastroenteritis.

Table 14.2. The differential diagnosis of enteritis and dysentery

Enteritis	Dysentery
Early appendicitis Irritable bowel syndrome	Inflammatory bowel disease (Crohn's disease, ulcerative colitis)
Small bowel disease (coeliac disease, Whipple's disease)	Diverticular disease Colonic neoplasms
Chronic laxative abuse	Villous adenoma of rectum Ischaemic colitis

Table 14.3. Antibiotic treatment of gastroenteritis

Food poisoning	Not indicated
Toxin-induced diarrhoea	Not indicated
Vibrio cholerae	Tetracycline, ampicillin, quinolone
Shigella spp	Ampicillin, trimethoprim, quinolone
Salmonella spp	Quinolone, ampicillin, cotrimoxazole
Campylobacter jejunei	Quinolone, erythromycin
Yersinia spp	Chloramphenicol, quinolone, aminoglycoside, tetracycline, cotrimoxazole
Clostridium difficile	Vancomycin, metronidazole
Amoeba histolytica	Metronidazole
Giardia intestinalis	Metronidazole
Cryptosporidium spp	?Spiramycin

Treatment

Rehydration is by mouth with the glucose electrolyte solution 'dioralyte' and by intravenous fluids: NaCl with K supplements.

Most infective gastroenteritis is self limiting and requires no specific antimicrobial therapy. Predisposing factors require the early pre-emptive use of antibiotics (Table 14.3).

Anti-diarrhoeal agents are best avoided, and spread is prevented by hygienic disposal of faeces and by handwashing.

In the UK, the Medical Officer of Environmental Health or C.C.D.C. should be notified.

Prognosis

Toxin-induced diarrhoea is a major cause of infantile death in preschool children in the underdeveloped world. Death is caused by dehydration.

Food poisoning rarely causes death. Botulism (see p. 155) and mushroom poisoning, although rare, have a very high mortality.

Enteritis and dysentery may be complicated by dehydration, prerenal renal failure, acute tubular necrosis, septicaemia and metastatic abscesses, including mycotic aneurysms. Toxic dilatation of the colon and colonic perforation can occur. There may be reactive arthritis (Reiter's syndrome) especially after *Shigella*, *Salmonella*, *Yersinia* and occasionally *Campylobacter* infections.

FEVER AND RASH

The presence of fever and a skin rash often indicates an underlying infectious disease but may also be a sign of an important non-infective disease. Diagnosis is dependant on the type of skin lesions present, their number and distribution. Assessment of lymphadenopathy, respiratory signs and travel history and further clues.

ERYTHEMATOUS RASHES (sunburn, red skin, blanches on pressure)

Scarlet fever

An acute streptococcal infection caused by erythrotoxin-producing strains, scarlet fever is acquired from a carrier or a case of streptococcal infection. The primary site of infection is the oropharynx, wounds, burns or the female genital tract.

Symptoms and signs
Sore throat, neck pain, fever, headache and myalgia are the symptoms of scarlet fever.

The signs are exudative tonsillitis, cervical lymphadenopathy, a red tongue with large papillae (raspberry tongue) or a coated tongue with protruding papillae (strawberry tongue), erythematous rash and circumoral pallor.

The skin desquamates at end of the first week.

Investigations
A throat or wound swab should be taken for culture.

Serology will show raised anti-streptolysin-O (ASO) and anti-deoxyribonuclease B (ADB) levels. White cell count will demonstrate leukocytosis and occasionally eosinophilia.

Treatment
Benzylpenicillin i.v. followed by phenoxymethylpenicillin to complete 10 days. Erythromycin is an alternative for those allergic to penicillins. The patient must be isolated at the outset.

Prognosis
The prognosis is excellent. Suppurative complications (peritonsillar abscess, retropharyngeal abscess, acute sinusitis, otitis media, pneumonia) are now rare.

Non-suppurative complications include acute rheumatic fever, acute glomerulonephritis, erythema nodosum and Henoch–Schönlein purpura.

Differential diagnosis

Common conditions include viral pharyngitis (adenovirus, influenza, enteroviruses, EBV, CMV, measles), *Mycoplasma pneumoniae* and *Candida*.

Uncommon conditions are diphtheria, secondary syphilis, angina of agranulocytosis and gonorrhoea.

Erythema infectiosum (Fifth disease, slapped cheek syndrome)

This is caused by parvovirus B19 and is an epidemic febrile illness of school children and young adults. There is a maculopapular rash which may recur together with flushed cheeks. Large joint arthritis is found in 10% of children and >50% of adults. Erythema infectiosum causes aplastic crises in chronic haemolytic disease, e.g. Sickle cell disease, and it mimics rubella. It is diagnosed serologically using radioimmunoassay or ELISA. There is no specific therapy. The prognosis is excellent but it may cause intrauterine infections leading to hydrops fetalis.

Erythema chronicum migrans (ECM)

ECM is the classic initial manifestation of Lyme disease, a systemic infection caused by the spirochaete *Borrelia burgdorferi*, which is transmitted by the tick *Ixodes*.

ECM is a large, erythematous, macular lesion spreading to 15–20 cm in diameter. The outer margin is bright and raised with central clearing. It spreads centrifugally and is associated with malaise, headache, myalgia, fever and lymphadenopathy. Later features of Lyme disease include neurological disease (meningitis, encephalitis, cranial neuropathies, motor and sensory radiculopathy), arthritis and cardiac disease (heart block).

Treatment is with tetracycline, penicillin or ceftriaxone.

Toxic shock syndrome

This is caused by the effects of an exotoxin produced by phage group 1 *Staphylococcus aureus*. It most often occurs in menstruating young women who are using tampons but can occur in either sex in association with focal staphylococcal sepsis. Onset is abrupt.

Symptoms and signs

Fever, with a temperature of 38.9°C or more, diffuse macular erythema are the main manifestations. Desquamation, especially of the palms and soles, occurs 1–2 weeks after the onset of illness. Hypotension occurs, with a systolic blood pressure of <90 mmHg and an orthostatic drop in diastolic pressure of >15 mmHg.

Multisystem involvement includes vomiting, diarrhoea and raised bilirubin, ALT and AST levels. There may be severe myalgia and a raised CPK level. The mucous membranes of the vagina, oropharynx and conjunctivae may be hyperaemic. Pyuria occurs and the urea and creatinine levels can be raised. Platelets are often <100 000 and the patient may be disorientated or have altered consciousness without focal neurological signs.

Investigations
Swab or culture for *Staph. aureus* is necessary.

Differential diagnosis
Streptococcal toxic shock syndrome, measles, rubella, leptospirosis, rickettsial infections, scarlet fever.

Management
Supportive measures include the administration of i.v. fluids, removal of the tampon and drainage of focal sepsis. Parentral flucloxacillin or vancomycin may be necessary.

Prognosis
The mortality rate is 3%, and there is a recurrence rate of 20% with subsequent menses.

Kawasaki syndrome (Mucocutaneous lymph node syndrome)
Kawasaki syndrome has an unknown aetiology and affects mainly children under 15 years. The pathology reveals a diffuse vasculitis, especially of the coronary arteries.

Symptoms and signs
Usually there is a fever lasting more than 5 days, bilateral conjunctival hyperaemia, dry red fissured lips, injected oropharynx and a strawberry tongue. The palms and soles are red with oedema leading to periungual desquamation. A polymorphic, erythematous, morbilliform rash, occurs. There may also be cervical lymphadenopathy and, occasionally, meningitis and diarrhoea.

Investigations
A full blood count will show mild anaemia, leukocytosis, thrombocytosis and, in convalescence, a neutropenia. The ESR is raised. Serial echocardiograms are required.

Treatment
This is with high dose aspirin, initially 80–100 mg/kg per 24 hours for 14 days, then 3–5 mg/kg aspirin for 8 weeks. Human non-specific immunoglobulin 400 mg/kg per 24 hours is given for 4 days. Corticosteroids should be avoided.

Prognosis
Arthralgia occurs in 30% at 2–3 weeks. Coronary artery dilatation and aneurysm formation develops in 20%, and the overall mortality is 5–10%.

Differential diagnosis
Scarlet fever, staphylococcal and streptococcal toxic shock syndrome, rickettsial infection, measles, leptospirosis, Stevens-Johnson syndrome, systemic lupus erythematosus (SLE), polyarteritis nodosa and juvenile rheumatoid arthritis, should be considered.

MACULOPAPULAR RASHES AND FEVER

Measles

This is an acute febrile exanthematous disease of childhood caused by an RNA paramyxovirus. It is highly contagious and is spread by droplet inhalation. The incubation period is 10–17 days.

Symptoms and signs
In the prodromal phase, fever, malaise, coryza and cough are present.

A brick-red, confluent macular rash spreads from the head and face to the neck, trunk and limbs (See Plate 1). The skin may also be oedematous. It is followed by fine desquamation. Koplik spots are seen on the buccal mucosa and may occur before the skin rash.

Marked conjunctivitis, coryza and irritability occur.

Investigations
Viral culture of throat washings and paired serology are indicated.

Differential diagnosis
Scarlet fever, toxic shock syndrome and severe rubella should be excluded.

Treatment
Antibiotics are used only if there is secondary bacterial infection.

Prevention. Active immunisation is with live attenuated measles vaccine, usually as part of MMR (measles, mumps, rubella vaccine). Passive immunisation in immunocompromised, non-immune patients is with human non-specific immunoglobulin.

Prognosis
Death from pneumonia and encephalitis are now rare but measles remains a major contributory factor in the death of the malnourished. Here septic complications, e.g. otitis media, mastoiditis, pneumonia and bronchitis, are common. Measles may also cause obstructive laryngitis and croup. Acute measles post infectious encephalitis is sometimes seen, as is subacute sclerosing panencephalitis (SSPE).

Rubella ('German measles')

This is an acute febrile exanthematous disease caused by an RNA togavirus. It is found worldwide causing mild febrile illness with a faint rash. Spread is by respiratory droplets and the incubation period is 14–23 days.

Symptoms and signs
There is a mild short-lived prodromal fever with occipital headache, sore throat and gritty eyes with conjunctivitis. Suboccipital and posterior auricular lymphadenopathy develop. The rash comprises pink macules on the face and trunk and fades within 3 days without desquamation.

Investigations

Paired serology: rubella haemagglutination inhibition test should be performed and rubella-specific IgM, should be sought.

Differential diagnosis

Other viral infections, e.g. adenovirus, enteroviruses (Coxsackie and Echoviruses), parvovirus B19, mild measles and scarlet fever.

Treatment

This is symptomatic only. Prevention is by active immunisation using a live attenuated vaccine (MMR).

Prognosis

The prognosis is usually excellent but complications include arthralgia and occasional large joint arthritis in adult females, thrombocytopenia and encephalitis in 1 in 6000.

Congenital rubella syndrome

Infection with rubella in the first trimester of pregnancy puts the fetus at risk of developing rubella syndrome. There can be multiple congenital defects, especially of the eyes and heart, together with deafness and psychomotor retardation. Viral infection of the liver, heart, lungs and brain may be persistent.

Enteroviral exanthem

These febrile rashes are caused by various members of the enterovirus group, e.g. Coxsackie A and B, and echoviruses. Enteroviral rashes are variable in extent and distribution, are non-pruritic, do not desquamate and heal without discoloration.

Other features include enantham (herpangina, ulcers on faces and palate, lymphadenopathy and lymphocytic ('aseptic') meningitis.

Investigations comprise isolation of the virus from the throat, stools and CSF, and also paired serology.

PETECHIA AND PURPURIC RASHES

Meningococcaemia

Neisseria meningitidis can cause a transient bacteraemia or septicaemia, with or without meningitis. Chronic meningococcaemia may rarely occur in a relatively well patient. Meningococcaemia can be a rapid and fulminant infection characterised by a spreading purpuric rash, shock, disseminated intravascular coagulation (DIC) and adrenal haemorrhage with acute adrenal failure (Waterhouse-Friderichsen syndrome).

Symptoms and signs

There may be severe myalgia and chills of sudden onset. The rash has a centrifugal distribution affecting the wrists, palms, lower legs, ankles and the soles of the feet. It is initially petechial or macular but rapidly expands to become purpuric or ecchymotic.

The patients may be febrile or hypothermic and can be extremely ill with hypotension and oliguria.

Investigations
These include blood cultures, microscopy and culture of CSF and counterimmunoelectrophoresis (CIE) of serum for meningococcal antigen.

Differential diagnosis
Gonococcaemia is associated with tenosynovitis, acral pustular or papular rash and arthritis. Bacteraemia may be caused by *Strep. pneumoniae* (asplenic patients), *Haemophilus influenzae* or *Staph. aureus*. In Rickettsial infection, there is often a history of contact with brushwoods and dog ticks or North American travel.

Infectious mononucleosis, rubella and measles with thrombocytopenia, infective endocarditis and fat embolism should also be excluded.

Treatment
Penicillin-G i.v. 1.2 g 3-hourly for 7–10 days or cefotaxime is appropriate, and if there is a history of penicillin allergy chloramphenicol should be given.

The patient should be isolated for the first 24 hours of treatment.

Prevention in contacts is with rifampicin, ciprofloxacin and meningococcal vaccine type A, C and W135.

Prognosis
Meningitis mortality is 2–10% but in septicaemia without meningitis it is 30%. Complications include cranial neuropathy, deafness, metastatic sepsis and immune complex mediated arthritis, iritis and pericarditis.

BULLOUS AND POX-LIKE RASHES

Varicella

The primary infection is chickenpox, a mild childhood illness but severe in immunocompromised patients and some adults, caused by the DNA-containing human (alpha) herpes virus 3 or varicella zoster virus (VZV). It is spread by droplets from human to human and the incubation period is 14–18 days. VZV becomes latent in the dorsal root ganglia of sensory nerves; reactivation presents as shingles in later life or if the patient becomes immuncompromised.

Symptoms and signs
There is a prodrome with fever, headache, malaise and a sore throat.

The rash comprises crops of rapidly evolving macules and papules which develop into vesicles and pustules with crusting (see Plate 2). They first appear on the trunk, face and proximal limbs, and may be itchy. There may be mouth ulcers (enanthem).

Investigations

The diagnosis is usually clinically obvious and no investigations are required. However, electron microscopy of vesicle fluid may reveal the virus, and there is a complement fixation test for VZV.

Differential diagnosis

This includes Kaposi's varicelliform eruption (herpes simplex infection of eczematous skin), cow pox (cattle, cat contact) and monkey pox (West and Central Africa).

Treatment

Acyclovir is rarely indicated for chickenpox in children, being limited to complicated cases and the immunocompromised. Varicella zoster immune globulin (VZIG), given within 96 hours of exposure to varicella or zoster, may prevent or attenuate the disease in susceptible close contacts. It is indicated for newborn children of mothers who develop chickenpox 6 days prior to or within 48 hours of delivery.

Prognosis

Chickenpox is rarely fatal but visceral dissemination, including varicella pneumonia and lymphocytic meningitis can occur, as can haemorrhagic chickenpox (in immunocompromised patients and in those with HIV disease). In children, Reye's disease may follow varicella.

OTHER INFECTIOUS DISEASES

Diphtheria

This is an acute infection by virulent *Corynebacterium diphtheriae* of the throat and upper respiratory tract. It is rare in countries such as Great Britain where children are usually immunized. The bacterium produces a toxin which can cause severe damage to the heart and nervous system.

Symptoms and signs

After an incubation period of 1–7 days, sore throat and malaise are the usual symptoms with dysphagia.

Signs include a greyish adherent membrane in the tonsillar area and pharynx. The membrane bleeds when attempts are made to remove it. There is often considerable oedema locally and of the neck.

Symptoms and signs are different when the nasal mucosa is affected; then there is usually a bloodstained nasal discharge only.

Diagnosis

The disease must always be suspected when there is a membranous pharyngitis, and it can be confirmed by isolation of *C. diphtheriae* from the pharynx or nose. Growth on Löffler's medium produces satisfactory results.

Complications

An acute cardiomyopathy with tachycardia, hypotension and ECG changes may develop in the second week. This can be fatal.

Respiratory obstruction is caused by mechanical obstruction of the larynx by membrane, and it may require tracheostomy.

A neuropathy affecting the ocular, bulbar and peripheral nerves may occur 2–10 weeks after the onset of illness. Respiratory involvement may require assisted ventilation. Gradual recovery is the rule.

Treatment

Antitoxin is given if the disease is suspected, 10–80 000 units, provided there is no reaction to an initial subcutaneous dose of 0.2 ml.

Penicillin and erythromycin help to eradicate the infection and prevent toxin formation. Throat swabs should be taken from close contacts and their state of immunity to the disease assessed. Penicillin or erythromycin is given to non-immune subjects who should also be vaccinated.

Whooping cough (pertussis)

This is a highly infectious disease caused by *Bordetella pertussis*. It causes a lower respiratory tract infection in childhood. Epidemics occur every 4 years or so in the UK and are encountered in areas of poor uptake of protective immunisation. It is seen most commonly in the under 5-year-olds and is more serious in infants.

Symptoms and signs

After an incubation period of 7–10 days there is an initial coryza followed by a cough which becomes severe, paroxysmal and accompanied by vomiting. The coughing paroxysm is often worse nocturnally and causes cyanosis. A whoop is the noise produced by inspiration following a paroxysm of coughing. The cough interrupts sleeping and eating and renders the affected child helpless.

Signs are few and are the result of pulmonary complications like pneumonia and pulmonary collapse. Occasionally subconjunctival haemorrhages or a frenal ulcer are found.

Investigations

A blood count shows a profound lymphocytosis. A bacteriological diagnosis can be obtained using nasal swabs.

Complications

These are serious and include pneumonia and lung collapse from secondary bacterial infection and mucus plugging, cerebral anoxia from prolonged coughing spasms which may cause fits and cerebral damage, and considerable weightloss because of vomiting and poor feeding.

Treatment

Careful nursing and frequent feeding are supplemented where necessary with antibiotic treatment of pneumonia. Control of paroxysms of coughing may be helped by cough suppressants but support and reassurance of the child are more helpful.

Prevention

A vaccine is protective (80%) but uptake has been impaired by problems arising from post-vaccination fits and occasional cases of encephalitis. The disease continues to be serious—400 deaths per year which could be prevented.

Mumps

This inflammatory disease is caused by a paramyxovirus infection leading to an acute painful inflammation of the parotid and occasionally other salivary glands.

Symptoms and signs

After an incubation period of 18–21 days there is severe malaise and fever, and tenderness in the neck and parotid glands (see Plate 3).

Signs include enlargement of parotid glands which obliterate the angle of the mandible, occasional painful enlargement of other salivary glands, e.g. submandibular, and a dry mouth with inflamed orifices of the parotid ducts.

Complications

Orchitis is seen in 20% of male sufferers. It may precede parotid involvement and lead to diagnostic confusion. Ophöritis in women is extremely rare.

CNS involvement (meningitis and encephalitis) is the most important complication. The former is much more common than the latter and encephalitis carries a mortality of 2–3%.

Pancreatitis (acute) is an occasional complication.

Diagnosis and treatment

The diagnosis is essentially clinical, but the virus can be isolated from throat washings and saliva, and antibody elevation can be detected. Treatment is supportive only, which includes oral hygiene, a soft diet etc.

Prevention

This is by vaccination which is usually given with measles and rubella vaccine (MMR) at the age of 18 months to 2 years.

Glandular fever (infectious mononucleosis)

This is a disease of predominantly young adults probably caused by the Epstein-Barr (EB) virus. Exact mode of transmission is uncertain but is probably by aerosol. Traditionally thought to be spread by kissing, there is little evidence to support this.

Symptoms and signs

Most infections are subclinical. In those with symptoms there may be fever, malaise, sore throat and cervical lymphadenopathy. A transient rash is seen in some patients and up to 50% have splenomegaly. Very rarely the spleen may rupture and cause death. Occasionally meningitis, encephalitis, myocarditis and pneumonitis occur but most patients recover fully in a few weeks.

Diagnosis
Diagnosis is made clinically but can be confirmed by the Paul-Bunell test. There is usually an increased mononuclear white cell count and there may be a modest thrombocytopenia.

Treatment
Most cases pass off untreated. With systemic involvement steroids may be used and acyclovir may help. There may be a reaction to amoxycillin and ampicillin and these antibiotics must never be used.

In a few cases infectious mononucleosis persists as a debilitating illness for a year or more.

HIV INFECTION AND AIDS

In 1981, the occurrence of *Pneumocystis carinii* pneumonia (PCP) and Kaposi's sarcoma (KS) in apparently immunocompetent homosexuals heralded the current pandemic of HIV infection and its ultimate sequela, acquired immune deficiency syndrome (AIDS). By 1983 the cause was identified as a human retrovirus, human immunodeficiency virus (HIV), which causes a progressive impairment of cell-mediated immunity. The resultant severe immunocompromise leads to many opportunistic infections, neoplastic growths and premature death.

HIV infection is pandemic but most prevalent in North, Central and South America, the Caribbean, Tropical Africa and South East Asia. It occurs in homosexual and bisexual males, i.v. drug abusers (IVDA), heterosexual contacts of infected patients, children born to infected females and recipients of infected blood and blood products, particularly in haemophiliacs.

HIV infection is spread by the venereal route, blood and blood product infusions, close contact with body fluids, and by blood-contaminated needles and syringes. It is not spread by ordinary social or domestic contact.

The incubation period is variable. The time from infection to detection of the antibody to HIV is 1–3 months. The time from infection to development of an AIDS-defining infection or tumour is 2 months to more than 10 years. Patients are infectious to others throughout but may be more so in the acute early stage and in the terminal stages of AIDS.

Pathology
HIV preferentially infects cells expressing the CD4 epitope, the T helper cell identity molecule. CD4-positive macrophages and monocytes are also susceptible to HIV infection. The CD4-positive lymphocytes are gradually and progressively depleted (Fig. 14.1).

Clinical classification
The Centers for Disease Control (CDC) classifies HIV infection as:

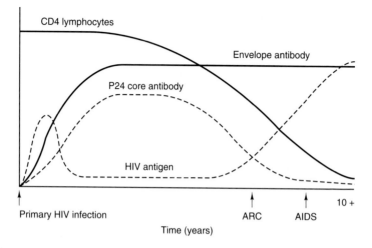

Fig. 14.1. Typical course of HIV infection.

Group I   Acute HIV infection
Group II   Asymptomatic
Group III   Progressive generalised lymphadenopathy
Group IV   Other diseases
Subgroup A Constitutional (Aids-related complex or ARC)
          B Neurologic
          C Infectious diseases
          D Secondary cancers
          E Other conditions

Group I (acute HIV infection)

Acute illness may occur within 2–3 weeks of primary exposure to HIV, presenting as either an acute infectious mononucleosis type illness or as an acute neurological disease (meningitis, meningoencephalitis, polyneuropathy).

Symptoms and signs
Fever, sweats, rigors, myalgia, arthralgia, headache, malaise, neck stiffness and sore throat may all be present as may lymphadenopathy, splenomegaly, pharyngeal erythema, palatal ulceration and a macular erythematous rash on the trunk.

Investigations
HIV antigenaemia (P24) is the investigation of choice but HIV antibodies remain the standard test now. Lymphopenia with normal CD4/CD8 ratio,

thrombocytopenia, atypical lymphocytes in blood film, mild liver dysfunction and CSF lymphocytosis may be present.

Differential diagnosis
EBV, CMV, toxoplasmosis, *Treponema pallidum*, rubella, HSV, hepatitis B and other causes of lymphocytic meningitis.

Treatment
Treatment is symptomatic.

Prognosis
Resolution is within 2–3 weeks. Lymphadenopathy, splenomegaly, lethargy, myalgia and fever may last several months. Patients remain HIV-infected for life ultimately with the development of AIDS.

Group II (asymptomatic HIV-seropositive)

This group is characterised by the absence of symptoms and signs of HIV infection. However, identifiable leukopenia, thrombocytopenia and diminished CD4 count may be present.

Group III (progressive generalised lymphadenopathy)

This group is defined as the presence of palpable lymphadenopathy at two or more extra-inguinal sites, persisting for more than 3 months, in the absence of other illness or condition which could explain the findings.

Pathology
Follicular hyperplasia develops early in HIV infection often within months of seroconversion.

Differential diagnosis
Lymphadenopathic Kaposi's sarcoma, Hodgkin's lymphoma, non-Hodgkin's lymphoma, toxoplasmosis, *Mycobacterium avium* complex infection, PCP, angioimmunoblastic lymphadenopathy.

Group IV

This is subdivided into:

Subgroup A (constitutional symptoms (aids-related complex)). One or more of the following will be present: fever for longer than 1 month, weightloss of more than 10% of initial bodyweight, diarrhoea for longer than 1 month, the absence of a concurrent illness or condition other than HIV infection.

Subgroup B (neurologic disease). For the CDC classification the indicated diseases are dementia, myelopathy and peripheral neuropathy.

Subgroup C1 (secondary infectious diseases). PCP, cryptosporidiosis, toxoplasmosis, extraintestinal strongyloidiasis, isosporiasis, candidiasis (oesophageal, bronchial, pulmonary), cryptococcus, histoplasmosis, mycobacterial infection *(MAC, M. Kansasii)*, CMV, severe herpes simplex virus infection, progressive multifocal leukoencephalopathy (polyoma JC virus).

Subgroup C2 (oral hairy leukoplakia). Polydermatomal HVZ, recurrent *Salmonella* bacteraemia, nocardiosis, tuberculosis, oral candidiasis.

Subgroup D (secondary cancers). Kaposi's sarcoma, non-Hodgkin's lymphoma, primary lymphoma of the brain.

Subgroup E (other conditions). Chronic lymphoid interstitial pneumonitis, infectious diseases not listed in subgroup 4C, neoplasms not listed in subgroup 4D.

Treatment of HIV infection and its complications (See Table 14.4)

Specific anti-HIV therapy. Azidothymidine (AZT, Retrovir) is introduced when CD4 <500 mm. Dideoxyinosine (DDI) is still on trial.

Prophylaxis against opportunistic infection. PCP is prevented with inhaled pentamidine, monthly and oral cotrimoxazole, daily. Acyclovir will prevent HSV and HVZ infections.
   Candidiasis is controlled with topical nystatin/amphotericin or oral-fluconazole.

Table 14.4. Treatment of opportunistic infections

PCP*	High-dose cotrimoxazole, i.v. corticosteroids
Tuberculosis	Rifampicin± isoniazid± pyrazinamide± ethambutol
MAI	Ciprofloxacin + clofazimine + rifabutin + amikacin
Cat scratch disease (Bacillary epithelioid angiomatosis)	Erythromycin
Syphilis	Penicillin
Cytomegalovirus*	i.v. ganciclovir,: i.v. foscarnet
Fungi—disseminated*	i.v. amphotericin ± flucytosine, itraconazole
Salmonellosis*	Ciprofloxacin
Giardiasis	Metranidazole
Isosporiasis*	Cotrimoxazole
Cryptosporidiosis	Nothing effective, ?spiramycin
Toxoplasmosis*	Sulphadiazine + pyrimethamine

* Many opportunistic infections require long-term therapy to prevent relapse.

Other clinical manifestations of HIV infection (See Tables 14.5, 14.6, 14.7, 14.8 and 14.9.)

Treatment of HIV-related Kaposi's sarcoma

Local therapy comprises radiation (800 cGy single dose), cryotherapy (liquid N_2), and intralesional chemotherapy (Vinblastine).

Systemic therapy is with vincristine, vinblastine, etoposide (VP16), adriamycin and bleomycin or alpha-interferon.

Table 14.5. HIV infection and the respiratory tract

Disease	Clinical manifestation	Chest X-ray
Pneumocystis carinii pneumonia (PCP)	Chronic pneumonia cough, dyspnoea, fever, cyanosis	Normal, focal infiltrate, interstitial infiltrate
Mycobacerium tuberculosis early	Cough, fever	Upper lobe (alveolar infiltrate)
Late	Cough, fever	Hilar, non-alveolar Mediastinal lympha-denopathy
Atypical	Cough, fever, weightloss	Diffuse interstitial infiltrate or normal
Viral CMV	Cough, fever	Interstitial infiltrate
Fungi *(Aspergillus, Cryptococcus, Histoplasma)*	Fever	Diffuse, nodular infiltrate Single nodules
Pyogenic bacteria *(Strep. pyogenes, Staph. aureus, Haemophilus, Branhamella, Legionella)*	Cough, fever, pleuritic pain	Consolidation Pleural effusion
Kaposi's sarcoma		Nodular infiltrate Pleural effusion Lymphadenopathy
Lymphoma	Fever, weightloss	Pleural effusion
Chronic lymphoid interstitial	Cough, dyspnoea	Interstitial infiltrate

Table 14.6. Dermatological manifestations of HIV infection

Infectious disorders

Bacterial	*Staph. aureus*—bullous impetigo, ecthyma, folliculitis, hidradenitis, abscess, cellulitis Primary and secondary syphilis Bacillary epithelioid angiomatosis (cat scratch bacillus *Afipia felis*)
Viral	Chronic persistent HSV, I and II Recurrent polydermatomal VZV (shingles) Molluscum contagiosum—pox virus Warts—human papilloma virus
Mycobacteria (atypical)	Ulceration Pustules, nodules—M.A.I.
Fungi (yeasts)	Intertrigo—Tinea Chronic fungal paronychia Nodules, pustules of systemic fungal infection Seborrhoeic dermatitis Ectoparasites—Scabies
Non-infective disorders	Drug eruptions Kaposi's sarcoma

Table 14.7. Gastrointestinal disease and HIV infection

Mouth	Oropharyngeal candidiasis Herpes simplex, herpes varicella zoster, hairy leukoplakia Papilloma virus, periodontitis, gingivitis, recurrent aphthous ulcers, Kaposi's sarcoma, non-Hodgkin's lymphoma
Oesophagus (dysphagia, pain on swallowing)	Candidiasis, herpes simplex, CMV
Stomach	Kaposi's sarcoma, non-Hodgkin's lymphoma
Hepatobiliary disease	Acalculous cholecystitis, gangrenous cholecystitis, granulomatous hepatitis, TB, chronic hepatitis B, sclerosing cholangitis (*Cryptosporidium*), hepatitis C

Table 14.8. Bowel disease and HIV infection

Malabsorption, diarrhoea, abdominal pain ± fever	*Salmonella, Shigella, Campylobacter* *Giardia intestinalis, Isospora belli, Cryptosporidium* Microsporidiosis, encephalitozoon CMV *Mycobacterium avium* *Strongyloides* AIDS enteropathy
Proctocolitis, diarrhoea ± blood and slime, fever	CMV colitis, herpes simplex, *Chlamydia, Cryptosporidium*, M.A.I., *Entamoeba histolytica*, rectal gonorrhoea, *Treponema pallidum*

Table 14.9. CNS manifestations of HIV infection

Brain	Primary HIV infection—Meningoencephalitis AIDS dementia complex Opportunistic CNS Infection: *Toxoplasma gondii* encephalitis Cryptococcal meningitis Progressive multifocal leukoencephalitis (polyoma JC virus) Herpes simplex encephalitis Fungal abscess Neurosyphilis *Mycobacterium tuberculosis* tuberculoma CMV ventriculitis Neoplasms Primary CNS lymphoma Metastatic lymphoma Kaposi's sarcoma Stroke Disease Embolic—marantic endocarditis Thrombotic—vasculitis, lupus anticoagulant Haemorrhagic—thrombocytopenia
Spinal cord	Vacuolar myelopathy—sensory disturbance, gait instability, hyperflexia Acute Myelopathy—lymphomatous compression, TB spinal abscess, herpes zoster myelitis
Peripheral nerves	Distal symmetric polyneuropathy—sensory glove/stocking numbness, paraesthesiae, dysaesthesiae (late onset) Inflammatory neuropathies—early onset, patchy motor and sensory Lumbosacral polyradiculopathy—CMV
Muscle	Polymyositis—proximal muscles, wasting, marked fatigue, pain AZT Related—rare

15

GENITOURINARY MEDICINE

Althea J. Scott, Patrick K. Taylor

Sexually transmitted diseases (STD) are conditions transmitted during sexual intercourse or close sexual contact. The scope of genitourinary (GU) medicine has expanded to include several other conditions not necessarily sexually transmitted. Despite worldwide increases in many of these diseases, the position in the UK remains fairly satisfactory, mainly because of the service established in 1917 as a result of the Venereal Diseases Regulations Act. Unlike most other hospital departments, patients may attend without a referral letter and confidentiality is still legally enforced under the updated 1974 Act.

The spectrum of disease has shifted from bacterial to viral infections and Figure 15.1 indicates current proportions of disease seen. Changing disease patterns are regularly monitored by the Department of Health. Partner notification (contact tracing) remains an important control aspect of asymptomatic carriers within the sexually active population. This situation is well known regarding the bacterial and venereal diseases but has only more recently been recognised in relation to chlamydial and wart virus infections, currently major causes of concern.

Control of all these diseases depends upon good medical management, including accurate diagnosis, effective treatment and follow-up, contact tracing and a period of sexual abstinence during treatment.

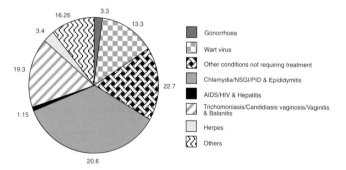

Fig. 15.1 Approximate proportions of disease seen in genitourinary clinics.

Table 15.1. Common causes of vaginal discharge

Physiological	Sexual stimulation, ectropion
Traumatic	
Physical	Self inflicted
Chemical	Douching
Infective	*Candida**, *Trichomonas**, *Gardnerella**, gonorrhoea, non-specific, puerperal, atrophic vaginitis, retained tampon
Candida often secondary to pregnancy, diabetes, antibiotics	
Neoplastic	
Benign	Polyp
Malignant	Carcinoma of cervix or corpus uteri

* The three commonest causes are summarized in Table 15.2.

VAGINAL DISCHARGE

Vaginal discharge is the most commonly presenting complaint in women. Investigation is by taking triple swabs in relevant transport media. A high vaginal specimen alone will readily identify the common causes of vaginitis (Table. 15.1) but an endocervical specimen is necessary to detect both gonorrhoea and chlamydia. Both organisms responsible also colonise the urethra and specimens from this site significantly increase pick up rates. Where the history is unclear or urinary pathology suspected a midstream specimen of urine (MSU) is of additional help. Women with STD have an increased risk of developing cervical intraepithelial neoplasia (CIN) and regular cervical cytological screening should be ensured.

Patients presenting with genital ulceration should have exudate from the lesion examined by darkfield microscopy for *Treponema pallidum* and a viral culture sent for herpes culture. It is a wise precaution to take blood for syphilis serology not only in these patients but in all clinic attenders, especially if prescribing antitreponemal antibiotics.

Having performed the above investigations it is justifiable to prescribe antibiotics without awaiting the results of the laboratory tests, should the clinical picture indicate necessity for immediate treatment.

The three commonest causes of vaginal discharge are summarised in Table 15.2.

URETHRAL DISCHARGE

In men urethral discharge is the most commonly presenting symptom indicating STD (Table 15.3). Microscopy can differentiate gonococcal from non-gonococcal urethritis with 90% accuracy. A urethral swab for gonorrhoea and a specimen for chlamydia should also be sent for microbiological examination. First voided urine samples provide very effective diagnosis of chlamydial urethritis. Presence of threads containing pus may be the only indication of infection if discharge is scanty or lacking.

Table 15.2. The three commonest causes of vaginal discharge

	Candida	Gardnerella	Trichomonas
Cause	Fungus	Bacterium	Protozoan
Incubation	12–24 hours	24–48 hours	7–28 days
Symptoms			
Dysuria	Often	Occasional	Often
Discharge	White, thick, 'cheesy' odourless	Yellow, thin, frothy, malodorous	Yellow, thin profuse, malodorous
Irritation	Present	Absent	Often
Signs			
Vulvitis	Often	Absent	Often
Cervicitis	Often	Often	'Strawberry cervix'
Investigations	Gram-smear, culture, check for glycosuria	Gram-smear, culture	Wet smear, culture
Treatment	Local cream and pessaries, clotrimazole, miconazole, nystatin oral antifungals (fluconazole)	Metronidazole	Metronidazole
Male contacts	Dysuria, balanitis, phimosis	Asymptomatic, balanitis	Asymptomatic carrier
(Treat male partner in all cases)			

Table 15.3. Common causes of urethral discharge

Physiological	Prostatorrhoea
Traumatic	
Physical	Masturbation
Chemical	Alcohol
Infective	
Gonococcal	
Non-gonococcal (NGU)	
NSU	Chlamydial or non-chlamydial
Other	*Trichomonas, Candida, Gardnerella,* viral, e.g. herpes, secondary to urinary tract infection (UTI), urethral stricture
Neoplastic (uncommon)	Urethral lesions

Gonorrhoea, an infection with *Neisseria gonorrhoeae,* and non-gonococcal urethritis comprise most cases of sexually transmitted urethral discharge. 50% of non-gonococcal cases are caused by *Chlamydia trachomatis.* 75% of female contacts attending are asymptomatic.

Symptoms and signs

Incubation is 1–10 days in gonorrhoea and 7–14 days in chlamydia. Only 5% of infected men are asymptomatic. Most men develop dysuria and mucoid or purulent urethral discharge. Proctitis is common in homosexuals. Pharyngitis may occur where oral intercourse is involved.

Gonorrhoea is asymptomatic in 70% of women and chlamydia in 90%. There may be dysuria or vaginal discharge. Diagnosis should always be confirmed bacteriologically.

Complications

Complications are comparatively rare and can be prevented by effective early treatment.

Local complications include prostatitis, acute epididymitis, periurethral abscess, urethral stricture and urethrophobia (constant fear of infection) in men.

Pelvic inflammatory disease (PID) is the most serious complication for women, and 10% will present evidence of involvement of one or both fallopian tubes, usually subacutely. Lower abdominal pain and tenderness is present with thickening and tenderness of the affected tube. Infertility can follow bilateral PID. Differential diagnosis is ectopic pregnancy.

Ophthalmia neonatorum is another complication. Both gonorrhoea and *C. trachomatis* are transmitted during birth, and the infected baby will develop conjunctivitis 2–10 days later.

Systemic complications of gonorrhoea are arthritis, septicaemia and endocarditis. Those of chlamydia infection are perihepatitis (Fitz Hugh-Curtis syndrome) and cervical dysplasia. Non-gonococcal urethritis (NGU) can lead to Reiter's disease (see Ch. 12).

Investigations

Men must not micturate for 3 hours before urethral tests.

1. Gram-stained smears and cultures from the urethra in men, and the cervix, urethra and vagina in women.
2. Enzyme-linked immunosorbent assay (ELISA) for chlamydia.
3. Two-glass urine test in men.
4. Wet vaginal smear to exclude *Trichomonas vaginalis* in women.
5. Smears and cultures from other sites if indicated, e.g. rectum, pharynx.

Treatment

Penicillin is the drug of choice in gonorrhoea giving over 90% cure rates. A suggested schedule might be amoxycillin 3 g stat orally with 1 g probenecid (to delay excretion). If there is penicillin allergy or non-treponemicidal therapy is required, ciprofloxacin 250 mg orally stat or spectinomycin 2 g i.m. stat is suitable.

Beta-lactamase-producing *N. gonorrhoeae* strains appear from abroad occasionally producing the enzyme beta-lactamase which destroys penicillin. Drugs of choice for these strains are ciprofloxacin 500 mg orally stat, spectinomycin 2 g i.m. stat or cefuroxime 1.5 g i.m. stat. *All* patients are then treated with oxytetracycline 500 mg 6-hourly for 1 week.

50% of all patients with gonorrhoea develop post-gonococcal urethritis (PGU) which is NSU occurring concomitantly with gonorrhoea. Most chlamydial and non-specific urethritis (NSU) infections respond to tetracyclines. The suggested schedule is oxytetracycline tablets 250 mg 6-hourly for 10 days. Erythromycin 500 mg 6-hourly for 14 days should be used in pregnancy or tetracycline allergy. Ofloxacin 200 mg 12-hourly for 10 days may be used as an alternative. Consorts of patients with non-specific infection should be treated routinely after exclusion of other infection.

Prognosis

Re-infection with *N. gonorrhoeae* and chlamydia following successful treatment occurs as many contacts are not traced. Relapses of NSU often occur for no apparent reason.

GENITAL WARTS (CONDYLOMATA ACUMINATA)

Genital warts are caused usually by sexual transmission of the human papilloma virus (HPV). There are over 50 types of HPV, four of these (types 6, 11, 16 and 18) showing preferential tropism for the genitoanal area. Types 6 and 11 occur mainly in benign lesions, and only rarely in cervical carcinoma, while with types 16 and 18 the reverse is true.

The argument continues as to whether genital warts cause cancer. The evidence to date is only suggestive of a role in CIN and little else. It is possible that HPV and smoking acting as cofactors may have some role.

Warts fall into three clinical types (acuminate, papular and flat) although there is often transition between them.

The mean incubation is about 3 months.

Symptoms and signs

Initially small lesions are often encouraged by discharge, and increase in size becoming filiform or hyperplastic.

Investigations

Routine cervical cytology and colposcopy if the cytology is abnormal.

Differential diagnosis. Condylomata lata, molluscum contagiosum, anal skin tags and haemorrhoids should be excluded.

Basis of treatment

The predisposing causes, e.g. discharge, should be removed. Trichloracetic acid or podophyllotoxin can be applied locally.

Cryotherapy, using metal probe or liquid nitrogen spray, or electrocautery for severe cases may be used.

Sexual contacts should also be examined.

Prognosis

Treatment may be prolonged and recurrences occur.

HERPES GENITALIS

Genital herpes is usually sexually transmitted. Most infections are caused by Herpes simplex type 2 but type 1 infections, usually associated with oral cold sores, are not uncommon.

Following an initial attack the virus quickly reaches the sacral ganglia where it lies dormant. Recurrent episodes may occur from reactivation of the virus.

Symptoms and signs

Following 4–5 days' incubation, prodromal itching or burning may occur at any genital site, preceding groups of vesicles which form painful ulcers. These become larger erosions which crust over before healing after 2–3 weeks. Painful regional lymphadenopathy occurs in 20% of cases.

Complications

Complications include urethritis, cervicitis, proctitis, urinary retention and disseminated infections (more severe in immunocompromised subjects). Most patients suffer recurrent episodes (less severe than the initial attack) because of reactivation of the virus. Some known trigger mechanisms for this are stress, illness (especially viral), trauma, photosensitivity (avoid sun beds or solariums). Many recurrences have no obvious precipitating factor. Frequency and duration of attacks varies, decreasing over several years and eventually ceasing completely.

Neonatal infection occurs if maternal lesions are present at birth. Transmission is during birth resulting in dermatitis, meningitis or encephalitis which can lead to brain damage. This is very rare and, with careful monitoring around term, a decision to perform caesarean section is sometimes taken to exclude fetal risk.

Investigations

Viral culture, darkfield examination and cervical cytology.

Differential Diagnosis

Table 15.4 shows the common causes of genital ulceration.

Basis of treatment

Attention to hygiene (normal saline bathing), prevention of secondary infection and analgesia (paracetamol, local anaesthetic creams) may be all that is necessary.

Table 15.4. Common causes of genital ulceration

Herpes	Scabies	Tropical STD (chancroid, donovaniasis, lymphogranuloma venereum)
Syphilis (primary, secondary, tertiary)	Folliculitis	
	Bechçet's syndrome (orogenital ulceration)	
Trauma		Carcinoma
Candida	Lipschutz ulcer	
Erosive balanitis	Drug eruptions	

In primary attacks, the treatment of choice (if started within 5 days of onset) is acyclovir 200 mg five times daily for 5 days. In recurrent cases many patients require no treatment; others do well with acyclovir cream 5% five times daily for 5 days when the prodrome occurs. In patients suffering severe attacks every 4–6 weeks, continuous prophylaxis is available with acyclovir tablets with the dosage titrated to levels just preventing attacks. Because of the expense of acyclovir, shorter courses of higher doses will probably be increasingly used.

The majority of patients have little trouble from recurrent attacks but some become bitter or obsessed with the disease, resulting in severe psychological problems which need counselling.

SYPHILIS

Syphilis is a sexually transmitted infection caused by the spirochaete *T. pallidum* acquired on direct contact with an early lesion. The incubation period is 9–90 days. Since treponemes are present in the surface lesions of early (but not late) syphilis, it is infectious only in the primary, secondary (following initial dissemination of treponemes to all body tissues) and early latent stages. (Table 15.5).

The essential process is that of an endarteritis obliterans leading to erosion of the surface of the lesion.

Latent syphilis

This follows the untreated secondary stage lasting between 2 years and a lifetime (average 10–15 years). There are no clinical signs, the diagnosis being made on serological grounds. Ultimately, routine serological tests may only be weakly positive or even negative.

Differential diagnosis
Dermatoses in secondary syphilis and other causes of genital ulcers (see Table 15.4).

Investigations
Darkfield microscopy is used to identify *T. pallidum* in serous exudate. Later stages need confirmation using serological tests (Table 15.6): VDRL for non-specific anti-treponemal antibodies, and TPHA and FTA-Abs for specific antibodies to pathogenic treponemes.

In latent and late syphilis, CSF examination (to exclude neurosyphilis) and X-rays of the chest (to exclude cardiovascular changes) and long bones are often advised.

Late syphilis

This is now relatively rare as effective early treatment halts progression of the disease. In 35% of untreated patients clinical signs of late syphilis will develop between 3 and 40 years after the initial infection. 15% will develop tertiary syphilis, 10% neurosyphilis, 10% cardiovascular syphilis and the remainder will continue as non-infectious latent cases.

Table 15.5. Stages of syphilis and their main symptoms

Stage	Symptoms
Acquired	
Early infectious (first 2 years of infection)	
Primary	Chancre (painless, indurated, ulcer), lymphadenopathy (local, painless, rubbery), rectal or vaginal chancres may not be noticed
Secondary (6–8 weeks after primary)	Malaise, mild pyrexia, lymphadenitis, rash (dull red/coppery maculopapular, non-itchy, often on palms and soles; can mimic any other rash), condylomata lata (fleshy warty lesions), mucous patches (ulcers), oral genitalia, moth-eaten alopecia
Early latent	No clinical signs, serology +ve, mucocutaneous relapses can occur
Late non-infectious	(3–40 years after initial infection)
Late latent	No clinical signs, serology +ve
Tertiary	Gumma
Cardiovascular syphilis	Aortic incompetence, aortic aneurysm, coronary ostial stenosis
Neurosyphilis	Tabes dorsalis, general paralysis of the insane, meningovascular
Congenital	
Early infectious (first 2 years of life, there is no primary stage)	
Symptomatic	Rash, mucous patches, condylomata lata, snuffles (nasal discharge, obstruction), failure to thrive, hepatosplenomegaly, periostitis, lymphadenopathy, meningitis
Latent	No clinical signs, serology +ve
Latent non-infectious (aged 2 years onwards)	
Latent	With or without stigmata
Symptomatic	(as for acquired infection)
	Gummatous (especially palate), cardiovascular, CNS
Stigmata (residual abnormalities due to early or late congenital infections presenting in later life)	
	Interstitial keratitis, Hutchinson's teeth, eighth nerve deafness, facial bone deformities

Congenital syphilis

Routine antenatal blood tests, and treatment of women during pregnancy has made congenital syphilis rare in the UK. It is most commonly seen in early maternal infections and placental transmission is after the fourth month of pregnancy to the fetus. If the mother is treated soon enough this usually treats the fetus at the same time.

Table 15.6. Current serological tests for syphilis

VDRL	TPHA	FTA-Abs	Probable diagnosis
+	-	-	Biological false positive (BFP) Repeat to exclude primary syphilis
+	-	+	Primary syphilis (? positive darkfield)
+	+	+	Secondary syphilis or beyond (usually untreated) VDRL titres often high in secondary syphilis
-	+	+	Treated, partially treated or past history of treated syphilis

Similar patterns occur in yaws, bejel and pinta

VDRL = venereal disease research laboratory test; TPHA = *T. pallidum* haemagglutination assay; FTA-Abs = fluorescent treponemal antibody absorption test.

Stages are similar to acquired syphilis but there is no primary stage. Investigations are as for acquired syphilis.

Treatment

The treatment of choice is procaine penicillin 0.9 megaunits i.m. daily for 14 days in early syphilis increasing to 21 days in late syphilis. Doxycycline or erythromycin may be used but for a longer duration in cases of penicillin allergy.

50% of patients with early syphilis develop the Jarish-Herxheimer reaction, of uncertain origin, about 6 hours after the first injection only, consisting of fever, malaise, headache and often rigors, lasting only a few hours. Patients should be warned of this. It is less frequent but may be more serious in late syphilis; therefore small doses of prednisone are given for 24 hours preceding and 2 days after the first injection to prevent this occurring.

In congenital syphilis babies should be given 200 000 units penicillin per 450 g bodyweight divided over a period of 10 days. Adults are treated as for late acquired syphilis.

Clinical and serological follow-up should be continued for at least 2 years.

Prognosis

In early syphilis the cure rate approaches 100% in patients who become serologically negative and remain so for 2 years.

HIV INFECTION AND AIDS (See Chap. 14)

16

ADVERSE DRUG REACTIONS AND ACUTE POISONING

Clive J. C. Roberts

ADVERSE DRUG REACTIONS

An adverse drug reaction is any unwanted effect resulting from a drug's use in treatment. This definition excludes deliberate and accidental overdose.

An understanding of the mechanisms helps in assessing the risk-to-benefit ratio—essential at the time of all drug prescribing. The toxicity in overdose must also be considered when there is a risk of self-harm, e.g. in giving amitriptyline or dextropropoxyphene to depressed patients.

Common examples of drug reactions include nausea with digoxin therapy, bronchospasm with beta-adrenoceptor blockers, ataxia and drowsiness with phenytoin, bleeding with warfarin, dry cough with captopril, cholestatic jaundice with chlorpromazine, gastric ulcer with non-steroidal-anti-inflammatory drugs (NSAIDs) and morbilliform rash with ampicillin. *Most drug reactions mimic naturally occurring conditions and are consequently difficult to detect early in drug development.* Occasionally drugs cause specific conditions not previously recorded, e.g. the recently discovered eosinophilic myalgic syndrome caused by tryptophan and the oculomucocutaneous syndrome caused by practolol. These also often go undetected because they are of low incidence and totally unexpected.

Epidemiology

Numerous studies have attempted to assess the size of the problem but the results depend on the methodology used. Figures commonly quoted are that adverse drug reactions account for 4% of hospital admissions, 1 in 1000 deaths in medical wards and occur in 10–20% of inpatients. In general practice it is estimated that adverse reactions may occur in up to 5% of patients. They are more frequent in the elderly (Fig. 16.1) because:

1. functional impairment leads to erratic drug taking
2. multiple pathology attracts polypharmacy

3. decreased hepatic and renal capacity leads to relative drug accumulation
4. impaired CNS and CVS function leads to increased sensitivity to drug effects.

The drugs most commonly implicated are oral anticoagulants, NSAIDs, corticosteroids, anti-hypertensives, antibiotics, diuretics and insulin.

Drug reactions result from specific sets of circumstances relating to the drug's pharmacology, to predisposing features in the patient and to the care taken in choosing the right drug at the right dose.

CLASSIFICATION

Predictable reactions (type A):

1. can be predicted from the known pharmacology of the drug
2. may be common within pharmacological groups
3. are due either to excessive action at the target receptor or to action at a non-target receptor (Table 16.1)
4. are related closely to the amount of drug in body
5. are determined by dose and by pharmacokinetic and pharmacodynamic factors (e.g. greatly reduced dose of warfarin needed in liver disease)
6. are common, accounting for 75% or more of all adverse effects
7. are largely avoidable with care.

In unpredictable (type B) reactions:

1. the effect is unrelated to established pharmacological effects
2. the effect may not be shared within pharmacological groups
3. the effect may be serious organ damage (e.g. pulmonary fibrosis with sulphasalazine)
4. there is a poor relationship to dose
5. are uncommon and difficult to detect in drug development
6. cannot be avoided if the drug is used (Table 16.2).
   Patient idiosyncrasy is a major factor.

The type A and B reactions account for the major commonly encountered adverse effects. The concepts employed in this classification are important. However, some reactions depend on dose but are not obviously related to their pharmacological effects (Table 16.3). Examples would be ototoxity with streptomycin and nausea with digoxin. Some therefore prefer to consider reactions as simply dose-dependent or dose-independent. Even this classification fails. For example the blood abnormalities and proteinuria which occurred in a small percentage of patients given captopril have now virtually disappeared following the recommended dose reduction. Lupus syndrome caused by hydralazine, although rare, occurs when high doses are used in poor metabolisers of the drug.

Fetal abnormality

Teratogenic drugs cause abnormalities of structural development of the fetus if given during the first 3 months of pregnancy. Amelia and phocomelia (absent

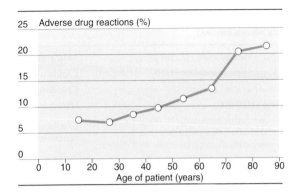

Fig. 16.1 The effect of age on adverse effect incidence.

Table 16.1. Some examples of predictable drug reactions

Excessive therapeutic effect	
Bone marrow depression	Azathioprine
Syncope	ACE inhibitors
Heart block	Digoxin
Hypoglycaemia	Chlorpropamide
Poor wound healing	Corticosteroids
Cardiac arrhythmias	Thyroxine
Effect at non-target receptor	
Micturition difficulty	Amitriptyline
Tremor	Salbutamol
Renal impairment	ACE inhibitors
Diabetes	Corticosteroids
Asthma	Beta-blockers
Constipation	Verapamil
Diarrhoea	Misoprostol

ACE = angiotensin-converting enzyme.

or deformed limbs) caused by thalidomide in the 1960s is the most memorable disaster. Teratogenic effects are difficult to detect and extreme caution must be exercised in using drugs during pregnancy. The unfamiliar prescriber should always check the manufacturer's literature. For example, some calcium channel blockers have been shown to be teratogenic in animals and are contraindicated in women of child-bearing potential.

Adverse effects on fetal wellbeing may occur. Many drugs cross the placenta and exert an effect in the fetus which may be harmful (Table 16.4). Easily predicted effects are from warfarin, sulphonylureas, carbimazole, corticosteroids,

Table 16.2. Some examples of unpredictable drug reactions (with incidences where known)

Retroperitoneal fibrosis (1/250)	Methysergide
Pseudomembranous colitis (1/1000–1/10 000)	Clindamycin
Aplastic anaemia (1/6000)	Chloramphenicol
Jaundice (1/10 000)	Halothane
Deep venous thrombosis (1/10 000) Myocardial infarction (1/10 000) Pulmonary embolism (1/20 000)	Combined oral contraceptive
Aplastic anaemia (1/10 000–1/20 000)	Phenylbutazone
Cholestatic hepatitis (2/100)	Chlorpromazine
Myositis	Simvastatin
Visual loss	Ethambutol
Hepatic damage	Sodium valproate
Marrow suppression	Mianserin

Table 16.3. Some examples of drug reactions which are difficult to classify

Gastric erosions	Aspirin and NSAIDs
Azoospermia	Sulphasalazine
Oral candida infection	Inhaled corticosteroids
Hyponatraemia	Carbamazepine
Dystonia and dyskinesia	Metoclopramide
Unproductive cough	ACE inhibitors

barbiturates and benzodiazepines. ACE (angiotensin-converting enzyme) inhibitors cause fetal death in some animal species and have caused oligohydramnios in human pregnancies as well as neonatal hypotension and renal failure. Clearly a high level of awareness of the risks when new drugs are introduced is mandatory.

Allergy and 'pseudoallergy'

Acute hypersensitivity reactions occur when release of histamine and other mediators follows the interaction of drug antigen and IgE antibody (B lymphocyte produced) on the surface of mast cells or circulating basophils. Rashes, oedema, bronchospasm and cardiovascular collapse may follow. Such reactions require previous exposure to the drug which, acting as a hapten, becomes antigenic after combining with a protein.

Table 16.4. Examples of drugs thought to be harmful in pregnancy

Known or suspected teratogens

Phenytoin, oral anticoagulants, griseofulvin	Various congenital malformations
Sodium valproate	Neural tube defects
Heparin	Osteoporosis
Tetracycline	Dental discoloration
Alkylating agents, methotrexate	High risk of congenital abnormalities
Penicillamine	Fetal abnormalities reported
Etretinate	Congenital abnormalities

Drugs causing adverse effects on the fetus

ACE inhibitors	Oligohydramnios, impaired renal function and hypotension
Streptokinase	Placental separation
Chlorpropamide	Neonatal hypoglycaemia
Benzodiazepines	Depressed neonatal respiration, drowsiness and hypotonia, withdrawal syndrome
Beta-blockers	Neonatal bradycardia
NSAIDs	Closure of ductus arteriosus in utero, possibly pulmonary hypertension, prolonged labour

Serum sickness syndrome is a less acute form of reaction which results from the damaging effects of circulating immune complexes. IgG or IgM antibody combines with antigenic drug and, if present in excessive amounts, may lodge in blood vessels giving rise to systemic and local inflammation. Interstitial nephritis is a common manifestation.

Delayed hypersensitivity is T lymphocyte mediated, e.g. contact dermatitis.

Some drugs can produce a reaction which mimics allergy on first encounter. Aspirin and other NSAIDs, for example, are capable of causing release of histamine and other mediators in susceptible individuals without immunological mechanisms being involved. The syndrome of flushing, urticaria, angiooedema, rhinitis, asthma and hypotension which follows resembles anaphylaxis. This 'pseudoallergy' may follow the administration of morphine, barbiturates, radiographic contrast media and other agents.

Dependence and withdrawal reactions

Psychoactive agents such as the benzodiazepines and barbiturates cause tachyphylaxis, psychological and physical dependence and when stopped can cause a withdrawal syndrome ranging from anxiety and insomnia to delirium and convulsions.

Other drugs may cause problems when discontinued. For example myocardial ischaemia may occur if beta-adrenoceptor agents are stopped suddenly.

FACTORS PREDISPOSING TO DOSE-DEPENDENT REACTIONS

Pharmacokinetic variation leads to reduced blood concentrations and therapeutic failure, or elevated concentrations and adverse effects. Pharmacodynamic variation (sensitivity of the receptor to a given concentration of drug) will have a similar effect. Genetic factors, disease processes, drug interaction and ageing are the main sources of variation and have effects at sites throughout the body and through many mechanisms (Tables 16.5 to 16.8).

Increased bioavailability

This term describes the fraction of administered drug which arrives in the systemic circulation. After oral administration it depends on proper pharmaceutical formulation, the fraction absorbed from the gastrointestinal tract and the proportion metabolised as it passes through the liver from the portal circulation (pre-systemic metabolism or 'first pass' effect). Drugs which are extensively and rapidly metabolised by the liver normally have reduced bioavailability. However, if that metabolism is impaired by enzyme inhibition (e.g. by cimetidine), liver disease or in the elderly or if blood is shunted around the liver, as in chronic liver disease, excessively high drug concentrations occur after oral administration (Table 16.6). This applies to several drugs from the following categories: beta-blockers, calcium channel blockers, opioids, antidepressants, sedatives.

Reduced hepatic clearance

The steady-state blood concentration of any drug is determined by the rate of clearance by its organ of elimination (usually the liver or kidney) irrespective of the distribution volume. Most liver injuries cause impairment of drug metabolism but inter-individual variation is so wide that changes may be minor. When synthetic function is impaired, as indicated by a fall in serum albumin or prolongation of clotting, serious drug accumulation of highly lipid-soluble agents may occur, e.g. CNS depressant drugs. Some drugs impair the clearance by the liver of others, e.g. cimetidine and azapropazone are both inhibitors of the metabolism of warfarin and phenytoin. Phenytoin is particularly likely to accumulate because its metabolism becomes saturated at high therapeutic doses. A disproportionate rise in drug concentration can result from a small change in dose or minor inhibition of enzymes. Some metabolic pathways are under genetic control, e.g. acetylation of drugs such as hydralazine and isoniazid can be classified as slow and fast. Slow acetylators tend to experience adverse effects (lupus syndrome and peripheral neuropathy respectively) whilst fast acetylators may suffer therapeutic failure.

Increased hepatic clearance

Induction of enzymes by barbiturates, rifampicin, carbamazepine, phenytoin and others result in reduced levels of warfarin and sulphonylurea anti-diabetic drugs. The result is decreased efficacy in the first place but if the dose has been

Table 16.5. Examples of adverse drug interactions with mechanisms

Reduced absorption	
of phenytoin	by sucralfate
of digoxin	by cholestyramine
Increased bioavailability	
of levodopa	by metoclopramide
of labetalol, propranolol, nifedipine and nortriptyline	by cimetidine
Decreased hepatic clearance	
of phenytoin, warfarin and tolbutamide	by azapropazone
of theophylline, pethidine, chlormethiazole, phenytoin, warfarin	by cimetidine
of azathioprine and warfarin	by allopurinol
Increased hepatic clearance	
of corticosteroids, warfarin, tolbutamide and the oral contraceptive	by barbiturates, phenytoin, carbamazepine, rifampicin and griseofulvin
Competition for renal excretion	
of chlorpropamide	by phenylbutazone
of methotrexate	by probenecid and NSAIDs
of digoxin	by quinidine
pH-dependent increase in renal excretion	
of aspirin	by antacids
Increased effects through electrolyte changes	
of digoxin	by diuretics
of diuretics	by corticosteroids
of spironolactone	by captopril
Increased effect by mutual potentiation at the target organ	
of beta-blockers	by verapamil
of warfarin	by aspirin
of anti-hypertensives	by nitrates
of phenothiazines	by benzodiazepines
Decreased effect by mutual antagonism at the target organ	
of insulin and tolbutamide	by thiazide diuretics and corticosteroids
of levodopa	by phenothiazines
of diuretics	by indomethacin
of valproate	by phenothiazines
of adrenergic neurone blockers	by tricyclic anti-depressants
Hypertensive crisis	
with MAOIs	and ephedrine etc. and tyramine-containing foods
with adrenaline	and beta-blockers

Table 16.6. Mechanisms of adverse drug effects in chronic liver disease with examples

Increased CNS sensitivity leading to risk of encephalopathy

    Morphine, benzodiazepines, phenothiazines

Impaired hepatic function leading to increased drug sensitivity

    Warfarin, chlorpropamide, aspirin

Exacerbation of fluid and electrolyte abnormalities

    Diuretics, NSAIDs, magnesium trisilicate mixture, carbenoxolone

Constipating agents leading to increased risk of encephalopathy

    Amitriptyline, codeine imodium

Increased bioavailability due to reduced metabolic capacity and portosystemic shunting

    Chlormethiazole, opioids, propranolol, labetalol, nifedipine, verapamil

Decreased elimination

    Phenytoin, theophylline, methotrexate

Possibly decreased protein binding

    Corticosteroids

Risk of hepatotoxicity leading to worsening of condition or diagnostic confusion

    Paracetamol, chlorpromazine, methyldopa, simvastatin, sodium valproate

titrated to the patient's requirement and the inducer is then stopped, overdosage may occur and cause bleeding or hypoglycaemia respectively.

Impaired renal excretion

The clearance of many drugs is proportional to renal function as measured by creatinine clearance. Dose adjustment in renal failure is an exact science taking account of the therapeutic margin of the drug, the degree of renal failure, the need for a loading dose and the distribution volume together with any risks particular to the condition (Table 16.7). It should be remembered that renal function tails off with ageing and that drug interaction may occur in the kidney.

Increased drug sensitivity

The elderly may become confused by normal doses of sedative drugs or hypotensive in response to vasodilators. They bleed more frequently with aspirin and suffer bone marrow depression more readily with mianserin and co-trimoxazole. Diuretics cause more electrolyte abnormalities in the aged. Organ failure—cardiac, respiratory, renal and hepatic—creates conditions in which specific reactions to drugs may occur, e.g. sedating drugs should not be given to patients with ventilatory failure, calcium channel blockers may exacer-

Table 16.7. Mechanisms of adverse drug effects in chronic renal failure with examples

Impaired elimination leading to predictable drug toxicity	Amiodarone, atenolol, benzylpenicillin, digoxin, metformin, glibenclamide
Increased sensitivity	Anti-psychotics, opioids
Exacerbation of renal impairment	ACE inhibitors, acyclovir, aspirin, cisplatin, colistin, gold, penicillamine, gentamicin, tetracycline, clofibrate
Exacerbation of metabolic derangement	Acetazolamide, carbenoxolone, loop diuretics, magnesium trisilicate mixture, NSAIDs, spironolactone
Increased incidence of rashes	Ampicillin, amoxycillin, pivampicillin, allopurinol, sulphonamides, sulphasalazine, nalidixic acid

Table 16.8. Some genetically determined drug reactions

Condition	Precipitating drugs	Adverse effect
Glucose-6-phosphate deficiency	Quinine, sulphonamides, nitrofurantoin, dapsone	Haemolysis
Porphyria (hepatic)	Barbiturates, griseofulvin	Attack precipitated
Malignant hyperpyrexia	Halothane suxamethonium	Hyperthermia, muscle rigidity, acidosis
Down's syndrome	Atropine	Increased response

bate cardiac failure, constipating drugs may be harmful in liver failure and potassium-retaining diuretics can be lethal in renal failure. Detailed knowledge and reference is required when treating these patients. Adverse drug interactions may also result in excessive drug sensitivity and some reactions are genetically determined (Table 16.8).

PREVENTING DRUG ADVERSE EFFECTS

The following principles of prescribing should reduce the risks:

1. Consciously assess the risk-to-benefit ratio when about to prescribe.
2. Identify pharmacokinetic and pharmacodynamic risk factors in the patient, e.g. liver disease, concurrent drugs etc.
3. Always ask about allergy.
4. Avoid drugs if at all possible in pregnant women or those seeking pregnancy.
5. Avoid polypharmacy in the elderly by establishing priorities.
6. Use new drugs only when the evidence for advantage is convincing.

7. Keep up to date with information in simple publications, e.g. *Current Problems, Drug and Therapeutics Bulletin* and *British National Formulary.*
8. Explain to patients the objectives and possible consequences of treatment.
9. Stop drugs which have become unnecessary.

DETECTING DRUG ADVERSE EFFECTS

Adverse effect monitoring during early development and clinical trials of drugs cannot identify all risks. Post-marketing surveillance is mandatory. In the UK doctors are encouraged to report adverse effects to the Committee on the Safety of Medicines using yellow forms which are supplied with the *British National Formulary.* All suspected reactions, however minor, are collected for new drugs (identified by ▼ alongside the entry) and serious adverse effects for established drugs. Detailed investigations are triggered when a suspicious number of reports is received. The system is not perfect but has been successful in identifying a number of important drug reactions.

ACUTE POISONING

According to The Office of Population, Censuses and Surveys (OPCS) statistics in 1986, 2121 people died in England and Wales from acute poisoning. Of these, 1069 were confirmed suicides. In 592 the cause was undetermined and in 460 a verdict of accidental death was recorded. Most of these are likely to have been acts of self-harm although successful suicide may not have been intended. Amongst the drug overdoses tricyclic antidepressants, paracetamol with or without dextropropoxyphene, barbiturates, salicylates and benzodiazepines are commonly recorded. Chlormethiazole, phenothiazines, morphine and diamorphine account for a significant number. About 85% of the deaths occur outside hospital. The average age of death is 40 years and the peak incidence 25–35 years. Approximately 35% more women than men are admitted to hospital after poisoning but almost twice as many men than women die after poisoning. Suicidal and parasuicidal behaviour is common in teenagers and the incidence in the over 60-year-olds is twice that in the younger age groups.

100 000 poisoned patients are admitted to hospital in the UK each year throwing a considerable burden on the acute medical and psychiatric services. As many as 20% of poisoned patients seen in accident and emergency departments are not admitted. Acute poisoning has been called the 'modern epidemic' and most house physicians will see numerous cases, virtually all of whom will be acts of self-harm.

Management of poisoning

Some poisonings (e.g. with chlormethiazole) are best treated by supportive measures and careful avoidance of meddlesome unnecessary procedures. Others (e.g. with paracetamol) require active administration of specific antidotes. Information on common poisonings is available in the *British National*

Formulary and in specific texts but the National Poisons Information Centres provide confidential information to doctors on the contents of proprietary products and also advice on the management of difficult cases.

Principles

1. Prevent further absorption of ingested poisons.
2. Sustain bodily functions and treat complications as they arise.
3. Administer antidotes or take measures to increase the elimination of the poison if appropriate.
4. Provide psychiatric or social assistance.

The order in which these principles are applied depends on the clinical state of the patient and the nature of the poison ingested.

Methods for reducing drug absorption

Gastric lavage and the administration of emetics retrieves a substantial amount of drug in only a small number of patients and then only when performed within 2 hours for most poisonings. These procedures are not without hazard. They should be employed only when a seriously toxic dose has been ingested within 4 hours or within 6–12 hours for salicylates, tricyclics or opiates which delay gastric emptying. They are contraindicated in corrosive or petroleum distillate ingestion or in known oesophageal or gastric disease. Gastric lavage should not be performed in uncooperative patients because of the risk of oesophageal perforation. The only acceptable emetic is syrup of ipecacuanha and this must not be given to patients whose consciousness is impaired. Salt must not be used as fatal hypernatraemia is well documented.

Administration of chelating agents (e.g. desferrioxamine for iron poisoning) or adsorbents (e.g. Fuller's earth for paraquat ingestion) have major importance in preventing absorption. Recently the use of activated charcoal has increased because it dramatically reduces the absorption of many drugs if given within 1 hour and significantly reduces it if given later. It also has a place in increasing drug elimination (see below). Activated charcoal does not adsorb alcohols, inorganic acids or alkalis, iron or lithium.

Intensive supportive treatment

Specific therapies do not exist for many poisonings, particularly central nervous system depressants. Lives can be saved by careful monitoring of vital functions and provision of support and treatment of complications (Fig. 16.2). Level of consciousness, heart rate, blood pressure, respiration and state of peripheral perfusion should be recorded regularly. Good nursing care is essential. Hypothermia should be identified by rectal temperature measurement with a low reading thermometer. If minute respiratory volume falls below 4 litres and blood gas levels change, artificial ventilation should be undertaken. Hypotension should be dealt with by first ensuring ventilation and hydration are adequate. The foot of the bed should be raised and only if these measures fail should infusion of dobutamine with dopamine be considered. Cardiac arrhythmias, dystonias and convulsions should be managed conventionally.

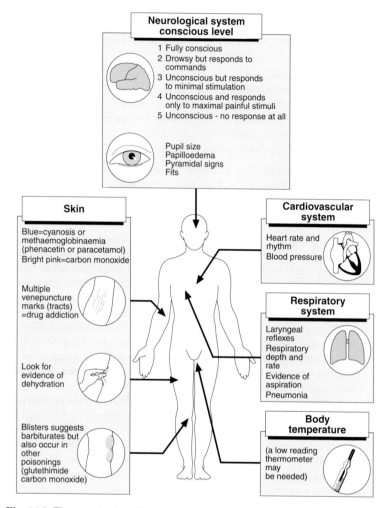

Fig. 16.2 The examination of a poisoned patient.

Methods for increasing drug elimination

Forced diuresis is of no value and can be hazardous but urinary alkalinisation increases the elimination of aspirin and is a useful part of therapy (see below).

Dialysis and haemoperfusion may increase the clearance of the drug from the blood but this is meaningless for drugs with wide distribution as the actual amount of drugs removed is small. These techniques are therefore rarely used. Dialysis effectively removes salicylates, lithium, methanol and ethylene glycol. Haemoperfusion involves the passage of blood through an adsorbent material such as activated charcoal or a polystyrene resin. This technique effectively removes barbiturates, carbamazepine, disopyramide and theophylline.

Repeat-dose activated charcoal enhances the non-renal elimination of many drugs. Not only drug which is secreted into bile, but also large amounts which diffuse into small intestinal secretions are held within the gut and their reabsorption prevented. Therefore for maximum efficiency charcoal should be given at a rate which keeps the small intestine filled. The technique has been shown to be effective for poisonings with aspirin, theophylline, phenobarbitone, carbamazepine, digoxin, meprobamate, phenytoin and others.

PARACETAMOL

Hepatic necrosis and acute hepatic failure sometimes associated with renal failure result from an overdose of paracetamol which is safe in therapeutic doses. The product of oxidative metabolism (N-acetyl benzoquinonimine) binds to hepatocyte proteins and damages the cells (Fig. 16.3). In normal doses this product is conjugated with glutathione and does no harm. In overdose the alternative metabolic pathways for paracetamol—sulphation and glucuronidation—become saturated and glutathione becomes depleted. Thus excessive amounts are produced and reduced amounts removed. Patients taking enzyme-inducing drugs, alcohol, the malnourished and those with pre-existing liver disease are at greater risk from paracetamol overdose. The two antidotes commonly used act as precursors to glutathione. N-acetyl cysteine must be given intravenously and causes occasional hypersensitivity reactions. Methionine is cheaper and can be given orally but is less reliable.

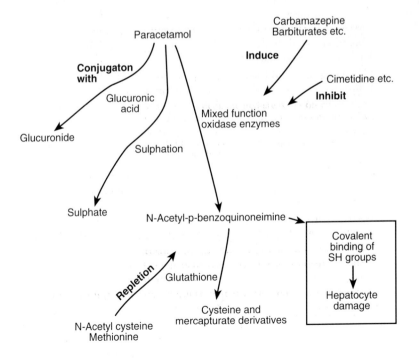

Fig. 16.3 Metabolism and mechanism of paracetamol toxicity.

Poisoning with paracetamol has a number of important distinctive characteristics:

1. It is common—perhaps the most common poisoning encountered in the UK.
2. It is dangerous—hepatic necrosis is recorded with as little as 10 g.
3. Symptoms develop late.
4. Measurement of blood concentration of drug accurately predicts toxicity.
5. Early administration of antidote saves lives.

All doctors should therefore be familiar with the procedure for dealing with this emergency as shown in Figure 16.4—and consider even liver transplantation.

SALICYLATES

Poisoning with aspirin and other salicylates is also common and dangerous. Symptoms and signs may be misleading and active treatment is indicated. As with paracetamol, measurement of the drug level has a predictive value and can be used as a guide to the need for active treatment. The lethal acute dose in an adult is 20–25 g.

The toxic effects of salicylates are complex and include acid–base disturbances, uncoupling of oxidative phosphorylation with inhibition of the production of high energy phosphates and disordered glucose metabolism. Initial respiratory alkalosis from increased rate and depth of respiration causes loss of bicarbonate and accompanying loss of sodium, potassium and water. This results in failure to buffer the subsequent metabolic acidosis caused by the interference with normal cell metabolism.

The symptoms and signs may not be apparent until the poisoning is well advanced. Nausea, vomiting and tinnitus progressing to deafness are common. Fever, flushed skin and sweating and hyperventilation may give way to excitability and agitation. The patient is usually dehydrated and blood tests may reveal hypokalaemia, hyponatraemia, alkalosis or acidosis, hyperglycaemia or hypoglycaemia and sometimes hypoprothrombinaemia. Pulmonary oedema and central nervous system depression are late and sinister signs.

Salicylate preparations tend to clump in the stomach. Gastric lavage up to 12 hours after ingestion is therefore worthwhile. The rate of elimination of aspirin can be greatly increased by repeated administration of activated charcoal and by urinary alkalinisation. The latter relies on ionisation of salicylate within the nephron tubule which renders it non-lipid-soluble and non-diffusible. Maintenance of hydration is also important but large volume diuresis is unnecessary and can be hazardous.

Plasma salicylate concentration should be determined. If less than 50 mg/100 ml oral rehydration is all that is required. However, a repeated estimation is advisable if the first was taken less than 6 hours from ingestion. If greater than 90 mg/100 ml or if there are CNS signs or pulmonary oedema, then haemodialysis is performed. Between these values 50 g of activated charcoal should be given every 4 hours. In young or middle-aged people, in the absence of hypotension, heart failure or renal impairment, urinary alkalinisa-

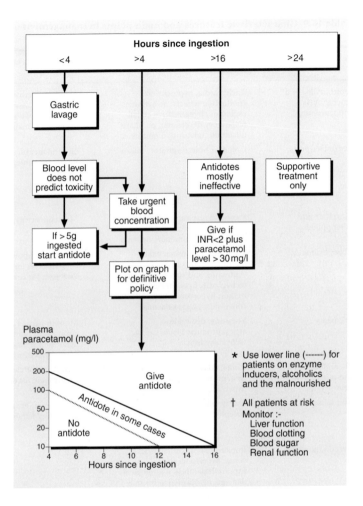

Fig. 16.4 Algorithm for treating paracetamol poisoning.

tion is carried out by infusing 500 ml 1.4% sodium bicarbonate over 1 hour followed by 500 ml 5% glucose with 20 mmol potassium chloride over 1 hour. Both are repeated until the plasma salicylate is below 40 mg/100 ml. Urinary output and pH must be monitored and the rate of infusion adjusted. If the procedure is prolonged, regular measurement of plasma electrolytes is required so that adjustments in the rate of potassium infusion can be made.

OTHER POISONINGS

Brief details of examples of other poisonings with drugs and some non-ingestants are given in Table 16.9.

Table 16.9 Characteristic features and main points in management of certain poisonings

Poison	Main effects	Supportive treatment
Amitriptyline and other tricyclic antidepressants	Tachycardia, hypotension conduction defects, arrhythmias excitation, hyperreflexia coma, respiratory depression, pupillary dilatation, micturition problems	Avoid anti-arrhythmics unless CVS embarrassment; treat convulsions with diazepam, hydrate and maintain oxygenation
Benzodiazepines	Coma without respiratory failure	General measures Beware pneumonia in elderly
Morphine and other opioids	Profound respiratory depression, coma, hypotension, pupillary constriction, pulmonary oedema	Maintain airway, oxygenation
Theophylline	Vomiting, abdominal pain, diarrhoea, tachycardia, ventricular and supraventricular tachycardia, hyper-reflexia, tremor, hyperventilation, convulsions, hypokalaemia	Potassium supplementation, beta-blockers for tachyarrhythmias, diazepam for convulsions
Digoxin	Vomiting, drowsiness, atrioventricular block, cardiac tachyarrhythmias	Monitor plasma potassium; atropine for bradycardia; lignocaine, amiodarone or atenolol for tachyarrythmia
Phenothiazines and other neuroleptics	Coma, convulsions, acute dystonic reactions with hyperreflexia, oculogyric crises	Diazepam for convulsions benztropine for dystonia
Iron salts	Haemorrhagic gastritis, encephalopathy, hepatic necrosis	Transfusion, treat convulsions and circulatory failure
Carbon monoxide	Impairment of consciousness, coma, hypertonia and hyperreflexia, focal neurological damage, myocardial ischaemia and infarction, cardiac arrhythmias, renal failure, muscle necrosis	
Ethylene glycol	Drunkenness, vomiting, coma, convulsions, cardiac failure, pulmonary oedema, acute renal failure	Correct metabolic acidosis Correct hypocalcaemia with i.v. calcium gluconate
Organophosphorous pesticides	Vomiting, sweating, salivation, pupillary constriction, bronchospasm, muscle twitching, diarrhoea, convulsions	
Cyanide	Headache, anxiety, dyspnoea, pulmonary oedema, confusion, coma, cardiovascular collapse	Maximum concentration oxygen, cardiovascular support

See text for aspirin, other salicylates and paracetamol.

Methods for increasing elimination	Antidote
None	Physostigmine, best avoided
None	Avoid flumazenil (antidote) in mixed overdoses (when deaths due to sudden unmasking of effects of tricyclics reported)
None	Naloxone in repeated doses
Repeated activated charcoal Resin haemoperfusion	
Repeated activate dcharcoal	Digoxin-specific Fab antibody fragments
None	
Intragastric and intravenous desferrioxamine according to serum iron	
100% oxygen with artificial ventilation Hyperbaric oxygen in severe cases	
Consider dialysis	Infuse ethanol to inhibit breakdown to toxic products
Remove contaminated clothes Wash skin	Atropine, pralidoxime
	Amyl nitrite and sodium thiosulphate Consider dicobalt edetate followed by dextrose i.v.

17

DISEASES OF THE ENVIRONMENT

Alan E. Read

Human beings are in constant battle with their environment and suffer from the effects of excessive heat or cold, as well as from dramatic changes in atmospheric pressure and from radiation. Defence mechanisms to protect against these hazards are, on the whole, well developed. In poor countries, the harmful effects of many of them are increased by a lack of adequate housing, heating, clothing, ventilation and nutrition. Furthermore, with the conquest of the sea-bed and space, new stresses and strains are regularly being discovered which test the body further. Only a brief review of some of these harmful influences is given in this chapter. They include the effects of heat, cold, alterations in atmospheric pressure, drowning and radiation.

HEAT

In the normal subject, the following mechanisms exist to facilitate the loss of heat produced from body metabolism and outside influences:

1. Vasodilatation of skin vessels and increase of blood flow to the skin allows heat loss by conduction and convection.
2. Sweating allows loss of heat by evaporation of sweat from the skin.
3. If heat loss is still insufficient, hyperventilation can be made to reinforce these methods of heat loss. Tissue damage occurs, however, if the body temperature rises above 41°C.

Fever

A temperature of greater than 37°C is a feature of many inflammatory, neoplastic and degenerative disorders. In such circumstances release of endogenous pyrogen (EP) takes place from inflammatory cells and these stimulate via interleukins hypothalamic centres which have an overall control of body temperature.

Table 17.1. Clinical features of hyperpyrexia

Coma, confusion
Impaired sweating (flushed dry skin)
Skin and mucous membranes: haemorrhagic tendency
Rectal temperature > 40°C
Oliguria, albuminuria, raised blood urea
Liver cell damage
Tachycardia, high pulse pressure
Hypotension, myocardial necrosis

HYPERPYREXIA (Table 17.1)

Although defence mechanisms are adequate, there are occasions when they fail and body temperature rises. This may occur:

1. if there is a high external temperature and humidity, particularly if the patient has not had a period of acclimatisation or wears the wrong clothing
2. in neurological disorders such as autonomic dysfunction, when vasodilatation may not occur
3. as a complication of serious overwhelming infection
4. when there is excessive heat production, as in a thyrotoxic crisis or in the rare genetic syndrome of malignant hyperpyrexia (see below).

Although symptoms such as painful muscle cramps and collapse may occur in non-pyrexial subjects who work under conditions of high ambient temperature, such symptoms are usually relieved by removing the patient to a cooler temperature and treating muscle cramps with sodium chloride infusions.

Heat stroke

Much more dangerous is the clinical syndrome of heat stroke which is accompanied by a raised body temperature.

Symptoms and signs
These include headache and vomiting, confusion and coma, a raised body temperature of up to 41°C or more and a hot and usually dry skin. This is accompanied by tachycardia and tachypnoea.

Investigations
These are relatively unhelpful, but there may be:

1. a leukocytosis in the blood
2. evidence of widespread myocardial damage on an ECG
3. abnormal liver function tests (LFTs)
4. a rising blood urea and a falling urine volume

5. evidence of diffuse intravascular coagulation (DIC) with thrombocytopenia etc. (see p. 358).

The symptoms result from organ damage, particularly in the brain, where there is necrosis of parts of the cerebral and cerebellar cortex.

Treatment

Heat stroke is a genuine medical emergency. The patient must be stripped of all clothing, placed in a cool environment with air fans around him. Any failure of the temperature to fall must lead to the immersion of the patient in ice-cold water. Phenothiazine drugs may be helpful in that they prevent shivering and heat generation. DIC may need further treatment.

Malignant hyperpyrexia

This is a very rare genetic disorder in which massive heat production from contracted muscles is triggered by general anaesthetic agents. The body temperature rises and central nervous system (CNS) damage occurs. The effect seems to be related to ineffective calcium handling in the defective muscles. Cessation of anaesthesia, intravenous dantrolene sodium and cooling are used to control the disorder. It is often fatal, and its known presence is an absolute contraindication to general anaesthesia.

Neuroleptic malignant syndrome

This is more common. A raised body temperature and muscle rigidity are accompanied by impaired consciousness. It is usually related to the taking of phenothiazine drugs, often early on in treatment. It is insidious in onset and the raised temperature is associated with a significant mortality.

COLD

A fall in the body temperature below 35°C is likely to occur in the following situations:

1. in healthy adults, usually as a result of exposure to severe cold without proper protection and with heat loss accentuated by alcohol, sedative and vasodilator drugs
2. in the elderly and infirm, it may occur more readily in those who have poorly heated houses and who have sustained some accident or stroke which renders them helpless or comatose
3. in a variety of endocrine disorders, particularly thyroid, pituitary and adrenal cortical failure.

Symptoms and signs

In severe hypothermia, the patient may be comatose, the pulse is slow and there is hypotension. The skin is pale and waxy and feels cold. Respiration is shallow. It is often difficult in such conditions to decide whether a patient has

Table 17.2. Clinical features of hypothermia

?Stroke	Pancreatic damage
?Endocrine dysfunction	Rectal temperature < 35°C
Bradycardia, J waves, dysrhythmia	Low blood pH, hypocalcaemia
Bronchopneumonia	Hypoglycaemia

some endocrine problem, but a careful history and examination for signs such as a thyroidectomy scar are all important (Table 17.2).

Investigations
1. The temperature is read serially using a low-reading rectal thermometer.
2. The blood pH, urea and electrolytes may show evidence of acidosis due to ischaemic tissue anoxia.
3. An ECG will confirm bradycardia and there may be a variety of cardiac dysrhythmias such as atrial fibrillation and characteristic J-waves (junction waves which occur between the QRS and ST segments).
4. It is important to monitor the blood sugar to counteract hypoglycaemia and to apply the appropriate tests for evidence of endocrine failure.
5. The serum amylase may be raised due to cold-induced pancreatic damage.

Treatment
Blood gases, urea and electrolytes are monitored, and repeated measurements are made of the rectal temperature with a low-recording thermometer to ensure that there is a response to treatment. Intubation may be required if there is severe respiratory failure. Re-warming is achieved by wrapping the patient in aluminium foil and nursing at room temperature. It is wise to keep procedures such as intubation to the minimum because of the risks of ventricular fibrillation. Bronchopneumonia is frequently present and early diagnosis and treatment with antibiotics may be required.

CHANGES IN ATMOSPHERIC PRESSURE

Exposure to low atmospheric pressure results from an ascent of high mountains or flight in an unpressurised aircraft. At 15 000 m (50 000 ft) the atmospheric pressure is reduced to about one-tenth of its normal value.

Pressure under water increases because of the overlying water mass; in order to sustain a diver air has to be supplied at increased pressure, or a diving bell resistant to water pressure has to be used. Increased atmospheric pressure in divers results in a number of acute disorders such as joint pains, unsteadiness and tremor, and barotrauma to the ears and sinuses as well as the more acute problems related to decompression.

Acute decompression sickness

If decompression occurs too rapidly in a diver ascending to the surface, then dissolved bubbles of gas are released into the tissues and bloodstream where they may cause tissue injury.

Symptoms and signs

1. There may be a patchy skin rash with pruritus.
2. In the joints and bones, pains known as 'the bends' or in milder cases 'the niggles' are the commonest symptoms. The knees, pelvic and shoulder girdles and elbows are most affected. The bones become tender and severe pain may be felt deep within the bone or muscle.
3. Pain may also occur in the chest, mimicking pleurisy and this is accompanied by severe dyspnoea.
4. In the nervous system, paresis and paraesthesia in the limbs may progress to complete paralysis of all four limbs with cerebellar signs, tinnitus, deafness and ocular paresis.

Treatment

Prophylaxis of this condition consists of ensuring that rapid decompression does not occur and that it is controlled in a decompression tank. Once the condition has occurred, treatment is by rapid recompression, otherwise there is a risk of severe and permanent neurological problems.

Decreased pressure of air gases

Ascent to levels of about 3000 m (10 000 ft) above sea level may be accompanied by an acute mountain sickness. This is a clinical syndrome associated with neurological and pulmonary symptoms due to the accumulation of fluid in the brain and in the lungs, i.e. cerebral and pulmonary oedema. Symptoms usually begin 1–2 days after ascending to a high altitude. They consist of headache which is often severe and occipital, vomiting and nausea, and accompanying dyspnoea with a dry cough. These symptoms may pass off, or with further ascent they may well progress to pulmonary oedema with breathlessness at rest, ataxia, drowsiness and eventual coma. It seems that hypoxia related to the ascent and the accompanying high blood PCO_2 causes fluid retention with movement of fluid into the cells from the plasma and interstitial fluid compartments.

Treatment

As the syndrome is due to rapid and too high an ascent, the basis of treatment entails slowing down the rate of climb and the use of the drug acetozolamide (Diamox). This is a carbonic anhydrase inhibitor which increases urinary bicarbonate excretion. It probably works by reducing cerebrospinal fluid formation and by producing an intracellular acidosis which stimulates the respiratory centre and prevents periodic episodes of apnoea and hypoxia. Dexamethasone is also effective in the management of established cerebral oedema. Pulmonary oedema is treated with diuretics and morphine in the conventional way.

Inert gas narcosis

This is another hazard for the diver who goes below about 50 m, as below this level nitrogen dissolves in nerve membranes and affects nerve function, leading to a deterioration in mental function. It can be prevented by replacing nitrogen with helium which does not have this effect on nerve membranes. This means that divers are kept in an oxygen–helium atmosphere when they are at extreme depths. Pure oxygen would seem to be the answer to all these problems, but it is itself toxic and interferes with surfactant production, causing a syndrome of pulmonary oedema and fibrosis. Therefore, it cannot be used to sustain divers at depth.

Lung rupture

This may occur if divers, on returning to the surface, fail to expel air from the lungs or have access to fresh intakes. The air in the lungs expands on ascent and may enter the pleural space, the mediastinum or the bloodstream, the latter with signs of air embolus. Divers are warned to exhale continuously as they ascend and to make sure that their ascent is not too fast.

Drowning

There are differences in the complications that occur depending on whether submersion is in fresh or salt water. In fresh water, drowning tends to be complicated by haemolysis and cardiac arrest, whereas with salt water disturbances of electrolyte metabolism are seen, particularly a raised serum potassium level. The temperature of the water is also very important, as patients are protected from tissue damage if they are immersed in cold water near $0°C$. These problems are of little importance when treating the patient which must be quick and effective.

Treatment

1. The airway must be cleared and artificial respiration and external cardiac massage started immediately.
2. The stomach must be emptied of swallowed water, and if the patient is comatose and has no gag reflex this must be delayed until an endotracheal tube can be passed to avoid aspiration.
3. Hospital treatment may be continued with assisted ventilation, and positive pressure ventilation may be required to treat pulmonary collapse.

Many patients will inhale water without producing serious cardiac or respiratory embarrassment, but it is important to remember that inhalation of relatively small amounts of fluid often produces delayed pulmonary complications some hours after admission. For these patients, ventilatory assistance and positive and expiratory pressure respiration may also be required, as may treatment with antibiotics to prevent serious infection.

DANGERS OF IONISING RADIATION

The horrors of nuclear war and the hazards resulting from the use of nuclear energy are an ever important threat to the world population—a threat brought into reality by the problems arising in Chernobyl in 1986. Radon gas which is a natural source of α radiation derived from granite has been suggested as an important cause of lung and other cancers and myeloid leukaemia.

The effects of ionising radiation are due to the fact that cell bombardment leads to the production of free radicles within cells and consequently to cell and tissue damage. X-rays and gamma radiation can act both as external and internal sources of neutrons. The effects of radiation depend on the size of the radiation dose. It has now been agreed that the unit by which this dose is measured is the Gray (1 Joule/kg) (1 Gray (Gy) is equivalent to 100 rads). Different radiations are compared by means of a unit of dose equivalence and the unit of dose equivalence is the Sievert (1 Sv = 100 rem).

In the case of acute exposure to radiation of the equivalent of 2–6 Gy or more there results a syndrome of acute radiation damage which is accompanied by anorexia, nausea, vomiting, fever and diarrhoea (Table 17.3). This is usually seen within 48 hours of exposure and may result in damage to the following structures:

1. Bone marrow. There is immediate damage to lymphocytes and resultant lymphopenia. Later, damage occurs to granulocytes and platelets from injury to stem cells. This results in bleeding and susceptibility to infection, usually 2–3 weeks after the radiation injury.
2. Gastrointestinal tract. Following initial vomiting, there may be a period of recovery followed within a few days by evidence of radiation damage to the GI tract. This results in mucosal atrophy, severe diarrhoea with electrolyte loss and dehydration.
3. Central nervous system. With fairly high dosage, 30–100 Gy, there may be evidence of nausea and vomiting with disorientation, coma and death due to direct effects of radiation on the CNS causing cerebral oedema.
4. Skin. There may be erythema blistering and secondary infection due to burning of the skin.

DELAYED EFFECTS OF IONISING RADIATION

1. Malignancy. There is an increased incidence of leukaemia, predominantly of the acute myeloid type. It tends to be more common in males and may occur anywhere up to 10 or more years after the initial exposure.
2. Solid tumours can also be produced by ionising radiation exposure, and here the tumour may occur 40 or more years after the original radiation hazard. Cancer of the skin is the most common but tumours in other organs such as the lungs or breast and lymphomas are well recognized.

Table 17.3. Acute and chronic effects of radiation

Acute	Chronic
Brain injury	Cataracts
Coma, convulsions	Neoplasia (thyroid, salivary glands etc.)
Skin burns, depilation	
Anorexia, nausea, vomiting, diarrhoea	Leukaemia
Bone marrow injury	Teratogenic effects in early pregnancy
Thrombocytopenia leading to bleeding	
Agronulocytosis leading to infection	Infertility

3. Fetal damage. Radiation of the fetus at the critical period 8–16 weeks after conception may lead to serious maldevelopment of the brain with mental retardation, and of course the hazards of leukaemia and solid tumours as seen in adults with radiation exposure.
4. Infertility. If the dose to the gonads is high enough, there may be a teratogenic effect and infertility.
5. Other organs where there may be localised but important damage include the eye where cataracts will be found.

Treatment

It is obvious that control of radiation exposure is vital if these serious consequences are to be prevented. The EC lays down the limits for annual exposure of radiation workers. This is now 50 MSv (5 rem) per year to the whole body, and there are also limits for exposure to specific organs where less than the whole body is exposed. It is assumed that a 40-year working life is applicable.

Treatment

This is entirely supportive and consists of the use of anti-emetics and sedatives for the acute symptoms, energetic replacement of fluid losses from vomiting and diarrhoea, and the combating of bleeding and infection with antibiotics, blood and platelet transfusions. Local surgery may also be required for the removal of necrotic tissue.

There is a suggestion that seriously radiated patients should have blood removed and stored so that this can be returned to them if bone marrow failure develops. Bone marrow may also be grafted.

THE OZONE LAYER

Protection from solar radiation is by means of an ozone layer in the upper atmosphere. Industrial activity resulting in the production of chlorine, bromine and other ozone-depleting gases has led to a partial loss of the ozone layer and increased ultraviolet irradiation of the earth. This was first noted in the southern hemisphere but is now occurring over the highly populated northern hemisphere. Skin ageing, skin cancer and cataracts are possible consequences. Protection of the skin by barrier creams is of great prophylactic importance.

18

INBORN ERRORS OF METABOLISM

Richard Harvey

The inborn errors of metabolism are a group of genetic disorders in which there is abnormal accumulation or deficiencies of particular substances in the body, usually as a result of malfunction of an individual enzyme or transport protein.

Most of these disorders are carried as autosomal or X-linked recessive traits because potentially lethal dominant genes tend to disappear through natural selection. The incidence of the clinical disorder reflects the prevalence of the causative abnormal gene, which often shows considerable variation, with markedly increased incidences of various disorders in isolated communities or in those which tend to intermarry. Thus there is a high incidence of lipid storage disorders (e.g. Tay-Sachs disease) in Jews, of glucose-6-phosphate dehydrogenase deficiency in Greeks and Italians and of variegate porphyria and hypercholesterolaemia in Afrikaaners.

Table 18.1. Factors which should suggest the possibility of inborn metabolic disease

Persistent vomiting (may suggest pyloric stenosis, but with acidosis rather than alkalosis)

Poor feeding, failure to thrive

Severe illness in neonatal period, suggestive of septicaemia

Unexplained drowsiness, fits, coma

Jaundice or hepatomegaly

Metabolic acidosis

Odd smell

Unexplained hypoglycaemia, hyponatraemia or neutropenia

Delayed development or mental retardation

Family history of death in early life

Consanguinity

Symptoms worse after feeds or improved on glucose/saline

Table 18.2. Abnormalities of miscellaneous plasma proteins/enzymes

Protein	Normal function	Deficiency state
Alkaline phosphatase	Bone mineralisation	Hypophosphatasia
Pseudocholinesterase	Participates in destruction of some synthetic choline esters	Suxamethonium (succinylcholine) sensitivity
C1 esterase inhibitor	Inhibits activity of the complement component C1	Hereditary angio-oedema
Alpha-1-antitrypsin	Inhibits damaging effect of trypsin on lungs	Familial emphysema
Caeruloplasmin	Oxidase activity Copper content 0.34%	Hepatolenticular degeneration (Wilson's disease)
Antihaemophilic globulin (AHG)	Blood clotting	Haemophilia A (classical haemophilia)
Immunoglobulins	Agammaglobulinaemia	All Ig classes very low Plasma cells absent
Selective IgA deficiency	—	Both plasma and secretory IgA deficient, other Ig classes normal
Thyroxine-binding globulin (TBG)	Transport of thyroxine	TBG deficiency

Clinical features	Inheritance
Abnormal bone mineralisation, often rather like rickets Hypercalcaemia sometimes Variable severity	Autosomal recessive
Succinylcholine is a popular muscle relaxant used in anaesthesia Normal persons given usual dose develop apnoea for 3–4 min In homozygous pseudocholinesterase deficiency apnoea often lasts over 30 min, necessitating artificial ventilation	Autosomal recessive Heterozygotes are mildly affected
Attacks of angio-oedema and/or atypical abdominal pains May be fatal if laryngeal oedema occurs Fresh plasma has been used to interrupt a severe attack Stanazolol (an anabolic steroid), in small oral doses, effectively prevents attacks	Dominant, varying penetrance
Development of emphysema in adult life Alpha-1-antitrypsin deficiency is found in up to 50% of patients with 'pure' emphysema Also liver disease	Autosomal recessive Heterozygotes are mildly affected
Low serum copper and increased copper absorption result in copper accumulation in tissues, with damage to liver (cirrhosis), kidneys (aminoaciduria etc.) and basal ganglia (involuntary movements) Exact pathogenesis still uncertain	Autosomal recessive
Easy bruising and bleeding, haemarthrosis etc	X-linked recessive
Recurrent pyogenic infections	X-linked recessive
Enteropathy with malabsorption, like coeliac disease, bacterial respiratory tract infections	Autosomal recessive
Thyroid function normal but total serum thyroxine low, so may lead to incorrect diagnosis of hypothyroidism TSH level is normal	Dominant

Diagnosis and screening

Most of the more serious inborn errors of metabolism present in early life and should be diagnosed as early as possible, partly because in some cases early treatment may be life saving or may prevent permanent brain damage, and partly because, even if no treatment is available, the risk in future pregnancies can be assessed and the parents counselled appropriately. Clinical features which suggest the possibility of an inborn error of metabolism are listed in Table 18.1.

Unfortunately it is impractical to screen all babies for all disorders. It is only worth finding an inborn error if it is potentially serious yet has an effective treatment available, and it is probably not worth looking in a newborn baby for disorders seen in fewer than 1 in 50 000 live births. Screening can obviously be more intensive in an ill baby (Table 18.1), and in families with an affected member, in children of consanguineous marriages or in mentally retarded individuals. In one screening programme in New England, 19 000 infants were screened, yielding 38 cases of hypothyroidism, 3 cases of phenylketonuria, 2 cases of homocystinuria and 1 each of galactosaemia and maple syrup urine disease. Screening costs were $0.80 for hypothyroidism and $1.20 for amino acid disorders.

Problems of carrier detection, prenatal diagnosis, counselling and the possibility of future genetic therapy are discussed in Chapter 19. Because of the relatively large number of inborn errors of metabolism, they have been grouped in this chapter in a series of tables which are self-explanatory (Tables 18.2-6). The rarest disorders have been excluded, and in some cases a single example has been included of a group of related disorders which are described more fully elsewhere in this book (e.g. haemophilia A).

Table 18.3. Inborn errors of amino acid metabolism

Condition	Defective enzyme	Biochemical and clinical consequences
Phenylketonuria	Phenylalanine 4-hydroxylase	Phenylalanine (PA) accumulates in the body fluids, phenylpyruvate and derivatives excreted in urine Severe mental deficiency, epilepsy, eczema Normal development possible if given low PA diet within first few months of life, continued long-term
Alkaptonuria	Homogentisic acid oxidase	Homogentisic acid accumulates in body fluids, and is excreted in urine Urine goes dark brown or black on standing, e.g. staining nappies Cartilage and sclerae may darken (ochronosis) and osteoarthritis appears from second or third decade Prognosis good without treatment
Homocystinuria	Cystathionine synthetase	Homocystine accumulates and is excreted in urine Mental retardation, dislocation of lenses and tendency to arterial and venous thromboses No proven treatment as yet
Albinism	o-diphenol-oxidase	Lack of melanin in skin, hair and eyes, resulting in nystagmus, photophobia, skin carcinomas Treatment is symptomatic (avoid sun, wear dark glasses)
Tyrosinosis	p-hydroxy-phenylpyruvic acid oxidase	Tyrosine accumulates and is excreted Rapid liver enlargement, cirrhosis and, usually, death in infancy due to hepatic failure Chronic types known—these develop renal tubular lesion with acidosis and vitamin-D-resistant rickets Prognosis poor however treated
Maple syrup urine disease	Branched chain ketoacid decarboxylase	Accumulation of valine, leucine and isoleucine with urinary excretion of their derivatives (characteristic smell) Severe cerebral degeneration with early death Milder form occurs which may be helped by diet low in the 3 amino acids
Goitrous cretinism	Tyrosine iodinase, Coupling enzyme, Iodotyrosine deiodinase	All types develop goitre and cretinism of variable severity Replacement therapy with L-thyroxine is completely effective

Table 18.4 Some inborn defects of transport mechanisms

Disorder	Site of defect	Biochemical abnormality
Cystinuria	Proximal renal tubule and small intestine	Defective tubular reabsorption and jejunal absorption of dibasic amino acids (cystine, lysine arginine, ornithine)
Hartnup disease	Proximal renal tubule and small intestine	Defective tubular reabsorption and jejunal absorption of most monoaminomonocarboxylic and acidic amino acids Deficiency of nicotinamide (derived from tryptophan) results in pellagra
Lignac-Fanconi or Debre-de Toni-Fanconi syndrome Cystinosis	Proximal renal tubule	Defective tubular reabsorption of most amino acids, urinary losses of glucose, phosphate (leading to rickets), bicarbonate (leading to acidosis), and deposition of cystine in tissues
Adult Fanconi's syndrome	Proximal renal tubule	Renal glycosuria, aminoaciduria, proteinuria and excessive urinary losses of phosphate, bicarbonate, potassium and water in various combinations
Renal tubular acidosis	Distal renal tubule	Impaired H^+ exchange in tubule resulting in acidosis, hyperchloraemia increased, calcium excretion
Hypophosphataemia (hereditary vitamin-D-resistant rickets)	Proximal renal tubule	Excessive urinary losses of phosphate resulting in low plasma phosphate
Pseudohypoparathyroidism	Proximal renal tubule	Tubules unresponsive to action of parathormone (parathyroids are normal) Abnormally low phosphate excretion high serum phosphate, low calcium
Nephrogenic diabetes insipidus	Distal renal tubule and collecting ducts	Tubules unresponsive to action of antidiuretic hormone Copious flow of dilute urine, which continues even if patient becomes dehydrated

Inheritance	Clinical effects	Treatment
Recessive	Formation of cystine calculi (about 1% of all urinary calculi, much greater proportion in children) Asymptomatic in many cases, these are usually heterozygotes	High fluid intake Alkalinisation of urine
Recessive	Pellagrous rash of face and extremities, (photosensitive) and cerebellar ataxia with falling attacks	Nicotinamide
Recessive	a. Acute childhood type: presents in first year of life with vomiting, thirst, failure to thrive Acidosis and vitamin-D-resistant rickets. Usually lethal in first decade b. Chronic type: usually presents about 2 years of age with vitamin-D-resistant rickets and photophobia (cystine deposits in eye) Cystine deposited in tissues, especially reticuloendothelial system Progressive renal damage and death from uraemia (usually in second decade)	Alkalis, vitamin D
Recessive	First symptoms in adult life (e.g. 30 years of age) with bone pain etc. due to osteomalacia	Vitamin D, other supplements if appropriate (e.g. potassium)
Various	Rickets or osteomalacia, sometimes asymptomatic	Alkalis, vitamin D
X-linked dominant	Presents as rickets around 1 year of age	Very large doses of vitamin D or dihydro-tachysterol
Dominant, varying penetrance	Onset in first or second decade Tetany, fits, cramps, paraesthesia, mental retardation Calcification in basal ganglia and subcutaneous tissue Short 4th and 5th metacarpals	Large doses of vitamin D Calcium supplements
X-linked recessive	Dehydration, mental retardation	High oral intake of water Chlorothiazide has antidiuretic effect in some cases

Table 18.4 Some inborn defects of transport mechanisms *continued*

Disorder	Site of defect	Biochemical abnormality
Renal glycosuria	Proximal renal tubule	Reduced tubular reabsorption of glucose
Iodine trapping defect	Thyroid	Inability to take up iodine from plasma
Congenital lactase deficiency	Small intestine	Inability to hydrolyse lactose This type much less common than acquired lactase deficiency
Congenital sucrase– isomaltase deficiency	Small intestine	Inability to hydrolyse sucrose and isomaltase

Table 18.5. Genetic disorders of collagen synthesis

Disorder	Defect
Marfan's syndrome (arachnodactyly)	Possibly poorly cross-linked collagen
Ehlers-Danlos syndrome	Seven different types, some with known defective enzyme (e.g. type VI, lysyl hydroxylase)
Osteogenesis imperfecta (fragilitas ossium, brittle bone disease)	Impaired synthesis of type I procollagen
Pseudoxanthoma elasticum	Uncertain — probably a defect in transcription
Cutis laxa	Uncertain, possibly lysyl oxidase deficiency

Inheritance	Clinical effects	Treatment
Dominant	None May result in mistaken diagnosis of diabetes mellitus Glucose tolerance test will distinguish the two	None required
Various	Goitrous cretinism	L-thyroxine
?	Symptoms develop within a few days of birth, as soon as feeding is established Misery, abdominal colic and acid diarrhoea (lactic acid formed from unabsorbed lactose)	Lactose-free diet
Recessive	Most present in infancy, with diarrhoea at weaning, some later Acid diarrhoea after sucrose and sometimes after starch	Sucrose-free, starch-reduced diet

Clinical features

Long thin limbs and fingers, high arched palate, dislocated lens, lax joints
Weak arteries leading to aneurysmal dilatation of aortic arch with resulting rupture, aortic valve incompetence
Dominant, varying penetrance

Various combinations of fragility and hyperelasticity of skin, easy bruising, 'cigarette paper' scars, hyperextensible joints with dislocations, poor tensile strength of aorta, gut and eye, leading sometimes to spontaneous rupture of any of these
Various different types of inheritance

Dwarfism, weak brittle bones, many deformities from fractures
Sclerae may be blue
May be severe type (fractures in utero, early death) or relatively mild

Small soft flat yellowish papules parallel to skin folds, especially sides of neck, axillae
Linear 'angioid' streaks in retina
Tendency to bleed spontaneously into gastrointestinal tract
Prone to hypertension, atheroma

Loose inelastic skin, hanging in folds
Hypermobility of joints
X-linked recessive or dominant

Table 18.6. Miscellaneous inborn errors of metabolism

Condition	Nature of disorder	Clinical features
Galactosaemia	Galactose-1-phosphate uridyl transferase deficiency	Normal at birth, but with milk (lactose) ingestion progressive accumulation of galactose causes hepatosplenomegaly and mental deficiency Cured by galactose-free diet if started early enough
Leucine-induced hypoglycaemia	Mechanism uncertain	Protein (leucine) ingestion causes hypoglycaemia, with fits and brain damage Prevented by adequate carbohydrate intake with proteins
Von Gierke's disease	Glycogen storage disorder (one of several types) due to glucose-6-phosphatase deficiency	Retarded growth, accumulation of glycogen in the liver and kidneys Frequent carbohydrate feeds, ?liver transplant
McArdle's syndrome	Deficiency of muscle glycogen phosphorylase	Muscle pain on exercise, relieved by oral glucose
Hurler's syndrome	Mucopolysaccharidosis (one of several types)	Dermatan sulphate and heparin sulphate progressively accumulate, with coarse facial features, hepatosplenomegaly, skeletal changes, mental retardation
Tay-Sachs disease Gaucher's disease and Niemann-Pick disease	Lipidoses (three of several types)	Accumulation of various lipids (specific for each type) in brain, liver, spleen etc. Usually recessive disorders occurring in Jews Most get dementia, epilepsy and blindness (cherry-red spot at macula) with early death, but in Gaucher's disease there is a chronic adult form consistent with a normal lifespan

19

GENETICS AND MOLECULAR MEDICINE

Peter Lunt

There are an estimated 10 000–100 000 separate transcribed genes in the human genome which has a total (haploid) DNA content of 3.3 x 10⁹ base pairs. The coding part of each gene which is transcribed into mRNA is arranged in several different sections known as 'exon sequences' or 'exons'. These are separated by non-transcribed 'intron sequences' or 'introns' which maintain the integrity and conformation of the gene for transcription and tissue-specific mRNA splicing. Other DNA sequences adjacent to genes regulate their overall transcription.

New or established 'mutation' allows potentially unlimited variation between individuals. Mutations in exons are usually deleterious, causing single gene 'Mendelian' disorders. Other DNA sequence variation may be neutral, beneficial or deleterious, and possibly through determining differences between people in response to similar environments, set their genetic susceptibility to common diseases or congenital defects. Genetic factors are likely if:

1. presentation is at a younger age than average
2. the disease has bilateral or multifocal onset
3. there is a positive family history.

Not all genetic material is in the nucleus; there are diseases caused by mutation in mitochondrial DNA. Also, in the recently recognised prion protein diseases, it seems that inherited mutation in a nuclear gene can code for an infective protein agent.

PATTERNS OF INHERITANCE

Familial disease follows one of several possible inheritance patterns: autosomal dominant (AD), autosomal recessive (AR), X-linked recessive (XR), X-linked dominant (XD), polygenic/multifactorial, chromosomal, mitochondrial or non-genetic.

The properties of these are summarised in Table 19.1, with examples in Table 19.4 and Figures 19.1, 19.2 and 19.3.

Table 19.1. Patterns of inheritance

Inheritance		Cause	Sex affected
Autosomal dominant	(AD)	Single faulty gene copy	M = F
Autosomal recessive	(AR)	Both gene copies faulty	M = F
X-linked recessive	(XR)	Faulty gene on X Chromosone	M but F possible★
Multifactorial	(MF)	Combination of several genes ± environment	Often unequal
Mitochondrial	(MT)	Mitochondrial DNA defect	M ≥ F

	Risk to offspring	Risk to sibs	Risk to wider family
AD	50%	50% if parent affected; low if not	Significant unless new mutation
AR	Very low (unless consanguinity)	25%	Very low (unless consanguinity)
XR	Nil to sons of affected; his daughters all carry 50% to carrier's sons	Up to 50% for brothers	Significant in female line
MF	Low (often 2–5%) †	Low (often 2–5%) †	Low; fails with distance †
MT	Up to 100% from mother; nil from father	Up to 100% if mother affected	Significant if female line

	Asymptomatic 'carriers'	New mutation	Severity within family
AD	Possible if late onset or reduced penetrance	Some cases; beware non-penetrance	Variable
AR	Both parents; 2/3 normal sibs; all offspring; low in population	Very rare	Uniform
XR	≥ 2/3 of mothers; 50% of carrier's daughters; all daughters of affected; 33–50% of sisters	Up to 1/3 of cases	Uniform
MF	–		Variable †
MT	Females if late onset or reduced penetrance	Occurs; deletions	Variable

Table 19.1. ★Rarely female carriers may manifest X-linked recessive conditions through homozygosity (father affected, mother a carrier), XO karyotype (Turner's syndrome), X-autosome translocation, or non-random X-inactivation (one X chromosome is inactivated in each cell in a female; usually this is randomly determined).

  † In polygenic inheritance, the genetic risk is raised the more cases there are in the family, the greater is the severity, or where the index case is of the less-commonly affected sex.

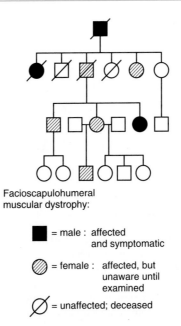

Facioscapulohumeral muscular dystrophy:

■ = male : affected and symptomatic

⊘ = female : affected, but unaware until examined

∅ = unaffected; deceased

Fig. 19.1 Autosomal dominant inheritance.

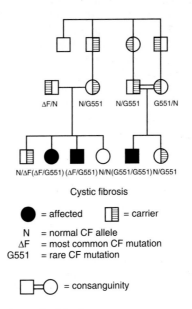

Cystic fibrosis

● = affected   ▣ = carrier

N = normal CF allele
ΔF = most common CF mutation
G551 = rare CF mutation

☐━○ = consanguinity

Fig. 19.2 Autosomal recessive inheritance.

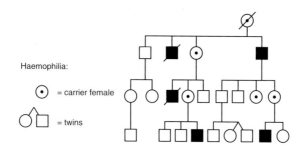

Fig. 19.3 X-linked recessive inheritance.

CHROMOSOME ABNORMALITIES

Chromosome abnormalities occur in 1/150 live births; and can result in either balance (from rearrangement) or imbalance (from duplication or deletion) of genetic material. Apart from sex chromosome abnormalities, imbalance is invariably associated with mental retardation and dysmorphism, and often with congenital malformation, poor growth, and early death. Some abnormalities survive only as mosaics, with a mixture of normal and abnormal cell lines.

Autosomal trisomies

These abnormalities have a whole extra chromosome. Trisomy 21 (t21, Down's syndrome) occurs in 1/700 births, but more frequently to older mothers (1/200 at age 38 years; 1/100 at age 40 years). In addition to moderate to severe mental retardation (IQ 25–50), associated problems can include hypotonia, congenital heart defects (especially AV canal, ventricular septal defect, Fallot's tetralogy) duodenal atresia, Hirschprung's disease, short stature, cataract, leukaemia and early-onset Alzheimer's disease. Maximum survival is usually 35–50 years. Mosaic trisomy 21 tends to be less severe. Other autosomal trisomies (t13 or t18) result in multiple malformations and neonatal or infant death. Mosaic trisomy 8 which usually causes some skeletal problems and only mild to moderate retardation, is an exception, being compatible with a normal lifespan.

Structural rearrangements

A subject with imbalance of genetic material often has a chromosome structural rearrangement. This may have originated in balanced form in either parent, whose karyotypes should therefore be studied.
Balanced rearrangements:

1. show no overall loss or gain of genetic material
2. are often inherited; a complete family study is advisable
3. rarely affect the carrier except where a breakpoint disrupts an expressed gene; such cases have proved invaluable for gene mapping (e.g. neurofibromatosis to 17q, polyposis coli to 5q)*

4. may produce offspring with unbalanced karyotype; either live born, or as recurrent miscarriage.

* 'p' = chromosome short arm; 'q' = chromosome long arm.

Sex chromosome anomalies

The overall incidence of sex chromosome aneuploidy is around 1/500 births. The incidence at conception is much higher, but over 90% of conceptuses with 45,XO abort spontaneously. Details are given in Table 19.2.

Fragile-X syndrome

This is the single most common cause of mental retardation in males (1/1200) after Down's syndrome. Using a low folate culture technique a 'fragile site' is seen on the distal long arm of one X-chromosome in about 80% of affected males and in 30–50% of carrier females. Inheritance is X-linked recessive; intelligence in female carriers may be reduced, but non-manifesting male and female carriers occur. The gene defect is an expansion of a tandemly repeated triplet base-pair sequence from one end of the 'fragile-X gene' which maps at or close to the 'fragile site' at Xq27. The severity of retardation tends to correlate with the size of insert.

Microdeletion syndromes

Several dysmorphic syndromes associated with retardation are caused by the deletion of contiguous genes from small sections of chromosome material, e.g. velocardiofacial/Di George syndrome (Table 19.3) on chromosome 22q. Detection may require the use of DNA probes to show an apparent lack of inheritance from one parent, or under a microscope to show hybridisation of a fluorescently labelled DNA probe from the deleted region to only one of a chromosome pair. The clinical phenotype may differ according to which parent's copy is lost, as for example at 15q11 in distinguishing Prader-Willi syndrome (hypotonia, obesity, hypogenitalism, and retardation) from Angelman syndrome (retardation, ataxia and characteristic EEG and facies). Alternatively, in these two conditions both copies of chromosome 15 may originate from one parent (uniparental disomy), and the outcome depend on which parent this is. This may reflect 'geonomic imprinting' whereby the paternal and maternal copies of certain genes may be expressed differently, according to early-determined differences in patterns of nucleotide methylation.

CONGENITAL ABNORMALITIES AND DYSMORPHIC SYNDROMES

A 'dysmorphic or malformation syndrome' is a recognised combination of morphological defects, usually of genetic origin. Often there are characteristic key major abnormalities (e.g. polydactyly, cleft palate, congenital heart defect) supported by associated minor features (e.g. transverse palmar crease,

Table 19.2. Sex chromosome anomalies

Syndrome	Turner	Klinefelter
Karyotype	45, XO (or mosaic)	47, XXY (or mosaic)
Sex	F	M
Incidence per 1000 M or F	0.4 (high fetal loss)	1.8
Stature	Short	Tall, eunochoid
Sexual development	Gonadal dysgenesis, absent pubertal development	Small penis and testes, gynaecomastia, female pattern of body hair
Fertility	Infertile, pregnancy with donor egg possible	Infertile
Average intellect	95% of expected	85–90% of expected
Personality	Normal	Shy, immature
Congenital anomaly	Coarctation, horseshoe kidney, lymphoedema, neck webbing, broad chest, cubitus valgus	Non-specific increase
Complications	Pigmented naevi, gonadoblastoma if XO/XY mosaic	Increased risk of breast cancer
Treatment	Oestrogen, growth hormone, gonadectomy if XO/XY	±Testosterone replacement systemically or local cream

increased eye spacing, café au lait patches); but all features are not usually present in any one individual. 10% of the general population have at least one minor dysmorphic feature; three or more increase the likelihood of an associated major malformation. Table 19.3 lists some of the more common dysmorphic syndromes encountered in general medicine.

MOLECULAR MECHANISMS IN DISEASE

Mutation can disrupt genes through:

1. Point mutation: amino acid substitution, removal or introduction of 'stop' codon.

Triple X	XYY	XX male	Testicular feminisation
47, XXX	47, XYY	46, XX	46, XY (XR gene)
F	M	M	F
1.2	1.0	0.04	?
± Tall	Tall	± Short	Normal female
Normal	Normal	As XXY, genitalia may be ambiguous	Absent uterus, normal secondary sex features
Normal, offspring usually 46, XX or XY	Normal, offspring usually 46, XX or XY	Infertile	Infertile
Mildly retarded	85–90% of expected	Variable	Normal
—	Impulsive/normal	—	Normal female
Not increased	Not increased	Can occur	Absent uterus
—	Prevalence 5 × in criminals	—	Gonadal tumours
—	—	—	—

2. Deletion: loss of whole or part of the DNA sequence of a gene; absence or truncation of the protein product.
3. Insertion: introduction of one or more extra base pairs. Unless a multiple of three base pairs, the triplet reading frame is put out of phase (frameshift) Disruption of a gene through insertion of a tandemly repeated three base-pair sequence may exhibit correlation between the size of the insert and the resulting phenotypic severity.
4. Regulator gene mutation: affects the level or timing of gene expression. Gene duplication may also affect gene expression.
5. Splice mutation: affects the splicing and joining of the transcribed exon sequences to make mRNA.

At cellular level mutation may act through:

Table 19.3. Some dysmorphic syndromes

Feature/system	Stickler syndrome	Velocardiofacial	Tuberosclerosis
Genetics	Dominant	Dominant microdeletion	Dominant
Chrom. location	12q	22q	9q, 16p
Gene	Collagen 2	?	?
Mutation	Point or deletion	Microdeletion	?
Facial	Small nose and chin	Broad nose, wide eye spacing	Adenoma sebaceum
Mouth	Cleft palate	Cleft or submucous cleft palate	
CNS		Retarded	Epilepsy, retarded
Hearing/vision	Deafness, myopia, detached retina		Retinal phakoma
Musculoskeletal	Arthritic hip, lax joints		Bone cysts
CVS		Fallot's, truncus, right aortic arch,VSD	Rhabdomyoma
Skin			Depig. patch, nailbed fibroma, shagreen patch
Other		Small thymus	Renal cyst

1. Reduced enzyme activity: most recessive inborn errors of metabolism.
2. Alteration of a structural protein: may affect membrane integrity, e.g. some dominant mutations.
3. Protein subunit alteration: dominant effect in multimeric protein.
4. Altered protein antigenicity: may facilitate immunoreactive disorders.
5. Oncogene activation: dominant promotion of uncontrolled cell division.
6. Oncogene suppressor mutation: reduces control of oncogene expression.
   e.g. Knudson 2-hit hypothesis for origin of malignancy: mutation in one

Neurofibromatosis	Myotonic dystrophy	Marfan syndrome	Sturge-Weber syndrome
Dominant	Dominant	Dominant	Sporadic
17q	19q	15q	—
Nerve growth regulator	Protein kinase	Fibrillin	—
Point or deletion	Expanded CTG tandem repeat	Point or deletion	—
Large head	Myopathic face, frontal balding, ptosis		Port-wine stain
		High-arched palate	
Glioma, mildly retarded	Mildly retarded		Epilepsy, tram-line calcified
Optic glioma	Cataract	Myopia, lens dislocation	Glaucoma
Scoliosis, pseudarthrosis	Grip myotonia, distal weakness	Tall, long digits, scoliosis, pectus, lax joints	
	Arrhythmia, (beware anaesthetics)	Aortic dissection, mitral prolapse	
Café-au-lait, neurofibroma		Thin	Port-wine stain
	Constipation		

copy of an oncogene suppressor is inherited as a dominant trait in all cells; a second somatic mutation occurring in the opposite copy of the gene produces a malignant cell line (e.g. familial retinoblastoma).

USE OF MOLECULAR GENETICS IN RISK ASSESSMENT AND DIAGNOSIS

In many Mendelian disorders, molecular genetic techniques now make possible genetic prediction for:

1. presymtomatic prediction in late-onset disorders
2. clarification of affected/unaffected status in cases of clinical doubt
3. prenatal diagnosis
4. carrier prediction in X-linked recessive, autosomal recessive and incompletely penetrant dominant disorders.

Genetic prediction relies on either an indirect or a direct method.

Indirect method. This is the ability to 'track' the faulty copy of a gene through a family by using indirect DNA probes which recognise normal DNA sequence variation at a site adjacent on the chromosome to the disease gene. This requires DNA samples from several members of a family.

Direct method. This is the ability to recognise the presence or absence of the specific mutation or mutation type causing the disease in a particular family. This may be possible using DNA from the test subject alone, or may require comparison with DNA from an affected family member.

Both methods require knowledge of the specific chromosomal regional localisation of the disease gene locus; most direct methods also require that the disease gene has been cloned and sequenced (Table 19.4)

Quite apart from predictive applications, the ability to recognise mutations within a specific gene is providing a definitive differential diagnostic test and absolute proof of diagnosis in a rapidly increasing number of genetic disorders (see Table 19.4).

Indirect methods for prediction: restriction fragment length polymorphisms (RFLPs) and other DNA markers

Once a disease gene is mapped to a specific chromosomal region, closely linked DNA marker loci can usually be identified using DNA probes. Marker loci are sites at which differences in DNA sequence in the normal population (termed 'polymorphisms'), and hence potentially between the two chromosome copies in any one individual, can be detected by chopping the DNA into fragments with bacterial restriction enzymes (nucleases). Where DNA sequence differences determine presence or absence of an enzyme chopping site, alternative length fragments, known as restriction fragment length polymorphisms (RFLPs) can be generated. Following the separation on an electrophoretic gel and 'Southern blotting' on to membrane filters the RFLPs can be recognised by hybridisation to a fluorescent or radioactively labelled DNA probe whose sequence is complementary to that of the marker locus. The many sites throughout the genome where occur multiple tandemly arranged repeats of short DNA sequences (e.g. CACACACA) provide other valuable polymorphic marker loci.

In any one family, provided that the marker and disease gene loci are sufficiently close together on the chromosome, one particular RFLP (marker locus allele), will consistently track with the mutated disease gene in that family, enabling prediction for at-risk family members (Fig. 19.4). The particular marker allele concerned will usually differ between different families. Only for

Table 19.4. Inheritance, chromosomal location, gene cloning and availability of DNA markers for some common genetic disorders

Disorder	Inheritance	Location	Gene cloned
Direct DNA test			
Acute intermittent porphyria	AD	11q	PBG deaminase
Adenomatous polyposis coli	AD	5q	FAP gene
Alzheimer's disease			
(early onset)	AD	21q	Amyloid precursor
Ehlers-Danlos syndrome (type 4)	AD	2q	Collagen 3
FSH muscular dystrophy	AD	4q	–
Huntington's chorea	AD	4p	Huntington
Marfan's syndrome	AD	15q	Fibrillin
Mytononic dystrophy	AD	19q	Myotonin kinase
Neurofibromatosis	AD	17q	NF gene
Osteogenesis imperfecta (type 1)	AD	7q or 17q	Collagen 1
Peroneal muscular atrophy			
(HMSN1)	AD	17p	–
Retinitis pigmentosa (some)	AD	3q	Rhodopsin
Retinoblastoma	AD	13q	RB gene
Stickler's syndrome	AD	12q	Collagen 2
Albinism (tyrosinase negative)	AR	11q	Tyrosinase
α-1-antitrypsin deficiency	AR	14q	α-1-antitrypsin
α-thalassemia	AR	16p	α-globin
β-thalassemia/sickle-cell	AR	11p	β-globin
Cystic fibrosis	AR	7q	CFTR gene
Phenylketonuria	AR	12q	PheHydroxylase
Christmas disease (factor IX)	XR	Xq26	Factor IX
Duchenne/Becker muscular			
dystrophy	XR	Xp21	Dystrophin
Fragile-X syndrome	XR	Xq27	FraX gene
G6PD deficiency	XR	Xq28	G6PD
Haemophilia A (factor VIII)	XR	Xq28	Factor VIII
Testicular feminization	XR	Xq12	Androgen receptor
Leber's optic atrophy	MT	MT	NADH dehydrogenase 4
Mitochondrial cytopathy	MT	MT	Mitochondrial genes
Linked DNA markers only			
Adult polycystic kidney disease	AD	16p	–
Hypertrophic cardiomyopathy	AD	14q	β-Myosin H chain
Tuberose sclerosis	AD	9q/16p	–
Friedrich's ataxia	AR	9q	–
Spinal muscular atrophy	AR	5q	–
Wilson's disease	AR	13q	–
Nephrogenic diabetes insipidus	XR	Xq28	–
Retinitis pigmentosa (some)	XR	Xp11	–

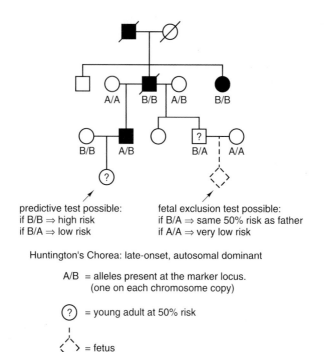

predictive test possible:
if B/B ⇒ high risk
if B/A ⇒ low risk

fetal exclusion test possible:
if B/A ⇒ same 50% risk as father
if A/A ⇒ very low risk

Huntington's Chorea: late-onset, autosomal dominant

A/B = alleles present at the marker locus.
(one on each chromosome copy)

(?) = young adult at 50% risk

⟨ ⟩ = fetus

Fig. 19.4 Clinical prediction by an indirect DNA marker.

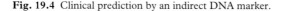

a marker locus extremely close to the disease gene may a mutation-linked marker allele correlate between families; but such 'linkage disequilibrium' can greatly assist with clinical genetic prediction and with research aimed at characterising the disease gene.

A prediction for any at-risk family member based on indirect markers requires study of several different members of the family (see Fig. 19.4). The ability to offer prediction and its accuracy are limited by:

1. the possibility of an alternative genetic diagnosis (heterogeneity)
2. the likelihood of meiotic crossover between marker and disease locus
3. the need to differentiate the 'high-risk' and 'low-risk' marker in the parent of the test subject
4. the availability of DNA samples from other members of the family.

Direct DNA methods for prediction and specific diagnosis

The limitations on indirect methods for prediction are avoided if direct methods are available for detection of the specific mutation or mutation type within the disease gene. This is already possible in several disorders following mapping, cloning and characterisation of the disease genes (Table 19.4). Direct DNA methods have unlimited potential, not only as absolute predictors of genetic disease or susceptibility, but as definitive tools for differential diagnosis.

In most cases direct methods require knowledge or a best guess of the family-specific mutation, and use DNA probes complementary to the mutation or, as in Duchenne muscular dystrophy, complementary to exons deleted from the gene. In cystic fibrosis (CF) the most common mutation is a three base-pair deletion (ΔF508) which can be detected with a short but specifically matching complementary DNA probe. Some rarer mutations in CF can also be tested for routinely using other mutation-specific DNA probes (e.g. G551D in Fig. 19.2). In sickle cell haemoglobin the β6: GAG$\rightarrow$GTG point mutation removes a restriction enzyme chopping site, and results in a specific RFLP recognised by a β-globin DNA probe.

In other conditions it is possible to test for a specific common mechanism of mutation, i.e. gene duplication in type I hereditary motor and sensory neuropathy, and expanded insertion within a gene of a tandemly repeated three base-pair sequence in myotonic dystrophy Huntington's chorea and fragile-X syndromes.

Other clinical applications of direct DNA probes

Monitoring spread or residual disease in cancer. Cells with malignant potential may show recognisable specific alterations of DNA (e.g. 9/22 chromosome translocation breakpoint in chronic myeloid leukaemia). DNA probes complementary to the altered sequence can be used to monitor remission or relapse, or, on biopsy sections, to assess the spread of malignant cells in a tissue.

Identifying infective agents. DNA probes with sequence complementary to DNA or RNA from specific bacteria or viruses can be used to identify the presence of these organisms in tissue sections by in situ hybridisation, or in blood or other body fluids following amplification of nucleic acids by polymerase chain reaction (PCR) techniques.

Future genetic susceptibility. With increasing understanding of the genetic basis underlying susceptibility to common diseases, screening within high-risk families or whole populations for specific higher-risk variant alleles will become feasible, and allow prophylactic measures to be taken.

GENE MAPPING

Knowledge of the exact chromosomal regional location of a disease gene is a prerequisite for the identification of closely linked marker loci for clinical application, and increasingly for the identification of specific mutations and for characterisation of the disease gene itself. This in turn leads to an understanding of the disease pathogenesis and to research for potential treatments. Gene mapping can be achieved through:

1. genetic linkage analysis to polymorphic marker loci in large families
2. genetic linkage analysis with a proposed and previously located candidate gene locus

3. chance finding of association with a chromosomal abnormality
4. in situ hybridisation to a chromosome spread, of a DNA probe with a sequence complementary to the transcribed mRNA
5. study of gene expression in human–rodent cell hybrids
6. looking for mutations in a candidate gene.

GENETIC COUNSELLING

Genetic counselling is the assessment and discussion of information pertaining to genetic risk with a person or couple who may be at risk of having inherited or of passing on a genetic disorder, often so that they can take informed decisions relating to personal prediction or to reproductive options. Assessment of risk may depend on the combination of a prior risk from their age and pedigree structure together with the results obtained from clinical, biochemical and molecular genetic investigations, particularly where predictive DNA tests are relying on indirect markers. Risk figures from the various parameters are usually combined using Bayesian statistical methods.

Accuracy of diagnosis

Accuracy of diagnosis is essential for correctly advising on inheritance pattern and recurrence risk, and especially for prediction from gene tracking with indirect probes.

Ethical issues: predictive testing

Predictive testing for a late-onset disorder (e.g. Huntington's disease) is offered only to a consenting adult and after due consideration; children should not be tested unless treatment could be offered.

Prediction for one family member should avoid unsolicited prediction for other members, e.g. in fetal exclusion testing (see Fig. 19.4).

Paternity testing may be required to validate inferred genotypes.

Prenatal tests

Invasive prenatal tests should only be offered if the outcome would influence management of the pregnancy. The legal limit for termination of pregnancy in the UK is 24 weeks' gestation.

The wider family

Family members who may be at risk of carrying or transmitting serious genetic disease but who are felt likely to be unaware of this should in general, and with a sensitive approach, be informed of their potential risk, together with an offer for further discussion and testing, particularly if prophylactic surveillance and therapeutic measures can be offered.

COMMUNITY AND POPULATION GENETICS

Prevalence of genetic disease

Many common diseases, perhaps affecting up to 30% of people, have a significant genetic component. Although individually serious single gene disorders are rare, they manifest in approximately 3–5% of the general population, the most common in whites being familial hypercholesterolaemia (AD: 1/500), fragile-X syndrome (XR: 1/1200 males) and cystic fibrosis (AR: 1/2000 births). In other populations the prevalence of a specific genetic disease may be much higher (e.g. sickle cell disease in Afro-Caribbeans).

Screening programmes

Screening for genetic disorders can be offered to family members at high risk, selected population groups or the whole population.

Population screening is only applicable if a positive result benefits the individual or his family, the false negative rate is low (high sensitivity), the false positive rate is low (high specificity), and the benefits outweigh the costs.

These criteria are met for neonatal screening for phenylketonuria and congenital hypothyroidism, and for haemoglobinopathy screening in specific racial groups. Population screening for CF in the UK, by which around 75% of carriers can readily be identified, is currently being evaluated. Screening for genetic susceptibility to common diseases may eventually allow prophylaxis or early treatment through lifestyle modifications and surveillance of those at risk.

Genetic disease and natural selection

Disease genes may be prevalent in a population because of the founder effect of isolated small populations, a high new mutation rate (e.g. neurofibromatosis), selective advantage for survival (e.g. sickle cell carriers vs. malaria) or associated increased fertility (e.g. Huntington's chorea).

The prevalence of a disease gene is otherwise maintained by the balance between new mutation and selection against the disease. For autosomal recessive genes at equilibrium the incidence of carriers approximates to $2 \times \sqrt{\text{disease}}$ incidence. For CF, the UK birth incidence of 1/2000 is achieved by a carrier frequency of $2/\sqrt{2000} = 1/22$. For a rare recessive condition with an incidence of 1/100 000 the carrier frequency would be 1/160.

MANAGEMENT OF GENETIC DISEASE

Avoidance: reproductive options

The possible options open to a couple at risk of having a child with a serious genetic disease are:

1. avoidance of pregnancy—contraception or sterilisation ($\pm$ adoption)
2. prenatal testing—chorion villus biopsy (CVB), amniocentesis, fetal blood sampling, ultrasound scan
3. IVF/GIFT and embryo selection—only possible for sex selection or for gene mutations detectable following DNA amplification by PCR techniques
4. artificial insemination by donor sperm
5. IVF/GIFT using donor eggs
6. accepting and taking the risk in a natura l pregnancy.

Prophylactic surveillance of those at risk

For genetic disorders amenable to prophylactic surveillance and treatment measures, predictive DNA testing of those at risk should be encouraged (e.g. familial adenomatous polyposis coli).

Treatment of genetic disease

Potentially this could be offered through:

1. biochemical compensation (e.g. dietary measures in phenylketonuria)
2. tissue-targeted protein replacement (e.g. to lungs in CF)
3. tissue or organ transplantation (e.g. bone marrow in thalassaemia, heart–lung in CF)
4. tissue-targeted gene replacement in child or adult
5. induction of expression of pseudogene
6. genetic engineering of embryo.

20

CARE OF THE ELDERLY

Gordon K. Wilcock

Many of the disorders that afflict our elders will be covered in the relevant chapters. Common symptoms in the elderly, rather than specific diseases, and one or two other important areas will therefore form the substance of this chapter.

CONFUSION AND DEMENTIA

Confusion is a very common presentation of disease in the elderly. It is important to differentiate between a confusional state that has been induced by another illness, e.g. a urinary tract or respiratory infection or a drug toxicity, and the more chronic conditions that causes dementia. The two can of course exist together as both are common (see p. 472).

ACUTE CONFUSIONAL STATES

These tend to occur suddenly, presenting over a relatively short period, e.g. days rather than weeks or months. The patient is often ill or has been recently prescribed different drugs or an increased dose of his or her usual medication.

The commonest infections are those of the respiratory and urinary tracts but infection anywhere could be responsible. Endocrine disorders, a raised blood urea level, electrolyte abnormalities and an elevated calcium level may also cause confusion. If a metabolic cause is discovered, the underlying reason should be sought.

Medication is a potent cause of confusion in the elderly and almost any drug should be suspected. Particularly important medications in this respect include antidepressants, anticonvulsants, anti-Parkinsonian treatment, beta-blockers, and hypnotics.

A number of other conditions may present with confusion, although less commonly. These include anaemia of any cause, especially if it has arisen relatively suddenly; neurological abnormalities such as a subdural haematoma, space occupying lesions, cerebrovascular events, and cardiac failure etc. Some of these usually present with a more chronic deterioration and are more likely to cause dementia than an acute confusional state.

A careful history, taken from a reliable third party if possible, physical examination and basic screening investigations will often establish the diagnosis. Treatment depends upon the underlying cause.

DEMENTIA

Dementia is diagnosed when the patient has global intellectual dysfunction. This of course means more than memory loss and can include difficulty in using language, difficulty with simple tasks such as subtracting serial sevens, disorientation in time and space, apraxias for day to day activities, and so on. The prevalence is around 2% of those aged 65–70 rising 10-fold to 20% by the age of 80 and over. With a few exceptions it is usually insidious and progressive.

In a small proportion of people there is a treatable component to the aetiology, e.g. hypothyroidism, vitamin B_{12} and folate deficiency, neurosyphilis etc. More usually it is caused by an irreversible condition such as Alzheimer's disease or multiple small strokes.

General principles of management of the agitated confused patient

Although wherever possible the physician will wish to treat an underlying medical condition that is causing confusion, more immediate steps may have to be taken to control disturbed behaviour. It is helpful to nurse the subject in a light and simple environment, and to relate to him or her with a kindly approach, carefully explaining what is about to happen, even if one feels the patient may not understand this.

If treatment is required for disturbance or wandering at night, chlormethiazole or triclofos sodium are often useful. Benzodiazepines should be avoided if possible, resorting to the short-acting preparations only if essential. Agitation or restlessness during the day may respond to small doses of thioridazine or promazine. These can also be used at night if necessary. Side-effects of phenothiazines include Parkinsonism, postural hypotension, photosensitivity, jaundice, and the development of tardive dyskinesia. The lowest dose should be prescribed and reviewed after a few days.

CONSTIPATION

Many old people are very conscious of their bowel habit, or lack of it, and become anxious if they do not have a daily evacuation. Reassurance that this is not always necessary may help, but rarely does. However, alteration in bowel habit, especially if accompanied by other symptoms, particularly weightloss, may indicate the presence of serious bowel pathology.

Causes of constipation

Many elderly people, especially women, have taken purgatives for most of their lives. It is this group that are often most difficult to treat. Like so many other problems in older people, however, constipation is often multifactorial in origin. Amongst the important contributory factors are impairment of mobility; drugs, especially those with an anticholinergic action, those which contain codeine or other opiate derivatives and some iron preparations; hypothyroidism, depression and some lesions of the gastrointestinal (GI) tract. A diet lacking in fibre may also play a part.

DEAFNESS

Deafness is often accepted as part of the normal process of ageing, and although there are many age-associated degenerative changes in the auditory mechanism and pathways, it is surprising how frequently there are simple contributory factors that are remediable. In general, older people lose the ability to hear the higher frequencies first, may suffer hypersensitivity to loud noises, and develop impairment of the ability to discriminate between different noises.

Assessment and management

Routine examination of cranial nerve function will ascertain whether or not there is likely to be a remedial cause, e.g. wax in the external auditory meatus. Wherever there is any doubt, hearing is best assessed by a qualified audiometrician.

A hearing aid can be difficult to use, but once understood can make an important contribution to the quality of life of the wearer. Modern technology has reduced the number of whistles and squeaks that the earlier aids used to add to the audible spectrum, and also allows improved performance in relation to the telephone, radio and television. Most modern aids are also able to make use of the induction loops that are installed in many public places, allowing the wearer to participate fully in public meetings etc.

It is important to face people with impaired hearing during conversation, as they become increasingly reliant upon the non-verbal cues that are such an important part of communication.

FALLS

Falls are a common medical problem of the elderly, responsible for many admissions to hospital and frequently result in fractures of the hip and wrist in osteoporotic females. There are many causes (Table 20.1), and not infrequently the aetiology is multifactorial. It is therefore essential to take a full history and conduct a comprehensive examination.

Enquiries should be made specifically about the following four points in the history: vertigo/giddiness, accident hazards, loss of consciousness, relation to posture. There are obvious pointers to specific aetiological factors. Postural hypotension most commonly results from the use of drugs, especially antidepressants, anti-Parkinsonian agents, diuretics and hypotensive agents. Other causes include hypocalcaemia, autonomic dysfunction secondary to diabetes mellitus, Parkinson's disease etc.

Treatment involves attention to the underlying cause, the use of compression stockings and if necessary fludrocortisone.

Table 20.1. Specific causes of falls

Cardiovascular system	Dysrhythmia, postural hypotension, myocardial infarction
Central nervous system	Cervical spondylosis, peripheral neuropathy, posterior column impairment, extrapyramidal disorders, cerebellar ataxia, epilepsy, visual impairment, TIA/stroke
Musculoskeletal system	Any form of arthritis, proximal myopathy

Treatment

This will depend upon the underlying cause. Where it is not possible to remedy the problem, instruction from a physiotherapist coupled with careful attention to the day to day environment is essential. In some cases an alarm system, activated by a button on a pendant hung around the neck or attached to the patient's wrist will help those who have fallen to summon assistance.

IMMOBILITY

As is the case for falls, this is often multifactorial in aetiology. Again, a single factor may be the last straw on a background of multiple pathologies.

Specific causes of immobility

A patient complaining of generalised weakness may well have a myopathy, especially that accompanying osteomalacia, electrolyte imbalances and malignancy. Frequently encountered neurological lesions include Parkinsonism, peripheral neuropathy and undetected cerebrovascular damage. There are many other potential neurological causes. Postural hypotension may also lead to an elderly person refusing to walk, as may other cardiovascular and also respiratory problems which reduce exercise tolerance. Minor foot problems are often overlooked and it is important not to forget that dementia and depression may also lead to immobility. Finally, many old people who have a history of falling will take to their bed or chair and refuse to move because they are frightened of further accidents.

Treatment

As is the case with so many problems in older people, diagnosis and treatment of the underlying cause is the most important factor. In addition, inpatient rehabilitation is usually necessary as even a few days in bed will make it very much more difficult for an elderly person to get back on his or her feet. This will allow the patient access to daily physiotherapy, occupational therapy and medical and social assessment.

An important part of the treatment of an immobile patient is the prevention of the development of pressure sores, venous thromboses, hypostatic pneumonia, constipation, contractures and the other consequences of being bed- or chair-bound.

INCONTINENCE OF URINE

Incontinence of urine is a frequent problem in older people. Unless there is an obvious cause it is very helpful to ask the nurses or a reliable carer to chart the pattern of the incontinence, relating it to time of day, meals, drinks etc. It is also important to ensure that one really is dealing with incontinence and not pseudoincontinence. The latter occurs when a person cannot get to the toilet in time, e.g. after a potent diuretic or with urgency of micturition from a urinary tract infection. This also arises when a patient is admitted to residential care and has difficulty finding the toilet, e.g. in the middle of the night.

Treatment

This depends upon the underlying cause. From a practical point of view these are best divided up in the elderly as follows:

1. Retention with overflow: commonest causes are prostatic hypertrophy in men, faecal impaction and drugs, especially those with an anticholinergic action such as antidepressants and anti-Parkinsonian treatment.
2. Stress incontinence and senile vaginitis: stress incontinence in the elderly usually requires a gynaecological referral as pelvic floor exercises are rarely successful in women over 80. A pessary may be helpful.
   Senile vaginitis is treated with a local oestrogen preparation although some patients respond better to an intermittent course of oral oestrogens.
3. Mental impairment: incontinence occurs commonly in people who are confused, whatever the cause. Sedative drugs taken at night may also impair the level of consciousness such that the patient sleeps through the need to void urine.
4. The uninhibited neurogenic bladder: this is a common cause resulting in the patient being unable to control spontaneous bladder contractions. It is best diagnosed with a cystometrogram. The incontinence is often accompanied by frequency and urgency. It may respond to flavoxate, but often environmental modification, e.g. a bedside commode, will prove more useful.

Many patients have incontinence for which the cause is not immediately apparent. Wherever treatment has failed it is important to consider whether or not referral to a specialist urodynamic unit would be helpful. Assistance from the incontinence advisory nurse will help in the management of the many elderly people whose problems are not remediable.

VISUAL IMPAIRMENT

Normal ageing changes affect the eye, for example the increasing difficulty with accommodation and the reduction in visual acuity that many people notice. Spectacles help the former; the latter rarely interferes with normal day to day vision significantly and is helped by adequate lighting.

Causes of visual impairment

There are many conditions which affect the sight of elderly people. Of these, three are particularly important as they occur commonly. Cataracts rarely cause total blindness and progress slowly. Once day to day life is significantly impaired on their account, however, the patient should be referred to an ophthalmic surgeon.

Glaucoma, often heralded by severe pain as well as blurring of vision, is an ophthalmological emergency requiring immediate referral for specialist treatment.

Retinal degeneration may be caused or aggravated by diabetes or hypertension, as in younger patients, and if this is the case should be treated similarly. It is more usually the result of senile macular degeneration which can be helped by visual aids, e.g., a magnifying glass, strong reading spectacles and good lighting.

Any sudden deterioration in visual ability should lead to specialist referral unless this is inappropriate, e.g. the field deficit resulting from a cerebrovascular accident.

It is important to remember that anyone who is partially sighted or completely blind may benefit from referral to an ophthalmologist who may be able to put them on the appropriate register, enabling them to claim additional statutory benefits.

RHEUMATIC DISEASES IN THE ELDERLY

The elderly suffer from a different spectrum of diseases (Table 20.2). The clinical presentation is often atypical, minor rheumatic disease on top of other

Table 20.2. Causes of rheumatic diseases in the elderly

Soft-tissue rheumatism, chiefly adhesive capsulitis

Osteoarthritis

Polymyalgia rheumatica

Crystal arthropathies: diuretic-induced gout, pseudogout

Trauma: unsteadiness, poor eyesight

Osteoporosis

Rheumatoid arthritis: tends to be more severe, may have a polymyalgic onset or present with diffuse swelling of the hands and forearms

Iatrogenic, e.g. haemarthrosis from anticoagulation, drug-induced systemic lupus erythematosus

Others: hypothyroid arthropathy, pain from Parkinson's disease, post-hemiparesis pain, septic arthritis

disorders cause a major disability, there are more problems with drug side-effects and polypharmacy, and the social consequences are worse.

Normal ageing changes may be mistaken for disease, e.g. the elderly hand resembles that in rheumatoid arthritis.

'Abnormal' investigations of no consequence are common in the elderly: radiographic osteoarthritis, chondrocalcinosis, hyperuricaemia, rheumatoid factor, antinuclear antibodies and mild elevation of the ESR.

Not all symptoms should be attributed to old age, and a careful diagnosis should be made. The priority is to maintain independence and avoid side-effects.

21

DERMATOLOGY

Clive B. Archer

Dermatology is essentially a general medical specialty, supported by basic science and clinical research activities and offers the opportunity to develop a wide range of surgical techniques. This image of dermatology is largely responsible for its present popularity as a career option amongst young doctors.

The number of different diseases in dermatology has been estimated at nearly 2000. One advantage of a visual specialty is that apparently similar diseases can be followed over long periods, during which different natural histories may emerge, a trend which, with the advent of endoscopy, is now unfolding in other medical specialities.

Commonly seen skin disorders include inflammatory dermatoses (psoriasis, the eczemas and urticaria), acne, and benign and malignant skin tumours. Most rashes are recognised by the pattern of the eruption, the history being used for fine tuning (e.g. in deciding on the distinction between an endogenous or exogenous eczema). Redness, or erythema, can be helpful in identifying inflammatory diseases but this sign may be difficult to assess in pigmented skin. If the diagnosis is not obvious it can be useful to consider which level of the skin is involved (e.g. is this an epidermal or dermal problem?) (Fig. 21.1). Table 21.1 shows a classification of skin diseases according to the main site of pathology within the skin, although in some disorders more than one level will be involved. A list of commonly used dermatological terms is shown in Table 21.2.

PSORIASIS

Psoriasis is an inflammatory, hyperproliferative disorder characterised by red scaly plaques (See Plate 4). It affects 1–2% of the population with equal sex incidence, occurs at any age (peak incidence 18–25 years) and tends to run a chronic course. It has a multifactorial inheritance, often skipping generations, and has been associated with several HLA-specific antigens, particularly the HLA-CW6 antigen. Trigger factors in genetically primed individuals include streptococcal infections, trauma and probably stress. Altered cell regulatory mechanisms in the epidermis may account for the increase in the mitotic rate and reduced epidermal cell transit time from the basal layer to the stratum corneum in active lesions. The actions of inflammatory mediators, such as

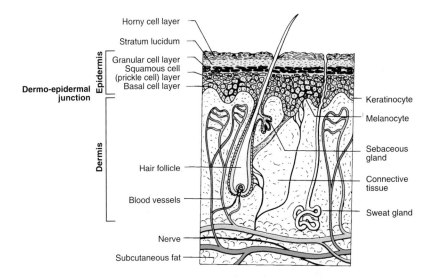

Fig. 21.1 Diagrammatic view of the skin.

Table 21.1. Dermatoses according to the level of pathology within the skin

Predominant change/ site of pathology	Disease
Epidermal changes (e.g. scaling, hyperkeratosis, crusting)	Psoriasis, eczema/dermatitis, superficial fungal infections, the ichthyoses
Epidermal appendages	Acne vulgaris, rosacea, hidradenitis suppurativa (apocrine glands in axillae and groin), alopecia areata
Dermo-epidermal interface and dermis	Pityriasis rosea, lichen planus, lupus erythematosus, erythema multiforme
Epidermal and dermo-epidermal cohesion (blistering disorders)	Pemphigus (e.g. vulgaris/foliaceus), pemphigoid, dermatitis herpetiformis, epidermolysis bullosa
Dermis	The urticarias, granuloma annulare, morphoea/scleroderma, dermatomyositis, xanthoma/xanthelasma, lymphoma (e.g. T cell lymphoma/mycosis fungoides)
Subcutaneous tissue	Erythema nodosum and other forms of panniculitis

leukotriene B4, platelet activating factor (PAF) and interleukins 1 and 8, on neutrophils and lymphocytes via cell adhesion molecules involved in cell trafficking is presently the subject of intense investigation.

Table 21.2. Dermatological terminology

Lesion	Any single small area of skin pathology
Macule	An area of colour change
Papule	A small[*] elevated (palpable) lesion
Weal (wheal)	An oedematous slightly raised lesion, often with a pale centre and reddish margin
Nodule	A large[*] elevated spherical lesion, often extending deeply into the skin
Plaque	A flat-topped palpable lesion
Vesicle	A small fluid-filled blister
Pustule	A small blister filled with neutrophils (pus)
Bulla	A large fluid-filled blister
Purpura	A visible collection of free red blood cells in the skin
Scale	Thickened fragments of the outermost layer of the epidermis, the stratum corneum
Crust	Dried plasma exudate
Excoriation	An abrasion caused by scratching
Lichenification	Area of increased epidermal thickness and increased skin markings as a result of chronic rubbing
Erosion	An absence of the epithelial surface
Ulcer	An absence of the epithelial surface with dermal damage (i.e. deeper than an erosion)
Scar	A permanent lesion resulting from repair by replacement with connective tissue
Telangiectasia	Dilated blood vessels visible on the skin surface

[*] It is not usually helpful to be dogmatic about precise measurements

Pathology

Inflammation in the dermis with a particular pattern of epidermal changes (elongation of rete ridges) and sometimes epidermal collections of neutrophils (microabscesses) is seen.

Symptoms and signs

The most common pattern is plaque psoriasis, usually affecting the elbows, knees, extensor aspects of the limbs and the scalp. Other patterns include guttate (frequently following a streptococcal sore throat in young individuals), flexural (moist red patches), pustular (localised to the hands and feet or generalised) and erythrodermic psoriasis.

In generalised pustular or erythrodermic psoriasis, sometimes occurring after erroneous administration of systemic corticosteroids, the patient may be very ill.

Nail changes include pitting, thickening and onycholysis, and in about 10% of cases there is an associated seronegative arthritis (see p. 371). Contrary to some earlier teaching, patients with psoriasis do sometimes complain of itching.

Investigations

Histology is not usually required to confirm the diagnosis. A throat swab, anti-streptolysin–O (ASO) titre, rheumatoid factor (RF) and X-rays of painful joints may be helpful.

Differential diagnosis

Common possibilities include eczema, pityriasis rosea and drug eruptions.

Treatment

Psoriasis can be actively and successfully treated in a number of ways, depending on its severity, persistence and the distribution of skin involvement.

Topical agents include moisturisers and emollients, tar compounds, appropriate corticosteroid ointments or creams, dithranol (anthralin) preparations and calcipotriol (a vitamin D analogue).

Ultraviolet light can be helpful in the form of sunlight, UVB or PUVA therapy (in which the skin is sensitised by the administration of an oral or topical psoralen).

Antibiotics are used for the treatment of streptococcal infections and, in severe cases, systemic drugs such as etretinate, methotrexate, hydroxyurea or cyclosporin A, with careful monitoring for side-effects, can be very beneficial.

Prognosis

Guttate psoriasis often clears spontaneously whereas plaque psoriasis is usually a chronic problem. There is a small mortality rate associated with generalised pustular or erythrodermic psoriasis, particularly in the elderly.

ECZEMA/DERMATITIS

These terms are often used synonymously. There are several types of eczema, characterised by the clinical appearance of itchy, red, scaly skin, sometimes with vesicles, exudation and crusting (Table 21.3).

Table 21.3. A classification of the eczemas

Endogenous	Exogenous
Atopic dermatitis	Irritant dermatitis
Seborrheic dermatitis	Allergic contact dermatitis
Discoid eczema	Infective eczema
Asteatotic eczema	Photo-dermatitis
Pompholyx	Drug-induced eczema
Varicose (venous) eczema	

Atopic dermatitis (atopic eczema) occurs in 2–3% of children, the onset of the disease being in the first year of life in 60%, and is frequently seen in patients with a personal or family history of atopic diseases (i.e. asthma, allergic rhinitis or atopic dermatitis). A gene defect has been established in atopy. This may underly a number of reported cell regulatory abnormalities in mononuclear leukocytes (monocytes and lymphocytes) in atopic dermatitis which may, in turn, lead to an exaggerated response of the skin to trigger factors in the environment, such as irritants (e.g. detergents, house dust) and antigens (e.g. cow's milk, house dust mite).

Seborrheic dermatitis is common and yeasts on the skin play an important causative role. Exogenous factors can worsen all types of eczema and may be causative in primary irritant or allergic contact dermatitis, the latter being a cell-mediated immune (type IV) response. Common sensitisers include nickel (as in costume jewellery), chromium, rubber, medicaments (including topical neomycin and preservatives), plants and pre-polymerised plastics and glues in industry.

Pathology

Oedema is present in the epidermis (spongiosis) with dilatation of blood vessels and infiltration with mononuclear cells in the dermis. Chronic changes include epidermal thickening (acanthosis).

Symptoms and signs

In atopic dermatitis the skin is often dry and extremely itchy. Scratching makes the eczema worse and produces lichenification, (see Plate 5). The severity fluctuates with time and secondary bacterial infection, usually with *Staphylococcus aureus*, can be recognised by exudation and crusting.

Any part of the body can be affected, often symmetrically; in infancy, the face and extensor aspects of the limbs are usually involved whereas in older children and adults eczema tends to affect the flexures (e.g. antecubital and popliteal fossae), the periocular regions and the nape of the neck.

Seborrheic dermatitis in infants affects the scalp and flexures (napkin dermatitis), frequently allowing the distinction from atopic dermatitis. Features of seborrheic dermatitis in adults include dandruff, paranasal and eyebrow scaling, and sometimes eczema in the presternal, interscapular, axillary and groin regions.

The circular lesions of discoid eczema usually occur on the extensor aspects of the limbs in adults. In pompholyx, patients often have large painful blisters on the palms and soles, with smaller itchy vesicles along the side of the fingers.

In the elderly, varicose eczema is common, affecting the lower legs and sometimes accompanied by venous ulcers.

Asteatotic eczema, associated with drying of the skin (e.g. following admission to hospital) usually affects the shins and the scaling takes on a 'crazy paving' appearance.

Contact dermatitis often involves the hands where it can be difficult to be sure of the aetiology based on the pattern of eczema alone. However, primary irritant dermatitis may initially involve the finger webs and the flexor aspects of the wrists, where the epidermis is thinner than on the palms.

Investigation

Patch testing to a standard battery of allergens and sometimes other potential sensitisers will often confirm a clinical diagnosis of allergic contact dermatitis. The distinction between allergic and irritant responses can be difficult and, to minimise false positive results, patch tests should be performed in a specialist dermatology department.

Skin and nasal swabs (before antibiotic therapy) can help to direct treatment, particularly in atopic dermatitis. Patients with atopic dermatitis usually have raised serum IgE levels with multiple positive prick test or radioallergosorbent test (RAST) responses to common antigens. However, these tests are not performed routinely since they are of limited diagnostic use, and patients (or their parents) may overinterpret the significance of an individual positive result, assuming for example that the eczema is 'caused' by the house dust mite, which may be one of many trigger factors.

A skin biopsy is not usually required.

Differential diagnosis

Psoriasis, pityriasis rosea, fungal infections (which are often unilateral) and drug eruptions.

Treatment

Eczema can be dramatically improved by the use of a combination of the following measures: moisturisers/emollients, topical corticosteroids ('the weakest that works'; 1% hydrocortisone is safe and can be obtained without a doctor's prescription), antihistamines (especially at night) for control of itching, and treatment of secondary infection.

In atopic dermatitis, additional measures include trial of a diet avoiding cow's milk antigen and eggs (of importance in only 10–15% of children), avoidance of house dust (an irritant) and house dust mites (an antigen), excessive drying of the skin, excessive heat and sweating, clothes which can irritate (e.g. wool and nylon) and close contact with 'cold sore' (herpes simplex) sufferers.

Seborrheic dermatitis responds well to the continued use of combined topical antifungal/corticosteroid preparations.

In contact dermatitis, strict avoidance of irritant and/or allergic factors is essential.

Prognosis

Atopic dermatitis improves with age, around 50% of those presenting in infancy resolving by the age of 10 years. Seborrheic dermatitis is usually responsive to therapy but tends to recur if treatment is stopped. The tendency to develop discoid eczema and pompholyx often resolves over a period of 2 years, whereas varicose eczema usually persists. Contact dermatitis can resolve completely on avoidance of exogenous factors, although this may not be so for certain sensitisers (e.g. chromate in cement workers).

ACNE

Acne vulgaris is a common disorder of the pilosebaceous units, affecting up to 90% of adolescents, in which hyperactivity of the sebaceous glands leads to seborrhoea (greasy skin) with blockage of follicular openings and the formation of comedones (black heads and white heads), inflammatory papules, pustules, nodules and cysts. Within the blocked follicle, normal skin bacteria (*Propionibacterium acnes* and *Staph. albus*) produce lipases causing the breakdown of triglycerides to irritant fatty acids which are thought to induce the clinical lesions.

Genetic factors may be important and the sebaceous glands seem to be hyperresponsive to circulating androgens. Acne can also be produced by drugs such as bromides, iodides, systemic corticosteroids and phenytoin.

Pathology

The pilosebaceous unit is distended and surrounded by inflammatory cells comprising neutrophils and lymphocytes, sometimes with foreign body giant cells, granulation tissue and fibrosis.

Symptoms and signs

Adolescents may present with blackheads (open comedones) in which the colour is caused by melanin pigmentation, whiteheads (closed comedones), papules, pustules, nodules, cysts and varying degrees of scarring, usually on the face, chest and back.

Differential diagnosis

Rosacea, perioral dermatitis (as induced by application of a fluorinated corticosteroid to the face), milia (small epidermal cysts), sarcoidosis or plane warts.

Treatment

Acne should be treated actively in order to avoid unnecessary scarring and psychological distress. Combinations of the following treatments are used:

1. simple desquamating agents or creams
2. topical or systemic antibiotics (e.g. oxytetracycline or erythromycin, 500 mg twice daily, usually about 6 months each, sometimes in rotation)
3. UVB light/sunlight (in moderation)
4. systemic antiandrogen drugs in females (e.g. Dianette)

5. isotretinoin therapy (teratogenic in females), with appropriate monitoring for side-effects, for severe cases with nodulocystic acne or those failing to respond to adequate dose of antibiotics
6. aspiration and injection of a corticosteroid for cysts.

The treatment of scarring by, for example, chemical peel or dermabrasion, is often unsatisfactory.

Prognosis

In most patients, acne resolves during the teenage years so that, in addition to providing active therapy, one can be reassuring. In some cases, acne persists into the mid-twenties or beyond; this was particularly common before the availability of isotretinoin.

ROSACEA AND PERIORAL DERMATITIS

Rosacea usually occurs in patients between 30 and 50 years of age, with a female : male ratio of 3 : 1. Intermittent flushing of the cheeks, nose, forehead and chin is triggered by being in a hot room, alcohol, spicy foods and, in some, exposure to sunlight. The redness may become persistent with telangiectasia, papules, pustules and lymphoedema. Rhinophyma (enlargement of the nose, usually in men) may occur and ocular effects include blepharitis, conjunctivitis and keratitis.

The differential diagnosis includes perioral dermatitis, which may complicate rosacea if a fluorinated corticosteroid has been applied. Treatment includes oxytetracycline (e.g. 250 mg three times daily for 2–3 months), topical metronidazole and avoidance of trigger factors.

Perioral dermatitis responds to similar therapy. Other potential side-effects of potent fluorinated topical corticosteroids are thinning of the skin (dermal atrophy) and systemic absorption.

OTHER SKIN DISEASES

Space does not allow a detailed account of the large number of other skin diseases. Tables 21.4–21.12 provide additional important information.

Table 21.4 lists the benign and malignant skin tumours which commonly present to the dermatologist. The role of sun exposure in the pathogenesis of basal cell epithelioma, squamous carcinoma and malignant melanoma is now more widely understood, following public information programmes aimed at producing early recognition and treatment. Reducing the incidence of skin cancer by encouraging a change in sun exposure habits will take longer to achieve.

Common infections and infestations are summarised in Tables 21.5–21.8. It is wise to consider the possibility of a superficial fungal infection in all cases of unilateral red scaly plaques, perhaps thought to represent psoriasis or eczema.

Some of the most interesting aspects of dermatology are seen when general medicine and the skin overlap (Tables 21.9–21.11). Skin lesions may be a manifestation of an underlying disease (as in acanthosis nigricans) or may be part of a systemic process (as occurs in lupus erythematosus).

In addition, it is important to be aware that there are a number of potential dermatological emergencies (Table 21.12) in which it is desirable for a dermatologist to be involved at an early stage.

Table 21.4. Benign and malignant skin tumours

Lesion	Clinical features/diagnosis	Treatment options
Melanocytic naevus	Brown or skin coloured, sometimes hair-bearing, usually regular shape/colour	Reassurance, excision
Seborrheic keratosis (seborrheic wart, basal cell papilloma)	Brown hyperkeratotic/warty lesion on face and trunk, usually in the elderly. Often multiple	Reassurance, cryotherapy, simple excision
Histiocytoma (dermatofibroma)	Firm pink or light brown dermal nodule, often on the leg	Reassurance, excision
Actinic (solar) keratosis	Red or light brown hyperkeratotic lesion(s) on sun-exposed skin (face, dorsa of hands). Small potential to become squamous cell carcinoma	Cryotherapy, topical 5-fluorouracil (5-FU), moisturiser
Keratoacanthoma (KA)	Domed lesion with central keratotic plug, growing rapidly (within 4 weeks) on sun-exposed skin; would spontaneously resolve over about 6 months. Must distinguish from a squamous cell carcinoma	Excision (for histology and to avoid puckered scar)
Basal cell epithelioma/carcinoma (BCC, rodent ulcer)	Pearly papule with telangiectatic vessels, sometimes ulcerated with rolled edge, mainly on head and neck. Potential for local erosion	Excision, curettage, radiotherapy
Squamous cell carcinoma (SCC)	Keratotic indurated lesion, usually growing over a few months. Potential to metastasise	Excision
Bowen's disease (squamous cell carcinoma-in situ)	Red scaly plaque, often on the lower leg. Diagnostic biopsy desirable	Excision, curettage, cryotherapy, topical 5-FU
Malignant melanoma (superficial spreading melanoma, nodular melanoma, acral lentiginous melanoma, lentigo maligna/Hutchinson's freckle, lentigo maligna melanoma)	Often arises on normal-appearing skin but a benign naevus may enlarge, change colour (e.g. turn black), bleed spontaneously or become itchy or inflamed. Some cases are familial (dysplastic naevus syndrome). Prognosis partly depends on depth of tumour so that early recognition is important	Wide excision (by a specialist)

Table 21.5. Superficial fungal infections

Disease	Cause
Dermatophyte infections	
Athlete's foot nail infections (tinea unguium)	*Trichphyton rubrum* *Trichophyton interdigitale* *Epidermophyton floccosum*
Tinea corporis	*T. rubrum*
Scalp ringworm (tinea capitis)	*Trichophyton tonsurans* *Microsporum canis, T. rubrum,* *T. verrucosum*
Candidal infections	
Napkin candidiasis Intertrigo (flexural)	*Candida albicans* infection, often complicating an irritant dermatitis
Candida paronychia	A hazard of regular immersion of the hands in water
Pityriasis versicolor	*Malassezia furfur* (pityriasis orbiculare in yeast-like form)

Table 21.6. Common bacterial infections of the skin

Disease	Cause
Impetigo (plate 6)	*Staphylococcus aureus* and group A streptococci
Erysipelas	Streptococcal infection (via minor abrasion) involving superficial lymphatic vessels
Cellulitis	Usually a streptococcal infection involving deeper layers of skin (distinction from erysipelas of little clinical importance)
Erythrasma	*Corynebacterium minutissimus*

Clinical features/diagnosis	Therapy
Sore, itchy moist white fissures in toe webs Mycology + (skin scrapings)	Topical antifungal
Thickened discoloured powdery nails Mycology + (nail clippings)	Oral antifungal (e.g. terbinafine griseofulvin)
Red scaly plaques, with an active red advancing edge and central clearing Often unilateral Mycology + (skin scrapings)	Topical ± oral antifungal
Hair loss, inflammation and scaling Mycology + (skin scrapings, hair roots) Wood's (UV) light fluorescence	Topical and oral antifungal (e.g.S griseofulvin)
Red shiny patches with 'satellite' lesions Mycology + (swab)	Allow moist area to dry, topical antifungal
Boggy inflamed nail fold, with pus Mycology + (swab)	Topical and oral antifungal (e.g. itraconazole)
Pink asymptomatic coalescing lesions on trunk with fine scaling and hypo- or hyper-pigmentation Mycology + (skin scrapings) Wood's light—pale yellow fluorescence	Topical selenium sulphide to whole trunk/arms

Clinical features/diagnosis	Therapy
Red, sometimes blistered, lesions develop into golden crusts May complicate atopic dermatitis Swab for micro-organisms and sensitivity	Topical (e.g. mupiricin) ± oral antibiotics (e.g. flucloxacillin, erythromycin)
Red oedematous area, often on a cheek or leg, with sharply demarcated border, and pyrexia and leukocytosis Organism often not isolated (swab, blood cultures), ASO titre	Systemic antibiotic (usually penicillin)
Red hot tender area of skin (e.g. surrounding a leg ulcer), accompanied by pyrexia and leukocytosis Palpable lymph nodes Swab and blood cultures (before antibiotics) may yield organism(s)	Systemic antibiotics (usually penicillin ± flucloxacillin)
Reddish-brown patches in axillae or groin region with fine scaling Swab and Wood's light—coral red fluorescence	Oral erythromycin

Table 21.7. Common virul infections of the skin

Disease	Cause
Herpes simplex (e.g. cold sores herpetic whitlow, eczema herpeticum, genital herpes)	Herpes virus hominis type 1 (usually in cold sores) type 2 (usually in genital herpes)
Herpes zoster (Shingles)	Herpes virus varicellae (reactivated chicken pox virus)
Warts	Human papilloma virus
Molluscum contagiosum	A pox virus
Pitynasis rosea	?viral
Acquired immune deficiency syndrome (AIDS)	Human immunodeficiency virus (HIV)

Table 21.8. Infestations

Disease	Cause
Scabies	Scabies mite (*Sarcoptes scabiei*) produces an allergic reaction
Lice	
Pedicularis capitis	Head louse
Pedicularis corporis	Body louse
Pedicularis pubis	Pubic louse

Clinical features/diagnosis	Therapy
Red vesicular sore then crusted lesions, often on lips or skin (e.g. finger or wrist) Eczema herpeticum may be a severe complication of atopic dermatitis May confirm diagnosis with a Tzanck smear or by electron microscopy of fluid	Symptomatic treatment ± topical acyclovir (systemic acyclovir for eczema herpeticum)
Dermatomal pain followed by linear red, macular, papular, vesicular then pustular eruption May be complicated by post-herpetic neuralgia	Symptomatic Systemic acyclovir in the elderly
Common warts (e.g. on hands), plane warts (often on face), plantar warts (verrucae), genital warts; usually self-limiting	Topical keratolytic agents, liquid nitrogen cryotherapy, podophyllin (for genital warts)
Reddish papules with umbilicated centre often on trunk or proximal limbs May be multiple Spontaneously remit	Expectant, sometimes topical phenol or cryotherapy (depending on age of child)
Red scaly asymptomatic oval macules on trunk, arms and upper thighs occurring a day after a solitary red 'herald patch' Spontaneous resolution in 6–8 weeks	Moisturisers ± weak topical corticosteroids
Kaposi's sarcoma: reddish-purple vascular nodules often multiple, associated with severe or persistent opportunistic infections	Excision or radiotherapy for Kaposi's sarcoma, if required Treatment of underlying disease

Clinical features/diagnosis	Treatment
Extremely itchy excoriated red papular rash particularly affecting finger webs, hands, wrists and pubic area Affected individuals may be asymptomatic Mite can be extracted from linear burrow	Usually gamma benzene hexachloride lotion overnight (to all occupants of the home)
Lots of school children have nits (eggs) sometimes with excoriation and secondary infection	Gamma benzene hexachloride or topical malathion
Itching, excoriation and secondary infection usually invagrants	Gamma benzene hexachloride or topical malathion
Itching and 'black dots' in pubic hair	Gamma benzene hexachloride or topical malathion

Table 21.9. Dermatological manifestations of systemic diseases

Disease/lesion	Clinical features/diagnosis/associated disorder
Acanthosis nigricans	Hyperpigmentation and hyperkeratosis of flexures (e.g. axillae) in absence of obesity Associated with adenocarcinoma e.g. carcinoma of stomach
'Pseudo' acanthosis nigricans	Changes of acanthosis nigricans in an obese person Associated with hyperinsulinaemia ± overt diabetes mellitus
Dermatitis herpetiformis	Extremely itchy, excoriated vesicles on elbow, scalp, buttocks and lower back Associated gluten-sensitive enteropathy may be asymptomatic but jejunal histology usually shows some degree of subtotal villous atrophy. Skin biopsy for histology and direct immunoflorescence (IMF) (perilesional skin) Responds to dapsone ± gluten-free diet
Erythema nodosum (Plate 7)	Painful red, circular smooth-surfaced lesions on the shins, resolving over a few weeks to leave a bruise-like appearance. May be caused by streptococcal infection, a sulphonamide, sarcoidosis or tuberculosis Investigations include a throat swab, ASO titre, Mantoux test (± Kveim test), viral titres
Generalised pruritus	In the absence of primary skin disease, generalised pruritus may be associated with iron deficiency anaemia, liver or renal failure, diabetes mellitus, primary biliary cirrhosis, hypo- or hyperthyroidism, polycythaemia vera and lymphoma
Granuloma annulare (Plate 8)	Reddish annular dermal lesions, with palpable edge, often over knuckles and on elbows Resolves spontaneously in 6–18 months Skin biopsy for histology Exclude diabetes mellitus; occurs in only 5% cases
Necrobiosis lipoidica (Plate 9)	Reddish-yellow shiny plaques on shins, with atrophy and telangiectasia May ulcerate Skin biopsy for histology Usually (but not always) associated with diabetes mellitus
Pretibial myxoedema	Red raised dermal lesions, often on shins Skin biopsy for histology Associated with hyperthyroidism
Pyoderma gangrenosum	Sometimes extensive, coalescing ulcers with undermined edge Skin biopsy may be helpful (not diagnostic) Associated with Crohn's disease, ulcerative colitis and rheumatoid arthritis Treated with prednisolone

Table 21.9 *cont.* **Dermatological manifestations of systemic diseases**

Disease/lesion	Clinical features/diagnosis/associated disorder
Systemic vasculitis (Plate 10) (e.g. Henoch–Schönlein purpura, polyarteritis nodosa)	Purplish palpable purpura (sometimes necrotic, ulcerated lesions) on limbs and buttocks Skin biopsy for histology ± direct immunoflorescence (IMF; early lesion) Investigate for antigenic stimulus (e.g. streptococcal infection) and degree of systemic involvement
Xanthelasma/ xanthoma	Xanthelasmata are flat yellowish lesions on eyelids Various types of xanthomata e.g. eruptive papules on buttocks (Plate 11) or tuberous xanthomata over elbows and knees Exclude hyperlipoproteinaemia

Table 21.10. Dermatological aspects of autoimmune/connective tissue diseases

Disease	Clinical features/diagnosis
Autoimmune diseases	
Addison's disease (adrenal insufficiency)	Melanin pigmentation in palmar creases and buccal mucosa
Alopecia areata	One or more bald patches on scalp with normal underlying skin Hair loss may occur at other sites, occasionally complete
Vitiligo	Symmetrical depigmented areas of skin Vitiligo, alopecia areata and Addison's disease may be associated with each other and with other autoimmune diseases, including pernicious anaemia and thyroiditis
Connective tissue diseases	
Lupus erythematosus (LE)	
Discoid LE (Plate 12)	Red, often atrophic, plaques on sun-exposed areas, especially the face (may cause scarring alopecia) Chronic tendency but only 5% progress to SLE Skin biopsy for histology and direct immunofluorescence (IMF-lesional skin) ANA +ve in 20%
Systemic LE (SLE)	Red, macular 'butterfly' rash* on nose and cheeks ± dorsa of hands and other sun-exposed areas, mainly in females. Provoked by sunlight and drugs (e.g. hydralazine, methyldopa, isoniazid, phenytoin)

Table 21.10 *cont.* **Dermatological aspects of autoimmune/connective tissue diseases**

Disease	Clinical features/diagnosis
	May also have rheumatological, renal, cardiac or haemopoietic symptoms and signs Skin biopsy for histology and direct IMF of lesional and non-lesional sun-exposed skin, e.g. on upper arm ('lupus band' test) ANA +ve, double stranded DNA antibody +ve Investigate other systems
Subacute LE	Sun-induced red lesions on face ± upper arms and trunk, associated by joint pains Skin biopsy for histology and direct IMF (lesional skin) Cytoplasmic antibodies (SSA/Ro, SSB/La) +ve
Morphoea	Usually localised firm white patches of skin, initially with an inflamed border Sometimes linear, occasionally generalised Skin biopsy for histological confirmation
Generalised scleroderma (systemic sclerosis)	Loss of mobility of the skin and other organs due to progressive fibrosis, leading to tight perioral skin with gastrointestinal and respiratory problems Females > males
CRST (CREST) syndrome	Hand features of CRST syndrome (calcinosis, Raynaud's phenomenon, sclerodactyly, telangiectasia) ± oesophageal dysfunction may occur alone or as part of generalised scleroderma Skin biopsy for histology, autoantibody screen, barium swallow
Dermatomyositis	Red, oedematous periocular rash (dorsa of hands sometimes affected) with proximal myopathy. CPK level elevated, characteristic EMG changes, skin biopsy ± muscle biopsy Chest X-ray and limited search for commoner forms of malignancy in the elderly

*Distinguish from rosacea which also produces a 'butterfly' rash

Table 21.11. Drug eruptions and skin ulceration

Drug–induced rashes

	Patterns of drug eruptions include morbilliform erythema, urticaria, exfoliative dermatitis, erythema multiforme (Stevens–Johnson syndrome), lichenoid/lichen planus-like eruption (Plate 13) vasculitis/purpuric eruption, pigmentation, fixed drug eruption and erythema nodosum
	Common agents include penicillins, sulphonamides and non-steroidal anti-inflammatory drugs
	History important

Ulcers

Leg ulcer	Venous leg ulcers, typically affecting the medial malleolar region(s), account for up to 90% of leg ulcers
	Important aspects of management are elevation and compression (e.g. with an elastic bandage or shaped tubigrip)
	Must distinguish from arterial (often painful) ulcers in which such measures would be inappropriate
	Other causes of ulceration include: diabetes mellitus, infection, rheumatoid arthritis, vasculitis, sickle cell anaemia, haemolytic anaemia, pyoderma gangrenosum and malignancy
Decubitus ulcer (pressure sore)	Commonly occur over sacrum
	Prevention by good nursing care important

*The ampicillin-induced rash in infectious mononucleosis does not necessarily imply penicillin allergy.

Table 21.12. Potential dermatological emergencies*

Disease/lesion	Cause
Angio-oedema	C1 esterase inhibitor deficiency (Hereditary angio-oedema), severe urticaria
Extensive burns	Various types
Toxic epidermal necrolysis (TEN)	Drug allergy, e.g. a sulphonamide
Staphylococcal antibiotics scalded skin syndrome (SSSS)	Toxin from *Staphylococcus aureus*
Erythema multiforme	Herpes simplex, drug allergy
Erythroderma/ exfoliative dermatitis	Psoriasis, atopic seborrheic or allergic contact dermatitis, drug eruption
Generalised pustular psoriasis	e.g. following systematic corticosteroids
Eczema herpeticum	Herpes simplex
Necrotising fasciitis	Deep infection, usually with beta-haemolytic streptococci Sometimes multiple organisms (bacterial synergistic gangrene)
Pemphigus (various types)	Autoimmune
Pemphigoid (builous pemphigoid)	Autoimmune
Arterial insufficiency —gangrene/ulceration	Arteriosclerosis, emboli

*Other potential dermatological emergencies include SLE, dermatomyositis, systemic vasculitis and pyoderma gangrenosum (see Table 21.10).

Clinical features/diagnosis	Therapy
Gross urticarial swellings with subcutaneous involvement, e.g. throat and tongue	i.m. adrenaline then IV hydrocortisone
Large areas of blistered denuded skin	Intensive care (good nursing, fluid balance, treatment of infection)
Large areas of blistered, denuded skin Skin biopsy for histology	Intensive care (good nursing, fluid balance, treatment of infection) N.B. Systemic corticosteroids may increase mortality
Blistered, denuded skin Skin biopsy for histology (to distinguish from TEN)	Sytemic antibiotics
Annular 'target' lesions with blistering of skin and lips Eyes and mucosa involved when severe (Stevens–Johnson syndrome) Skin biopsy for histology	Topical ± oral corticosteroids
Large areas of erythema with variable desquamation	Bed rest, emollients/ moisturisers, mild topical corticosteroids Treatment of fluid loss
Erythematous psoriasis with sterile pustules	As above ± oral etretinate
Excoriated vesicles in atopic dermatitis Occasionally encephalitis Confirm by Tzank smear or electron microscopy of vesicular fluid	Systemic acyclovir
Red spreading cellulitis with necrosis Swab ± skin biopsy for culture (including anaerobes) and sensitivity	Surgical debridement, systemic antibiotics
Erosion on skin and mucous membranes Skin biopsy for histology and direct IMF (perilesional skin) Autoantibody titre (indirect IMF)	Prednisolone, azathioprine
Tense blisters on skin, with red haemorrhagic base Skin biopsy for histology and direct IMF (perilesional skin)	Prednisolone, azathioprine
Necrotic digits; painful necrotic ulceration Ultrasound studies, arteriography	Surgery

22

PSYCHIATRY AND MEDICINE

Howard G. Morgan, Montagu G. Barker

This chapter focuses on the ways in which psychiatric illness may complicate or mimic physical disorders. It assumes that other more lengthy texts will be consulted on matters such as basic clinical symptoms and signs, classification of psychiatric illness and its treatment. Likewise the use of drugs cannot be referred to except in outline.

Psychiatric illness is usually multifactorial in origin. The final picture of illness is often the interaction of biological, psychological and relationship difficulties in the setting of certain life events.

PSYCHIATRIC ASPECTS OF ORGANIC DISEASE

THE ORGANIC BRAIN SYNDROMES

The psychiatric syndrome associated with physical or biochemical disorder of the brain is characterised by the following clinical features:

1. memory loss, most marked for recent events
2. impairment of consciousness
3. disorientation (time, place, person)
4. intellectual impairment (deficient grasp, reasoning, social disinhibition)
5. non-specific features: hallucinations (particularly visual), mood disturbance (lability, depression, disinhibition), delusional ideas, neurological signs
6. marked variability, usually worse at night.

The acute organic brain syndrome

The characteristic features of the organic brain syndrome occur but clouding of consciousness and disorientation predominate. When these lead to anxiety, bewilderment, misinterpretations and visual hallucinations this is called delirium. Causes are listed in Table 22.1.

Table 22.1. Causes of acute organic brain syndrome

Causes	Clinical Examples
Metabolic	(Electrolyte imbalance) uraemia, liver failure, diabetes, anoxia
Infective	Simple fevers in children, tonsillitis, meningitis, encephalitis, AIDS, infections in the elderly
Traumatic	Head injury
Degenerative	Cerebrovascular ischaemia
Dementia	Alzheimer's disease
Alcohol	Withdrawal in dependent individuals
Nutritional	Thiamine deficiency, e.g. complicating alcoholism
Anaemia	Addisonian anaemia

Clinical example: delirium tremens

Aetiology
Absolute or relative alcohol withdrawal in a person who is physically dependent upon alcohol. Concomitant infection is also frequently implicated, as is trauma such as head injury.

Symptoms and signs
Confusion, disorientation, gross ataxia, coarse tremor of hands, agitation, intense fear, visual and tactile hallucinations, and paranoid ideation develop, 48 or 72 hours after alcohol withdrawal.

Complications
Physical injury, status epilepticus, hyperthermia, dehydration, electrolyte imbalance.

Investigations
Chest and other infections, dehydration, injury, cardiovascular collapse should be sought. Prophylaxis against epileptic fits is advisable when there is a history of previous fits.

Differential diagnosis

Alcoholic auditory hallucinosis. This may be independent of the withdrawal syndrome and occurs in the setting of clear consciousness. It may last days and even become chronic.

Head injury is common in persons who have taken excessive alcohol.

Hepatic failure may also present with confusion and clouding of consciousness (see p. 297).

Treatment

Adequate sedation (chlordiazepoxide or diazepam) is important. Chlormethiazole should only be used in the case of inpatients because of dependency and risk of fatal respiratory depression if taken with alcohol.

Fluid and electrolyte imbalances and hypoglycaemia must be corrected. Intramuscular vitamin B complex must also be given.

It is necessary to treat infection, prevent injury and use anticonvulsants if fits occur. Magnesium may also reduce central nervous system (CNS) excitability. The minimum possible restraint should be used, and a darkened room avoided. Relatives should be asked to sit with the patient to minimise disorientation. The mortality may be as high as 15%.

The chronic organic brain syndrome (dementia)

Aetiology

There is cerebral atrophy with neuronal loss. It is termed senile atrophy in patients over 60 years, and presenile atrophy under that age; 3–5% of individuals over 65 years have significant dementia.

Symptoms and signs

The characteristic features of the organic syndrome occur, but consciousness is usually unimpaired except in acute episodes of confusion or delirium which may be precipitated by super-added complications such as chest infections, anaemia, or merely removal from familiar surroundings. Impairment of recent memory is evident, at first with preservation of distant memory. Deterioration of intellectual function is often progressive with loss of judgement, sexual or social disinhibition and aggression. Localised neurological dysfunction and irregular step-wise deterioration suggest a vascular cause.

Causes

It is important to search carefully for treatable cases particularly in the young. *Alzheimer's disease* is much more common in women usually starting after the age of 70 years. Memory loss is an early feature, and dressing apraxia due to early involvement of parietal lobes is common, sometimes with extrapyramidal signs.

Pick's disease. A rare condition which usually commences between 50 and 60 years of age, Pick's disease is inherited as an autosomal dominant. It tends to be associated with early social disinhibition and dysphasia, with later onset of memory loss.

Multi-infarct dementia. Depressive features may be marked at an early stage, presumably related to retained insight.

Alcoholic dementia. Cortical atrophy, intellectual deficit and severe personality changes may occur at a late stage of alcohol dependence.

Trauma. In head injuries the severity of dementia correlates well with the duration of the post-traumatic amnesia. The 'punch-drunk syndrome' in boxers leads to pyramidal, extrapyramidal and cerebral signs, with impotence and sometimes morbid jealousy.

Metabolic/nutritional causes include hypothyroidism, hypoglycaemia, renal dialysis, hepatic failure, vitamin B_{12} deficiency, Cushing's syndrome, hypoxia from any cause.

Infective. Neurosyphilis (GPI) (see p. 148), depression, grandiose ideas, and occasionally paranoid psychosis occur.

AIDS. Dementia is relentlessly progressive.

Neoplastic disease. Cerebral tumours can cause intellectual impairment but also lead to focal signs; with frontal tumours these may develop late.

Neurological diseases (e.g. multiple sclerosis), Parkinson's disease and Huntington's chorea are other causes of dementia.

Investigations

Normal Pressure Hydrocephalus. These are appropriate for a secondary cause, e.g. serum B_{12} measurements. In Alzheimer's disease there is strong positive correlation of EEG abnormality with cognitive impairment. The degree of ventricular dilatation on the CT scan correlates with the severity of dementia.

Differential diagnosis

Depression may be present with poor concentration and resulting memory impairment (pseudodementia). Schizophrenia may simulate dementia by producing autistic behaviour and self-neglect.

Hysterical amnesia and chronic intoxication with medication, e.g. in epilepsy, should also be considered.

Clinical example: the amnesic syndromes

These are characterised by a severe recent memory defect in which registration seems unimpaired but recall is rapidly lost. There may be confabulation and confusion of temporal sequence of events. Causes include vascular accidents around the hippocampus, subarachnoid haemorrhage, trauma (particularly of the temporal lobes), infection (encephalitis and meningitis), metabolic (cerebral hypoxia), carbon monoxide poisoning, and toxic agents (carbon monoxide poisoning, glue sniffing, alcohol poisoning).

The Wernicke-Korsakoff syndrome

This is commonly caused by thiamine deficiency complicating alcohol abuse but also occurs in hyperemesis gravidarum. Initially it resembles Wernicke's encephalopathy with confusion, ataxia, nystagmus, ptosis, and disorders of conjugate gaze. This may then lead to the Korsakoff's syndrome in which, in spite of clear consciousness, there is gross impairment of recent memory.

The patient may confabulate to cover gaps in memory. Treatment consists of urgent administration of vitamin B_1 complex intramuscularly, including thiamine up to 50 mg per 24 hours.

The prognosis is better with a short history and early treatment. Chronic disability occurs although gradual improvement may result over an extended period.

Hepatic encephalopathy

This often complicates liver failure (see p. 297).

Renal encephalopathy

This is a progressive organic brain syndrome caused by uraemia with super-added effects of underlying disease, e.g. cerebrovascular insufficiency, and secondary psychological reaction. Early clinical features include fatigue and poor concentration but later episodes of confusion or delirium occur, leading finally to coma.

When renal dialysis is carried out rapidly there may be headache, confusion, fits and even coma, possibly related to cerebral oedema or reactive hypoglycaemia. Some patients develop a chronic progressive dementia possibly related to the accumulation in the brain of aluminium derived from dialysate.

EPILEPSY

Ictal (the attack)

When the fit is generalised, the clinical picture is unequivocal. However, focal episodes may mimic a psychiatric disorder in several ways (see Table 22.2).

1. Focal: simple. There may be no loss of consciousness and the episode may constitute no more than an 'aura'. This may include dysphasia, deja and jamais vu, forced thinking, compulsive symptoms, distortion of time sense, dreamy states, anxiety which may be extreme, anger, depression, feelings of pleasure, laughter, visual and auditory illusions, hallucinations which may be autonomic in nature such as the rising gastric sensation in temporal lobe epilepsy.

2. Focal: complex. When actual loss of consciousness occurs there may be automatism which is a state of clouded consciousness during the seizure with retention of posture, together with simple and complex movements lasting less than 5 minutes in 80% of cases. An episode of automatism lasts less than 1 hour. Awareness and subsequent recollection are impaired. At first there may be simple oral movements such as lip-smacking, and these may lead to pushing, pulling, turning or running. In *absence* attacks (petit mal fits) there may be both oral and other forms of automatism.

Post-ictal

Automatism is more likely to be complex but if aggressive it tends to take the form of pushing or fending off. Rarely is it directed or organised and it does not take the form of a purposeful, violent or criminal act. An acute confusional psychosis with visual hallucinations and delusional ideas may also occur, leading to aggressive behaviour.

Inter-ictal

In post-traumatic epilepsy when there is frontal damage there may be disinhibited aggressive behaviour. Concomitant brain damage may cause perseverative paranoid personality traits.

Depression in epilepsy is common. Up to 7% of patients with epilepsy associated with organic brain damage eventually commit suicide.

Chronic drug intoxication may be misdiagnosed as dementia. Chronic schizophreniform psychosis is particularly associated with temporal lobe epilepsy. All the cardinal signs of schizophrenia may develop and the onset may be long delayed after the epilepsy itself began.

Table 22.2. **Differential diagnosis of psychiatric complications of epilepsy**

Panic attacks	Sleep-walking
Non-ictal rage or violence	Organic confusional state
Pseudoseizures (hysterical reaction)	Catatonic schizophrenia
Fugue state	

ENDOCRINE DISORDERS (See Table 22.3)

AIDS

Initial denial may be followed by anxiety, depression with suicidal ideas, anger or hypomania. When dementia occurs it leads to progressive global intellectual loss, sometimes complicated by delusional ideation.

SOMATIC ASPECTS OF PSYCHIATRIC ILLNESS

Illnesses which are primarily psychiatric in nature often mimic physical disease by presenting with physical symptoms and signs, some of which are disabling and serious.

AFFECTIVE DISORDERS

For somatic features see Table 22.4

Differential diagnosis

1. obsessional/compulsive disorder: specific checking and ritualistic behaviour such as hand-washing is the presenting symptom
2. alcoholism
3. drug dependence (opiates, benzodiazepines): accentuation of anxiety occurs in withdrawal
4. schizophrenia
5. physical disorders: organic causes of many kinds may need to be ruled out.

HYSTERICAL REACTION

Symptoms and signs

Hysteria represents an unconscious psychological reaction to conflict or a threat in which symptoms and signs of organic disease are often closely simulated. It leads both to primary gain by relief of anxiety and to secondary gain such as avoidance of the feared situation. Great care should be taken before invoking such a diagnosis because of its great unreliability. Hysterical reaction and organic disease are not mutually exclusive diagnoses: they often occur together. Furthermore, a hysterical reaction should never be diagnosed merely on the basis that organic disease has been excluded. It is necessary to establish psychological meaning as to why a hysterical symptom appears.

Table 22.3. Psychiatric aspects of endocrine disorders

Disorder	Common	Less common
Thyrotoxicosis	Anxiety, hyperactivity	Depression, agitation or apathy Organic confusional state in severe toxicity
Hypothyroidism	Organic brain syndrome with memory impairment Dementia in adults or mental handicap in children if untreated Depression which may require antidepressive therapy	Paranoid hallucinatory psychosis, mania, coma
Cushing's disease	Depression, anxiety, stupor, episodic acute excitement	Paranoid delusions, auditory hallucinations, elation, acute confusional state
Addison's disease	Mild memory impairment Organic-type features such as confusion, especially when hypoglycaemia is present	Depression, apathy, irritability
ACTH and corticosteroid therapy	Euphoria when dosage is high and prolonged, or in predisposed individuals	Depression, psychosis with a mixed picture of disorientation and depression or mood elevation Delusional ideas, hallucinations, catatonia
Hypopituitarism	Depression, apathy, memory impairment	Confusion, delirium, coma which can be fatal in the absence of hormone replacement
Phaeochromocytoma	Acute anxiety-type symptoms with severe headaches often precipitated by emotional arousal or physical exertion	
Insulinoma	Episodic behaviour such as aggression that is out of character May be confusion or loss of consciousness	

The clinical picture may be of two types:

1. *Conversion* refers to the process whereby emotional conflict is transformed into physical symptoms or signs such as paralysis, anaesthesia, blindness, tremor. Careful physical examination may reveal important inconsistencies compared with those of true physical disease, e.g. sensory loss of atypical distribution etc.

Table 22.4. Somatic features of anxiety and depressive states

Neurological	Motor restlessness, tension headaches, action tremor of hands
Gastrointestinal	Poor appetite, weightloss, nausea, frequent bowel action, constipation, abdominal discomfort, dysphagia
Respiratory	Over-breathing (in panic disorders this may lead to paraesthesiae, tetany and feelings of faintness leading to accentuation of anxiety), subjective difficulty in achieving adequate air intake
Cardiovascular	Palpitations, tachycardia, chest discomfort
Genitourinary	Frequency or urgency of micturition, impotence, loss of libido
Autonomic	Sympathetic overactivity (cold sweaty peripheries, dry mouth, dilated pupils, tachycardia)

2. *Dissociation* occurs when one part of mental activity is split off from the rest, as in amnesia. This is characterised by its global nature, involving both recent and distant memories, perhaps even to the extent of loss of knowledge of personal identity. It is therefore strikingly different in its precise characteristics from amnesia from organic brain damage in which recent memory loss is the most marked feature.

Initially the patient with hysterical symptoms may be very disturbed, but later can show a remarkable lack of concern (belle indifference).

Differential diagnosis
Organic disease and malingering.

Treatment
It is important to remember that organic disease and hysterical symptoms may co-exist.

Prognosis
This depends upon the underlying cause and how easily it can be resolved.

PSYCHOLOGICAL DISORDERS OF FOOD INTAKE

ANOREXIA NERVOSA

The incidence in females exceeds that in males 15 to 1. Onset is usually in adolescence but a small proportion begin at pre-puberty.

The illness is probably a response to difficulty in negotiating the many potential problems of adolescence.

Symptoms and signs
The patient feels well, has abundance of energy, but there is a marked loss of weight, deliberate reduction of food intake, selective calorie avoidance and subterfuges (exercise, self-induced vomiting, purgation, misuse of diuretics).

Examination reveals loss of subcutaneous fat and muscle bulk although power remains good and tendon reflexes are brisk in the absence of complications. Bradycardia, cold extremities and peripheral cyanosis are typical when severe weightloss has occurred. Secondary sexual hair is retained and there may be fine truncal lanugo hair.

Amenorrhoea (usually following weightloss) in females and loss of sexual interest and impotence in males will be seen.

Psychological symptoms include a highly specific fear of becoming fat with a phobia for normal weight and weight increase, fears of loss of control of the self and behaviour, secondary depression, obsessional features and anxiety, and conscientiousness with rigid eating habits. The patient often denies being ill and resents any intervention aimed at producing weight gain.

Complications

Hypokalaemic alkalosis results from persistent vomiting and abuse of purgatives or diuretics. Gross muscle weakness may follow as may tetany with muscle spasm, general paraesthesia and stridor. There may be moderate normochromic anaemia.

Family tensions may be severe. Depression is often seen and there is increased risk of suicide.

Tricyclic antidepressants or phenothiazine may cause epileptic convulsions (because the epileptic threshold is lowered). Chlorpromazine may cause hypothermia or cholestatic jaundice.

Different diagnosis

Physical disorders which may mimic anorexia nervosa include malabsorption syndrome, Crohn's disease, neoplasia, diabetes mellitus, thyrotoxicosis and tuberculosis.

Psychological disorders which may mimic anorexia nervosa include depressive illness, anxiety state, phobic anxiety for swallowing, obsessional neurosis and paranoid psychosis (with fear of food contamination).

Treatment

Restoration of adequate nutrition is essential. If the bodyweight falls below 70% of average for height and age immediate admission to hospital may be imperative, particularly when the weight fall has been rapid and there is also electrolyte disorder or dehydration.

The patient may need bedrest with firm control of dietary intake. Otherwise a negotiated treatment plan on an outpatient basis may be feasible. Relatives should also be offered support.

Prognosis

Of hospital treated patients, 40–60% recover, 20–30% have a relapsing illness, and 20–30% develop a chronic illness. Up to 5% die in 5 years from severe weightloss, suicide, ileus or intestinal dilatation related to electrolyte deficiency, infection and the toxic side-effects of medication.

BULIMIA NERVOSA

This is characterized by a disordered control of food intake even though the bodyweight may remain within normal limits. Onset is in late teenage years or early twenties. Females greatly outnumber males. Some cases may be examples of weight-normalised anorexia nervosa.

Symptoms and signs

There is a powerful urge to overeat, leading to episodes of bingeing which may be massive. Periods of food denial, vomiting or purgative abuse follow. There is a fear of becoming fat.

Callosities on the back of the hand are used to self-induce vomiting, which leads to severe erosion of dental enamel due to the regular presence of acid gastric contents in the mouth.

Bilateral painless swelling of the parotid glands may be present.

Investigations

Electrolyte levels should be checked regularly. ECG may show evidence of hypokalaemia.

Differential diagnosis

Anorexia nervosa, or functional (psychogenic) vomiting which occurs in the absence of specific worries about body-weight.

Treatment

Reduction of frequency and severity of binges by prolonged personal support, achieving regular food intake (use of dietary diary), management of mood disorders, and the use of cognitive behavioural therapy or group therapy are the mainstay of treatment.

Prognosis

Relapse and chronicity are common when the condition is related to wider personality problems of impulse control and social difficulties.

SUBSTANCE ABUSE

ALCOHOL DEPENDENCE

At first it may have only a psychological component but later there also develops physiological dependence involving tissue tolerance, leading to unpleasant physiological symptoms on withdrawal.

Genetic, social and cultural factors are important. Predisposing occupations involve free and ready access to alcohol as well as its regular social use, e.g. publicans, armed forces, commercial travellers, or high stresses together with relative affluence, e.g. doctors particularly those who begin drinking heavily as students. Persons with high levels of anxiety who use alcohol as an anxiolytic are also at increased risk of developing excessive dependence. Highest rates of alcohol abuse occur in the 20–30 year age groups.

Of hospital medical inpatients, 8% of females and 29% of males have a drink problem.

Symptoms and signs
The 'alcoholic dependence syndrome' has several components:
1. narrowing of drink repertoire
2. salience of drink-seeking behaviour
3. responsibilities become neglected
4. increased tolerance to alcohol
5. repeated withdrawal symptoms (typically with tremor and sweating, worse on waking in the morning)
6. relief drinking, often in the morning to reduce the degree of withdrawal symptoms
7. subjective awareness of compulsion to drink
8. reinstatement after abstinence.

Alcohol-related disabilities
Physical disabilities related to alcohol abuse include liver disease, chronic pancreatitis, acute gastritis, peptic ulcer, oesophagitis, macrocytosis without anaemia, megaloblastic anaemia, ischaemic heart disease, cerebrovascular accidents, cardiomyopathy, peripheral neuropathy, Wernicke's encephalopathy, head injury and cerebellar degeneration.

Psychological disabilities related to alcohol abuse include depression, (greatly increased risk of suicide and non-fatal self-harm), anxiety (especially during alcohol withdrawal), acute auditory hallucinosis usually lasting a few days only, visual hallucinosis which may lead to the full picture of delirium tremens, recurrent violent behaviour, memory impairment (short-lasting episodes or in the chronic form as Korsakoff's syndrome) and dementia.

Social disabilities related to alcohol abuse are work difficulties (absenteeism, unemployment), marriage difficulties and breakdown, erratic behaviour at home, social isolation, vagrancy and criminality.

Investigations
The serum gamma glutamyl transpeptidase (GGT) level is raised in 75% of alcohol-dependent individuals; a raised blood level and macrocytosis will also be present.

Differential diagnosis
Alcohol abuse should be considered in a wide range of physical conditions as listed above.

Treatment
1. Minor tranquillisers (diazepam) are given in reducing doses if withdrawal symptoms are severe. Chlormethiazole can be addictive and cause respiratory depression if taken with alcohol.
2. Intramuscular parentrovite.
3. Any concomitant infection must be treated.
4. Prophylactic anticonvulsants should be prescribed when there is a previous history of epileptic fits during alcohol withdrawal.

5. Prophylaxis against physical injury, especially in ataxic patients.
6. Treatment of the addiction itself on an individual or group basis is essential.
7. Involvement of the spouse can be crucial.
8. Use of community treatment agencies such as Alcoholics Anonymous.
9. Antabuse (toxic acetaldehyde produced when alcohol is ingested) should be used only under specialist advice.

Prognosis

The best outlook is associated with social stability, co-operative attitude, first treatment episode and stable personality. Safe levels of drinking (taking 1 unit as equivalent to half a pint of beer, one tot of whisky, a half glass of sherry or one glass of wine): weekly consumption below 14 units for women and 21 for men.

OTHER ADDICTIVE AGENTS

Opiates (morphine, heroin) are smoked, taken orally, injected subcutaneously, intramuscularly or intravenously. Rapid development of habituation and tissue tolerance means that the dosage tends to escalate progressively. Withdrawal symptoms include rhinorrhoea, lacrimation and sweating, abdominal cramps and diarrhoea.

Complications include those related to dirty needles (local thrombophlebitis, septicaemia, bacterial endocarditis, HIV infection and AIDS), overdose that can be lethal, depression and suicide.

Treatment by methadone substitution is often effective.

Barbiturates are increasingly used by young multiple drug abusers. In overdose, respiratory and cardiovascular depression can be severe and fatal. Local injection may lead to necrotic skin lesions and localised phlebitis. Withdrawal fits are common.

Amphetamine abuse leads to increased arousal and excitability. Prolonged excessive intake may lead to paranoid psychosis. Withdrawal may be complicated by severe depression.

Cocaine produces effects similar to amphetamines. It is usually inhaled nasally (snorted) and it can produce paranoid delusions as well as other psychotic complications.

Hallucinogens such as mescaline and LSD produce vivid visual hallucinations, as well as disorientation for place. Physical withdrawal symptoms do not occur, although unpleasant flashback-type memories may be encountered.

Solvent sniffing occurs mainly in children and adolescents, often as a group activity. It may lead to liver and CNS damage and may present with stupor or unconsciousness. Asphyxia from the use of a plastic bag is an added hazard.

Diagnostic pointers include solvent odour, evidence of solvent or glue on hands and face, and 'glue sniffer's rash surrounding the mouth.

Benzodiazepines when prescribed regularly in high dosage over a prolonged time, may lead to dependence with distressing accentuation of anxiety and tremor and insomnia on withdrawal. They should therefore only be used in short courses and in doses which are as low as possible. Lorezapam, which has a very short half-life, has proved itself to have powerful addictive complications. Withdrawal from benzodiazepines may initially require inpatient treatment.

SOME IMPORTANT TOPICS

The violent patient

Points to remember in management:

1. Establish a diagnosis (e.g. alcohol withdrawal state, epilepsy, delusional state).
2. Staff should remain calm and non-critical.
3. Avoid confrontation. Talk and listen to the patient. If restraint is necessary use the minimum degree of force required to control violence, and aim to calm rather than provoke.
4. Use clothing rather than direct body restraint if possible. Never press on neck, chest or abdomen.
5. Remove the patient's shoes and beware of the potential hazard of neckwear.
6. Great care is required when administering intramuscular or intravenous drug injection. Use a safe drug such as diazepam (particularly valuable in alcohol withdrawal).

Violence, of course, may not necessarily indicate that an individual is ill.

Suicide and non-fatal deliberate self-harm

Suicide. Suicide risk factors are summarised in Table 22.5. All psychiatric conditions carry some increased risk but depressive illness, alcohol and drug dependence by far outstrip the rest.

Non-fatal deliberate self-harm (DSH). This very commonly presents in hospital in the form of drug over-dosage or self-laceration. Typically it is most common in young adults, and in females more than males although the incidence in the latter has increased in recent years. All of those patients are at increased risk: 1% commit suicide and 20% repeat DSH in the following year.

Table 22.5. Factors associated with increased risk of suicide

Males > females; older age group; divorced > widowed > single; social class I or V

Living alone; socially isolated; intractable adverse life events; unemployment/retired

Past psychiatric history, especially affective illness, alcoholism; family history of affective illness; previous self-harm

Recent event: bereavement/separation/loss of job; poor physical health; current evidence of depressive illness; abuse of alcohol; alienated, with loss of sympathy/support from others

---

Detailed evaluation of the mental state is therefore important in all DSH patients before they are allowed home. Depressive features and persistent suicidal ideas should be taken seriously along with other risk factors (Table 22.5).

Postpartum mental disorders

The birth of a child is a major life event often associated with significant psychiatric morbidity. Two-thirds of women experience 'maternity blues' with symptoms of irritability, weepiness and withdrawal on the fourth and fifth day postpartum, but recover within 24 hours; 1 in 500 women postpartum suffer from the severe psychotic illness known as puerperal psychosis within the first 10 days. Moderately severe postnatal depression affects about 1 in 10 women during the first 3 months.

Symptoms and signs

Puerperal psychosis. The clinical picture is often one of sleeplessness, restlessness, morbid preoccupation with the baby's health, delusional ideas which may be grandiose or bizarre in other ways. The mood fluctuates from acute depression to mania and high excitement; the risk of harm to the baby and suicide is great.

Postnatal depression. Postnatal depression is often not apparent until after discharge from the maternity unit. The classical features of a depressive illness are present; these include early morning waking with anxiety and panic in the early hours improving later in the day. Recurrent preoccupation with minor symptoms and blemishes on the baby may draw attention to the mother's morbid fears. Severe maternity blues, a family history of depression or a previous history of an affective illness along with concomitant major life events, such as a house move or recent bereavement, indicate high-risk individuals.

Anxiety states

Obsessive compulsive disorders. High anxiety, often fears of losing control and being aggressive. Insight is retained, and it is important to distinguish this from psychotic illness (specialist advice should be readily sought regarding differential diagnosis).

Treatment

Where there is any risk of suicide or harm to the baby, close supervision is essential but must be in conditions which allow continued contact between mother and baby. The treatment is that of the particular illness, e.g. mania, depression or schizophrenia. Rapid relief of symptoms is important: when acute depression, mixed depression and elation, or excessive restlessness with perplexed mood occur, electroconvulsive therapy (ECT) might be given early in addition to appropriate medication. In most patients with postnatal depression, treatment with antidepressants at home, along with supportive counselling and psychological treatments, will be sufficient.

Prognosis

Early vigorous intervention and treatment is essential. Most patients with a puerperal psychosis will recover completely, although up to 20% will have a further puerperal depression.

Postnatal depression is often missed, leading to a significant number becoming chronically ill over many months. With active treatment the majority recover, particularly the mother has a good previous personality and social support.

23

TROPICAL MEDICINE

Stuart Glover

MALARIA

Malaria is an acute and chronic disease caused by the obligate intracellular protozoan of the genus *Plasmodium*. There are four species of human malaria; *P. vivax, P. falciparum, P. ovale* and *P. malariae*. Malaria parasites are transmitted to humans by female anopheline mosquitoes, the definitive host for plasmodia.

Malaria is widespread in the tropics and subtropics causing an estimated 1 million deaths annually; 2000 cases are diagnosed each year in the UK. There were 8 deaths in the UK from malaria during 1989 and 1990. *Falciparum* malaria accounts for 52% and *vivax* for 40% of the malaria diagnosed in Britain. It can on rare occasions be acquired at international European airports, during very brief stopovers in malarious airports (runway malaria), by blood transfusions and organ transplantation. Neonatal malaria is rare.

Pathology

Plasmodial trophozoites alter the deformability of red blood cells which become sequestered in the microcirculation of the brain, myocardium, gut and kidneys with resultant ischaemia and organ dysfunction. With maturation of trophozoites to schizonts, red cells will rupture, contributing to anaemia. Tumour necrosis factor (TNF) levels rise with schizont release.

Symptoms and signs

The incubation period is 10–15 days for *falciparum* and as long as 24 months for *vivax*. The onset of symptoms is delayed by prior chemoprophylaxis, partial therapy and natural immunity.

Primary attacks in non-immune individuals are abrupt, causing:

1. cold stage (vasoconstriction): rigors, vomiting, rising temperature
2. hot stage (vasodilatation): dry and hot skin, severe throbbing headache, high fever >40°C, restlessness and delirium
3. sweating stage: drenching sweat, rapid defervescence.

Fever is variable and irregular in *falciparum* and may even be absent. A tertian (every 48 hours) pattern occurs in established *vivax* and *ovale* malaria. Fever may cause delirium.

Other signs include splenomegaly, hepatomegaly with mild jaundice (caused mainly by haemolysis), anaemia and tachycardia with relative hypotension. Retinal haemorrhage is evidence of cerebral malaria, even in non-comatose subjects.

Investigations

Blood films, thick and thin, show intracellular trophozoites ('ring forms'); also crescent shaped gametocytes may be seen. Full blood count reveals anaemia, thrombocytopenia and monocytosis. Eosinophilia does *not* occur in malaria.

Urinalysis for haemoglobinuria, urea and electrolytes for renal function, liver function tests (LFT) and blood sugar monitoring are also required.

Differential diagnosis

Irrespective of the clinical presentation or whether or not prophylactic antimalarial drugs have been taken, a history of travel to an endemic area makes it mandatory to rule out malaria.

Malaria can and does mimic many other diseases such as typhoid fever, brucellosis, viral hepatitis, arboviral infections (dengue fever), viral haemorrhagic fevers (Lassa fever), tick typhus, Q fever etc.

Treatment

For *P. vivax* and *P. ovale* malarias are treated using the '10 tablet chloroquine course' (day 1: chloroquine base 600 mg stat; chloroquine base, 300 mg 8 hours later; days 2–3 chloroquine base 300 mg; then primaquine 15 mg daily for 14–21 days).

The treatment of *P. malariae* malaria is as for *P. vivax* but there is no need for primaquine.

Uncomplicated *P. falciparum* infections where the patient is able to swallow tablets are treated in chloroquine-resistant areas (now widespread) with quinine 600 mg 8-hourly for 7–14 days and oxytetracycline 250 mg 6-hourly for 7 days, or with mefloquine 1000 mg in a single dose.

Complicated *P. falciparum* infections where the patient is unable to swallow are treated in chloroquine-resistant areas with quinine dihydrochloride 20 mg/kg loading dose i.v. infusion over 4 hours, followed by 10 mg/kg i.v. infusion over 4 hours every 8 hours until the patient is able to swallow and complete a 7-day course.

Other aspects of treatment include management in an intensive care unit with monitoring of the pulse, blood pressure (BP), central venous pressure (CVP), urine output, blood gases, blood sugar, renal and hepatic function, haemoglobin, platelet count, coagulation status, and conscious level (Glasgow Coma Scale), and prophylaxis and treatment of fits in cerebral malaria.

Prophylaxis

1. Countries where *P. falciparum* is resistant to chloroquine: chloroquine 300 mg base, weekly plus proguanil (Paludrine) 200 mg daily.
2. Countries with multi-resistant *P. falciparum* (Thailand, Laos, Kampuchea, South Vietnam, Papua New Guinea):
   a. Maloprim (pyrethamine 12.5 mg, dapsone 100 mg one tablet weekly *plus* chloroquine 300 mg base weekly;
   b. Mefloquine 250 mg weekly.
3. Personal protection includes using mosquito nets impregnated with permethrin, window screens, insect repellants (diethyl toluamide), burning mosquito coils, and wearing sensible after-sunset clothing—long sleeves and trousers.

Prognosis

Vivax and *ovale* malaria are rarely fatal but relapses may occur unless treated with primaquine. Malaria *malariae* is associated with nephrotic syndrome. *Falciparum* malaria, if untreated, can be rapidly fatal in non-immune individuals.

A poor prognosis is associated with delayed diagnosis, hyperparasitaemia, hypoglycaemia, convulsions, pulmonary oedema, acute renal and hepatic failure, haemoglobinuria and retinal haemorrhages.

Pregnant, primiparous women, children and asplenic patients are at increased risk of severe *falciparum* malaria.

Complications of *P. falciparum* malaria include cerebral malaria which has a 20–50% mortality, acute renal and hepatic failure, hypoglycaemia, hyperpyrexia and fluid and electrolyte imbalance. Renal involvement may be associated with oliguria and haemoglobinuria (Blackwater fever). Gram-negative septicaemia (Algid malaria) may occur.

SCHISTOSOMIASIS (BILHARZIASIS)

Schistosomiasis is an extremely common parasitic infection caused by several species of intravascular trematodes or blood flukes. Three main species of schistosomes infect humans: *Schistosoma haematobium* is prevalent in Africa, the Middle East and Goa, and forms in the vesicle venous plexus. *S. mansoni* is found in Africa, Arabia, Brazil, Suriname, Venezuela, the Caribbean, the Nile Delta and infects the inferior mesenteric veins. *S. japonicum* is restricted to China, the Philippines and Indonesia (Sulawesi) and infects the mesenteric veins.

Humans are the definitive host and main reservoir of *S. haematobium*, *S. mansoni* and *S. japonicum* but several mammals also host the latter. Various species of snail act as intermediate hosts.

Pathology

Adult worms remain in intravascular locations for years producing large numbers of ova. These ova penetrate the gut or bladder wall to be excreted to the environment, or become trapped within the organ walls where granulomata develop, or embolise to the liver, lungs or central nervous system (CNS) where obstructive granulomata form.

Symptoms

Cercarial dermatitis or swimmers' itch may develop within a few hours of metacercariae penetrating the skin.

Acute schistosomiasis or Katayama fever occurs 3–8 weeks post infection. It is immune complex mediated. Fever, prostration, diarrhoea, arthritis, lymphadenopathy, hepatosplenomegaly and massive eosinophilia can be fatal.

Established schistosomiasis (See Table 23.1)

FILARIAL INFECTIONS

Lymphatic filariasis is caused by the nematode parasites *Wuchereria bancrofti*, *Brugia malayi* and *B. Timori*. The adult macrofilariae live in lymph glands and vessels causing inflammation and subsequent obstruction. Adult females produce microfilariae which circulate in the blood and which are transmitted by a variety of biting mosquitoes.

Loiasis is caused by infection with the filarial worm *Loa loa* which is transmitted by horse flies of the genus *Chrysops*.

Onchocerciasis is a chronic filarial disease caused by *Onchocerca volvulus* and is transmitted by black flies of the genus *Simulium*. The disease affects the skin, eyes and lymph nodes.

Symptoms and signs (See Table 23.2)

Investigations

Blood films may show microfilariae and eosinophilia. A nucleopore membrane can be used to filter the blood to facilitate diagnosis. Serology will show antifilarial antibodies. Tropical pulmonary eosinophilia with lung shadowing may be evident on chest X-ray.

Skin snips can be examined for onchocerciasis.

Prognosis

Onchocerciasis can cause blindness. Lymphatic filariasis causes elephantiasis, genital oedema and chylothorax.

Treatment

Diethylcarbamazine (DEC) is given for 21 days increasing from 1 mg/kg to 6 mg/kg in divided doses every 3 days. Onchocerciasis is treated with ivermectin 150 µg/kg in a single dose. Re-treatment may be needed.

Table 23.1. Schistosomiasis

	S. Mansoni	*S. Haematobium*	*S. Japonicum*
Symptoms	*Gastrointestinal:* None or abdominal pain, diarrhoea, dysentery,	*Bladder:* None or terminal haematuria, dysuria, nocturia frequency, suprapubic pain	*Gastrointestinal:* Diarrhoea, dysentery, abdominal pain *CNS:* headaches, convulsions
Signs	Rectosgmoid polyps hepatosplenomegaly, ascites, oedema, cor pulmonale	Anaemia, chronic renal failure (obstructive uropathy)	Hepato-splenomegaly, raised intracranial pressure, cor pulmonale
Investigation	Eosinophilia Stools: lateral spined ova Sigmoidoscopy: rectal 'snips' Barium enema Serology	Eosinophilia Urine and stools: terminal spined ova Rectal biopsy Cystoscopy: 'sandy patches' IVU Serology	Eosinophilia Stools: ova Rectal biopsy Serology CT scan: Brain Intracranial granulomata which may be calcified
Treatment	Praziquantel 40–60 mg as a single dose† Oxamniquine*	Metrifonate†	Praziquantel
Prognosis	Colorectal cancer Pipe stem fibrosis of the liver Portal hypertension Oesophageal varices Cor pulmonale Chronic *Salmonella* carriage Spinal cord damage	Iron deficiency anaemia Hydronephrosis Hydroureter Fibrous/granulomatous ureteral strictures Bladder wall calcification Bladder papilloma/cancer *S. typhi* carriage in urine Urethral stricture	Oesophageal variceal haemorrhage Liver failure Appendicitis Space-occupying lesions in brain—convulsions

*15-30 mg/kg /day over 2-3 days
†10-mg/kg 3 doses at 2-week intervals

ENTERIC FEVER

In the 10-year period 1981–1990 approximately 1700 cases of typhoid fever were diagnosed in England and Wales; 89% were contracted abroad, mainly on the Indian subcontinent, and of those less than 15% were infected in the Mediterranean and Middle-East. In the same period, there were 1000 cases of paratyphoid A and B.

Table 23.2. Symptoms and signs of filariasis infections

Species of filarial parasite	Geography	Symptoms and signs
W. bancrofti (nocturnal periodicity)	Asia, Middle-East, Africa, South and Central America, the Caribbean	Acute filarial fever, funiculitis, epididymitis, orchitis, hydrocele, lymphadenitis, genital/limb oedema, elephantiasis, chyluria
W. bancrofti (diurnal subperiodicity)	Pacific islands, Polynesia	As above
B. malayi (nocturnal periodicity)	South-East Asia, Japan, China	Lymphadenitis (inguinal), retrograde lymphadenitis, distal elephantiasis, genitals spared
B. malayi (diurnal subperiodicity)	Malaysia	As for *B. malayi*
B. timori	Indonesia	Filarial abscess
Loa loa	West Africa	Calabar swellings, adult worms under skin and in conjunctivae
O. volvulus	Africa, Yemen, Central and South America	Dermatitis, nodules, keratitis, iritis

Pathology

Salmonella typhi causes enteric fever: *S. paratyphi* types A, B and C cause paratyphoid fever. These micro-organisms are exclusively human pathogens causing acute disease or chronic faecal carriage. Transmission is by food, milk, shellfish or water contaminated with sewage or by a single human carrier.

After ingestion and during the incubation period of 10–14 days, organisms penetrate the intestinal mucosa and spread to the regional lymphatics. Bacteraemia follows with spread of salmonellae to Peyer's patches in the small intestine.

Symptoms and signs

The onset is insidious with malaise, myalgia, anorexia, chills, headache, a dry cough, constipation and rising fever. *Typhoid fever is not usually a diarrhoeal illness*. If untreated, apathy, abdominal pain and distension are seen in the second week and deterioration with delirium in the third.

There is a stepladder rise in temperature. Rose spots which are pink macules seen over the chest and abdomen, cropping over 1–2 weeks and lasting 3–4 days occur in about 50% of cases. They are caused by septic emboli. Splenomegaly is present in 40%. There may also be confusion and psychiatric symptoms such as catatonia or psychosis.

Investigations

Blood, urine and stool cultures are obtained, and a full blood count shows leukopenia and lymphocytosis.

Differential diagnosis

Malaria, brucellosis, occult bacterial abscess, amoebic liver abscess, infective endocarditis, viral haemorrhagic fever etc.

Treatment

Based on the sensitivity of the organism, ciprofloxacin, co-trimoxazole or amoxycillin/ampicillin can be used for 14 days. Intravenous dexamethasone is suitable for hypertoxic typhoid fever.

Prognosis

The prognosis is excellent with prompt recognition and appropriate therapy but complications include relapse in 5–10% of patients within 2 weeks of completing therapy, gastrointestinal haemorrhage and perforation in a small percentage, pneumonia, thrombophlebitis, and myocarditis and pericarditis. Metastatic sepsis in the meninges, bones and joints may develop, as may toxic psychosis. Some go on to become chronic faecal carriers.

BRUCELLOSIS

Brucellosis is a zoonosis, endemic in Mediterranean countries and the tropics. There are 20–30 cases diagnosed annually in Britain, mostly in returning travellers. It used to be an occupational hazard in vets, abattoir workers and farmers.

Pathology

Brucellae are gram-negative coccobacilli. The four important species are: *B. abortus* (cattle), *B. melitensis* (sheep, goats, camels), *B. suis* (pigs) and *B. canis* (dogs).

Brucellae are spread by direct contact with animal products of conception, inhalation of infected droplets and ingestion of unpasteurised milk and cheeses. Brucellosis is a disseminated infection, and organisms multiply within the cells of the reticuloendothelial system. Granulomata form in the liver and spleen, and abscess formation occurs in the lymph nodes and the vertebrae.

Symptoms and signs

In acute brucellosis, the incubation period is usually 2–4 weeks but can be as long as several months. The onset may be acute or insidious with fever, chills, night sweats, myalgia, arthralgia and severe fatigue. Splenomegaly occurs in

Table 23.3. Serological investigations of brucellosis

	Acute brucellosis	Chronic brucellosis	Past brucellosis
Agglutination test (IgM)	>1/320	Low titre (<1/80)	Variable 1/10 – 1/640
2-Mercaptoethanol (IgG)	>1/320	Low titre (<1/80)	Low titre (<1/40)
Anti-human globulin test	Negative	>1/160	Low titre (<1/80)

Cross reactions occur with antibodies to *Yersinia enterocolitica* 09 and vaccine *Vibrio cholerae*.

10–20%, lymphadenopathy in 10%; there is minimal hepatomegaly and variable fever.

Chronic brucellosis causes malaise, lethargy and depression. Splenomegaly is occasionally seen.

Investigations

Prolonged culture of blood, bone marrow, liver and lymph nodes is useful. Serology includes an agglutination test to measure IgM antibodies and 2-mercaptoethanol test to measure IgG antibodies. Anti-human globulin test is useful in chronic *Brucella* infection (Table 23.3).

Differential diagnosis

Epstein-Barr virus (EBV), cytomegalovirus (CMV), enteric fever, Q fever, tuberculosis, histoplasmosis, malaria, trypanosomiasis, kala-azar, connective tissue disorders, lymphoma and sarcoidosis all need to be considered.

Treatment

Treatment, lasting 4–6 weeks, is with oxytetracycline 500 mg 6-hourly plus streptomycin i.m. 0.75–1.0 g per 24 hours or with doxycycline 200 mg per 24 hours.

For chronic cases oxytetracycline or doxycycline plus rifampicin, or co-trimoxazole plus oxytetracycline or rifampicin or streptomycin is given for 6–12 weeks.

Prognosis

Unrecognised brucellosis may become chronic. Acute brucellosis may be complicated by granulomatous hepatitis, meningitis, arthritis, spondylitis of lumbar, thoracic and cervical vertebrae, paravertebral and psoas abscesses, endocarditis and epididymo-orchitis.

AMOEBIASIS

Amoebiasis is a widespread human and primate infection of the gastrointestinal (GI) tract by the protozoan *Entamoeba histolytica*. Most common in the tropics and subtropics, the infection is acquired by ingestion of cysts and is associated with poor sanitation, inadequate food hygiene and male homosexual practices.

Pathology

Amoebic dysentery affects the caecum and colon. Mucosal ulcers extend into the submucosa as 'collar stud' abscesses and infection may spread to the liver and occasionally to the lungs and brain. A granulomatous mass may rarely develop in the caecum (amoeboma).

Symptoms and signs

Many patients are asymptomatic or symptomless cyst excretors (carriers). Amoebic dysentery has an insidious onset with mild to severe bloody diarrhoea. Abdominal pain is mild and there is rectal tenesmus but no fever and little systemic toxicity. It can become fulminant, e.g. in pregnant women, the immunocompromised, or with steroid therapy.

Liver abscess affects 20–60-year-olds, M>F. Usually it is a single abscess in the right lobe of the liver. Concurrent amoebic dysentery is absent. There is sudden onset of pain over the liver, referred to the shoulder tip or scapula. Fever, anorexia and weightloss occur. Tenderness over the liver and right basal pleural effusions develop.

Investigations

In amoebic dysentery, proctoscopy is needed for a rectal smear and microscopy reveals motile, haematophagous trophozoites which contain red blood cells. The serology is IFAT–positive in 75% of cases.

For liver abscess, scanning—ultrasound or CT—shows a fluid-containing cavity. The serology IFAT–positive in 95%. Cellulose acetate precipitation (CAP) test becomes positive after 10–14 days and negative after treatment.

Differential diagnosis

Amoebic dysentery
Inflammatory bowel disease (ulcerative colitis, Crohn's colitis), pseudomembranous colitis, ischaemic colitis, bacillary dysentery and bacterial colitis have similar clinical features.

Amoebic liver abscess
Pyogenic abscess, hydatid cyst of the liver and hepatoma must be considered.

Treatment

Amoebic dysentery, liver abscess and amoeboma are treated with oral metronidazole or tinidazole for 5–10 days. Dehydroemetine is cardiotoxic. Percutaneous aspiration may be needed if the abscess fails to resolve, or if rupture is imminent.

A colectomy is required for fulminating amoebiasis.

Cyst excretors should be treated with diloxanide furoate for 5 days.

Prognosis

Most patients with amoebic dysentery respond to therapy, and haemorrhage, perforation, peritonitis and amoeboma are uncommon. Metastatic amoebiasis of the liver, lung and brain can occur. Amoebic infection can extend from the anal canal to the skin, vulva, vagina, cervix, penis or give rise to chronic postoperative sinuses.

TRYPANOSOMIASIS

Trypanosomes are flagellated protozoan parasites. *Trypanosoma brucei rhodesiense* and *T. brucei gambiense* are subspecies and cause East African and West African trypanosomiasis respectively, collectively known as 'sleeping sickness'. *T. cruzi* causes American trypanosomiasis, Chagas' disease.

AFRICAN TRYPANOSOMIASIS

Approximately 20 000 cases are reported annually to the World Health Organization. Transmission is by various species of tsetse fly (*Glossina*). West African trypanosomiasis occurs in forests and riparian woodland and affects local populations, while East African trypanosomiasis is associated with savanna and mammals—antelope, bush buck, hartebeest. Tourists and game wardens are at risk.

Pathology

A trypanosomal chancre develops at the site of inoculation and causes blood and lymphatic dissemination, and eventual meningo-encephalitis. West African trypanosomiasis is a chronic protracted disease lasting for years. East African trypanosomiasis is of rapid onset, with death in <6 months due to myocarditis or early meningo-encephalitis.

Symptoms and signs

There is variable fever, headache, malaise, myalgia and arthralgia.

A trypanosomal chancre, seen at the site of tsetse fly bite, is painful, indurated and up to several centimetres in diameter. There is a transient erythematous rash called circinate erythema.

Splenomegaly, hepatomegaly and lymphadenopathy occur, as does peripheral oedema. A variety of neurological signs including tremors, chorea, cranial neuropathy, ataxia, psychosis, somnolence and coma are present.

Investigations

Giemsa-stained blood film and tissue fluid show trypanosomes. Serology; IFAT (Immuno-Fluorescent Antibody Test); ELISA (Enzyme Linked Immuno-Sorbent Assay).

CSF examination will show raised pressure, lymphocytic pleocytosis, morular cells of Mott (foamy plasma cells), a raised protein and the presence of trypanosomes.

Differential diagnosis

Rabies and viral encephalitis must be excluded.

Treatment

Suramin is used for both types. Pentamidine is suitable for West African trypanosomiasis and if the CNS is involved, melarsoprol, an arsenical, is used. Recently, eflornithine has been advocated for West African trypanosomiasis.

Prognosis

Trypanosomiasis is fatal if untreated, usually from myocarditis or encephalitis. Intercurrent infection leading to bronchopneumonia is common. Death can be the result of drug toxicity—melarsoprol has a 5% fatality rate.

AMERICAN TRYPANOSOMIASIS—CHAGAS' DISEASE

Infection with *T. cruzi*, a widespread zoonosis of Central and South America affecting 10–12 million people, is transmitted via the faeces of triatomine bugs of the Reduviidae family. Parasites enter the body via bite sites, mucosal surfaces or conjunctivae. Transmission by blood transfusion, laboratory accident and via the placenta have been described.

Pathology

There is inflammation and subsequent fibrosis of the heart and GI tract. The cardiac conduction system and the myenteric plexus of the GI tract are affected.

Symptoms and signs

Acute disease is mostly asymptomatic. Others experience malaise, headaches, irritability and myalgia. Entry via the eye causes palpebral oedema, conjunctivitis and local lymphadenopathy (Romana's sign). A chagoma, an inflamed ulcer at the point of entry, may be seen. Fever, subcutaneous oedema and splenomegaly all occur.

In chronic disease, cardiac symptoms include dyspnoea on exertion, swollen ankles, palpitations, dizziness and syncope. Gastrointestinal symptoms include dysphagia, regurgitation, flatulence, constipation and abdominal distension.

However, cardiac involvement may be asymptomatic with first degree AV block, right bundle branch block and ST-T wave abnormalities on the ECG. Arrhythmias, e.g. ventricular ectopics and ventricular tachycardia, may develop, as may myocardial failure.

Pulmonary infarction is sometimes seen in the GI tract, megaoesophagus, megacolon, and dilatation of the stomach and small intestine occurs.

Investigations

These include microscopy of blood film for trypanosomes, Giemsa stains of blood films, haemoculture and serology.

Differential diagnosis

This is very wide and includes glandular fever, toxoplamosis, myocarditis, acute glomerulonephritis, acute schistosomiasis, tuberculosis, brucellosis, meningo-encephalitis etc.

Treatment

Treatment is with nifurtimox or benzonidazole for acute Chagas' disease.

Prognosis

In acute Chagas' disease there is a 10% mortality from myocarditis and meningo-encephalitis. In chronic disease, between 20 and 50% of patients develop heart failure with a high risk also of sudden death.

Megaoesophagus leads to aspiration pneumonia and malnutrition while megacolon can lead to sigmoid torsion etc.

LEISHMANIASIS

Visceral, cutaneous and mucocutaneous syndromes are caused by organisms of the genus *Leishmania*. Disease manifestations depend on the species of parasite, geographical location and immune status of the patient. Approximately 10 million people are infected annually, of whom 400 000 have visceral leishmaniasis. *Leishmania* are transmitted by biting sandflies. (Table 23.4). The zoonotic reservoir includes dogs, foxes, rodents and man.

In cutaneous leishmaniasis, single or multiple painless papular-ulcerative lesions (Aleppo, Baghdad or Delhi boil) may last up to a year. They heal spontaneously, leaving atrophic, depigmented scars.

In diffuse cutaneous leishmaniasis, large numbers of parasites spread throughout the skin.

Mucocutaneous leishmaniasis occurs only in Latin America months to years after recovery from a cutaneous ulcer caused by *L. braziliensis braziliensis*. There are destructive lesions of nasal and oropharyngeal mucosa.

Visceral leishmaniasis (VL or kala-azar) is caused by the *L. donovani* complex. Parasites disseminate to the reticuloendothelial system. VL is characterised by progressive splenomegaly, hepatomegaly, pancytopenia, fever, weightloss and a tendency to secondary bacterial and mycobacterial infections.

Investigations

These include biopsy of cutaneous lesions to demonstrate intracellular amastigotes (Leishman-Donovan bodies).

Serology (IFAT or ELISA) and splenic, liver and bone marrow histology are needed.

Treatment

This is with pentavalent antimonial drugs, e.g. sodium stibogluconate (Pentostam), for 10 days or meglumine antimonate (Glucantime).

Prognosis

95% will be cured by antimonial drug therapy but with visceral leishmaniasis there may be intercurrent infection, especially of the respiratory and GI tracts. Intestinal and vaginal haemorrhage occur, as does tuberculosis with post kala-azar or dermal leishmaniasis. Reactivation may occur in the immunocompromised and HIV-infected patients.

LASSA FEVER

This is a serious acute febrile illness caused by an arenavirus which is excreted by the rat *Mastomys natalensis* in its urine, thereby contaminating food, abrasions etc. Person-to-person spread occurs via all body fluids. It is found in West Africa.

Symptoms and signs

After an incubation period of 2–3 weeks, fever, headache, prostration and severe pharyngitis accompany lymphadenopathy, vomiting, diarrhoea and chest pain. A maculopapular rash develops on the trunk after 10–14 days and mucosal bleeding occurs. Oliguria and hypotension with renal failure and coma are extremely bad signs.

Investigations

Although largely a clinical diagnosis, leukopenia, impaired platelet function and isolation of the virus are, together with antibody studies, the important investigations.

Table 23.4. Transmission of Leishmaniasis

Form of disease	New world parasite	Old world parasite
Cutaneous		
Simple	*L. braziliensis guyanensis*	*L. major*—Mediterranean
	L. braziliensis panamensis	*L. tropica*—Mediterranean
	L. mexicana mexicana	India, Greece
Diffuse	*L. mexicana amazonensis*	*L. Aethiopica*—Africa
Mucocutaneous	*L. braziliensis braziliensis*	
Visceral	*L. Donovani chagasi*	*L. Donovani donovani*—India, China, East Africa
		L. donovani infantum—Middle-East, China, Africa, Mediterranean

Treatment

This is symptomatic, but special care is required to preserve hydration. Ribavarin reduces mortality. Secure isolation facilities to protect medical and nursing staff should be available in Europe and the USA.

WORMS AND FLUKE INFESTATION

See Tables 23.5 and 23.6.

Table 23.5. Helminths (worms) Round worms

Name	Life cycle
Ascaris lumbricoides	Common in tropics from faecal contamination (eggs) of food and water. Larvae traverse lungs, pharynx and then gut
Ancylostoma duodenale *Nectator americanus* (hook worm)	Worms about 1 cm long. Larvae from gut enter skin, travel to lung and develop in small bowel. Common in tropics
Strongyloides stercoralis (Strongyloidiasis)	Worms approx 2 mm long. Inhabit gut. Transmitted as per hook worm. Pulmonary larval phase occurs. Found in tropics and in AIDS
Enterobius vermicularis (threadworms)	Usually in children. Threadlike worms cause intense perianal pruritus. Auto infection maintains the infestation
Filaria *Trichinella spiralis* (trichinosis)	Worms are the result of consuming undercooked meat, the meat containing larvae which penetrate lumen of gut and disseminate widely
Toxocara canis or cati (toxocariasis)	Humans infected from dog and cat faeces. Larvae then disseminate. 15% of soil samples in England show larvae. Migrans causes a febrile lesion with eosinophilia. There may be hepatosplenomegaly

Effects/diagnosis	Treatment
Occasional pulmonary infiltrates and fever Can obstruct gut or bile ducts or be vomited *Diagnosis:* Eggs ++ in faeces	Mebendazole 100 mg b.d. for 3 days Prevented by not using human faeces on crops
Anaemia due to gut blood loss from adult worms Hb may be 5 g or less Congestive heart failure may occur *Diagnosis:* Eggs ++ in faeces	Mebendazole 100 mg b.d. for 3 days Encourage wearing of shoes and safe disposal of faeces
Usually none May be diarrhoea and malabsorption Occasional urticaria Massive infestation in patients who are immunosuppressed Causes an often fatal septicaemic disorder *Diagnosis:* Larvae in duodenal aspirate Eosinophilia	Thiabendazole 25 mg/kg Up to 1.5 g is given twice daily for 3 days. Prevention: as for hook worm ? prophylactic thiabendazole for at risk patients who are immunosuppressed
Pruritus ani Sometimes vulvo-vaginitis *Diagnosis:* Scotch tape swab from perineal skin for eggs or recognition of egg-laying female worms	Mebendazole 100 mg as a single dose given twice after a week's interval Prevent finger sucking, nail biting and encourage hand washing after use of toilet
Fever, orbital oedema, muscle pains and eosinophilia May be CNS and heart involvement *Diagnosis:* Muscle biopsy for encysted larvae	Thiabendazole 25 mg/kg up to 1.5 g twice daily for 5 days
Ocular form: Causes loss of vision due to retinal or lens lesions Visceral larva *Diagnosis:* ELISA toxocara antibody tes	Diethylcarbamazine in a 21-day course. *Note*: ocular disease may not respond as the causative worm is dead Prophylaxis: regular de-worming of dogs Collection of dog faeces

Table 23.6. Trematodes (flukes) and cestodes (tape worms)

Name	Life cycle
Schistosomiasis	see p. 539
Fasciolas hepatica (fasciolasis)	Fluke (3 cm x 1.5 cm) invades biliary tree A miracidia from faecal larvae— penetrates a freshwater snail and then encysts on watercress and other aquatic flora before being eaten by sheep or man
Taenia saginata (beef tape worm)	Worm (bisexual) inhibits small gut; segments passed in faeces From undercooked beef Common in Africa, South America and Middle-East
Taenia solium (pig tape worm)	Uncooked pork
Diphyllobothrium Latum (fish tape worm)	Uncooked fish
Echinococcus granulosus (hydatid disease)	The dog tape worm, usual intermediate host sheep—thus direct contact with dogs or contaminated pasture and sheep causative Common in sheep-rearing areas

★Cysticercosis—human infection with an intermediate stage of *T. solium*—can occur by ingestion of worm eggs or by regurgitation of gravid segments (eggs) into the stomach. Encystation occurs in the tissues, and in the muscles they may calcify. Occasionally epilepsy, hydrocephalus and visual disturbances can occur. CNS involvement is diagnosed by CT scanning and positive serological test. Praziquantel in a 14-day course is effective.

Effects/diagnosis	Treatment
Upper abdominal pain Fever, chills, hepatomegaly and occasionally jaundice *Diagnosis:* Eggs + in stools Eosinophilia	Bithionol 40 mg/kg given as a twice daily dose for 15 days Isolation of sheep from watercress beds
Usually none Sometimes patient notices segments or larger pieces of worm *Diagnosis:* stool segments	Praziquantel 10 mg/kg as single dose If no segments passed for 4 months, the patient is cured Prophylaxis: thorough cooking of beef
Nil *Diagnosis*: microscopy of segments	As for *T. saginata* with purging 2 hours after treatment
General symptoms may occur with fatigue etc. and there may be vitamin B_{12} deficiency due to consumption of B_{12} in the gut *Diagnosis*: Eggs in faeces	Praziquantel as for *T. saginata*
Large and sometimes multiple cysts in liver, lung, bone etc. causing cystic swellings Occasional rupture into bronchus or abdomen with amyphylaxis and collapse *Diagnosis*: Eosinophilia and CT scanning	Mebendazole and albendazole may help Surgery may be required for solitary hepatic and pulmonary cysts and secondary abscess is an important complication

INDEX